Automated Hematology Analyzers: State of the Art

Editors

CARLO BRUGNARA
ALEXANDER KRATZ

CLINICS IN LABORATORY MEDICINE

www.labmed.theclinics.com

March 2015 • Volume 35 • Number 1

ELSEVIER

1600 John F. Kennedy Boulevard • Suite 1800 • Philadelphia, Pennsylvania, 19103-2899

http://www.theclinics.com

CLINICS IN LABORATORY MEDICINE Volume 35, Number 1
March 2015 ISSN 0272-2712, ISBN-13: 978-0-323-35658-9

Editor: Joanne Husovski
Developmental Editor: Colleen Viola

Reprints. For copies of 100 or more, of articles in this publication, please contact the Commercial Reprints Department, Elsevier Inc., 360 Park Avenue South, New York, New York 10010-1710. Tel. 212-633-3874, Fax: 212-633-3820, E-mail: reprints@elsevier.com.

Clinics in Laboratory Medicine (ISSN 0272-2712) is published quarterly by Elsevier Inc., 360 Park Avenue South, New York, NY 10010-1710. Months of issue are March, June, September, and December. Business and Editorial offices: 1600 John F. Kennedy Blvd., Suite 1800, Philadelphia, PA 19103-2899. Periodicals postage paid at NewYork, NY and additional mailing offices. Subscription prices are $250.00 per year (US individuals), $419.00 per year (US institutions), $135.00 per year (US students), $305.00 per year (Canadian individuals), $510.00 per year (Canadian institutions), $185.00 per year (Canadian students), $390.00 per year (international individuals), $510.00 per year (international institutions), $185.00 (international students). Foreign air speed delivery is included in all Clinics subscription prices. All prices are subject to change without notice. POSTMASTER: Send address changes to *Clinics in Laboratory Medicine*, Elsevier Health Sciences Division, Subscription Customer Service, 3251 Riverport Lane, Maryland Heights, MO 63043. **Customer Service: 1-800-654-2452 (US). From outside of the US and Canada, call 1-314-447-8871. Fax: 1-314-447-8029. E-mail: journalscustomerservice-usa@elsevier.com (for print support) or journalsonlinesupport-usa@elsevier.com (for online support).**

Clinics in Laboratory Medicine is covered in *EMBASE/Exerpta Medica, MEDLINE/PubMed (Index Medicus), Cinahl, Current Contents/Clinical Medicine, BIOSIS and ISI/BIOMED.*

Contributors

EDITORS

CARLO BRUGNARA, MD
Professor of Pathology, Harvard Medical School, Department of Laboratory Medicine, Boston Children's Hospital, Boston, Massachusetts

ALEXANDER KRATZ, MD, PhD, MPH
Associate Professor of Clinical Pathology and Cell Biology, Columbia University College of Physicians and Surgeons; Director, Core Laboratory and Point of Care Testing Service, Columbia University Medical Center, New York Presbyterian Hospital, New York, New York

AUTHORS

MICHAEL PIERRE BERNIMOULIN, MD
Haematology Division, Hôpitaux Universitaires de Genéve, Geneva, Switzerland

CAROL BRIGGS, FIBMS
Head Evaluation Unit, Department of Haematology, University College London Hospital, London, United Kingdom

CARLO BRUGNARA, MD
Professor of Pathology, Harvard Medical School, Department of Laboratory Medicine, Boston Children's Hospital, Boston, Massachusetts

GEORGE S. CEMBROWSKI, MD, PhD
Associate Professor, Laboratory Medicine and Pathology, Mackenzie Health Sciences Centre, University of Alberta Hospital, Edmonton, Alberta, Canada

DEVON S. CHABOT-RICHARDS, MD
Assistant Professor, Department of Pathology, University of New Mexico, Albuquerque, New Mexico

GWEN CLARKE, MD, FRCPC
Clinical Professor, Laboratory Medicine and Pathology, University of Alberta; Canadian Blood Services, Edmonton, Alberta, Canada

GIUSEPPE D'ONOFRIO, MD, PhD
Professor of Hematology and Clinical Pathology, Research Center for the Development and Clinical Evaluation of Automated Methods in Hematology, Catholic University of Sacred Heart, Rome, Italy

CAROL D'SOUZA, FIBMS
Principal Lecturer, Biomedical Sciences, Faculty of Science & Technology, University of Westminster, London, United Kingdom

LYDIE DA COSTA, MD, PhD
Professor, AP-HP, Robert Debré; Sorbonne Paris Cité; Inserm U1149, Bichat-Claude Bernard, CRI; Laboratoire d'excellence des globules rouges, Paris, France

TRACY I. GEORGE, MD
Professor, Department of Pathology, University of New Mexico, Albuquerque, New Mexico

RALPH GREEN, MD, PhD, FRCPath
Distinguished Professor, Department of Pathology and Laboratory Medicine; Medical Director, UC Davis Medical Diagnostics, University of California, Davis Health System, Sacramento, California

JOHN M. HIGGINS, MD
Department of Pathology, Center for Systems Biology, Massachusetts General Hospital; Department of Systems Biology, Harvard Medical School, Boston, Massachusetts

ALBERT HUISMAN, PhD, PharmD
Department of Clinical Chemistry and Haematology, University Medical Center Utrecht, Utrecht, The Netherlands

JOSEPH E. KISS, MD
Division of Hematology-Oncology, Department of Medicine, The University of Pittsburgh Medical Center, and The Institute for Transfusion Medicine, Pittsburgh, Pennsylvania

THOMAS PIERRE LECOMPTE, MD
Professor, Faculty of Medicine, Haematology Division, Hôpitaux Universitaires de Genéve, Geneva University, Geneva, Switzerland

SAMUEL J. MACHIN, FRCP
Professor, Haemostasis Research Unit, Department of Haematology, University College London, London, United Kingdom

ELISA PIVA, MD
Department of Laboratory Medicine, University-Hospital of Padova, Padova, Italy

MARIO PLEBANI, MD
Professor of Clinical Biochemistry and Clinical Molecular Biology, Department of Laboratory Medicine, University-Hospital of Padova, Padova, Italy

LINDA M. SANDHAUS, MD, MS
Associate Professor of Pathology, University Hospitals Case Medical Center, Cleveland, Ohio

ANTHONY N. SIRECI, MD, MSc
Assistant Professor of Clinical Pathology, Department of Pathology and Cell Biology, Columbia University, College of Physicians and Surgeons, New York, New York

FEDERICA SPOLAORE, MD
Department of Laboratory Medicine, University-Hospital of Padova, Padova, Italy

SUE ELLEN VERBRUGGE, PhD
Department of Clinical Chemistry and Haematology, University Medical Center Utrecht, Utrecht, The Netherlands

SEBASTIAN WACHSMANN-HOGIU, PhD
Professor in Residence, Department of Pathology and Laboratory Medicine, Center for Biophotonics, University of California, Davis, Sacramento, California

EDWARD C.C. WONG, MD
Director of Hematology, Division of Laboratory Medicine, Children's National Health System; Associate Professor, Departments of Pediatrics and Pathology, George Washington School of Medicine and Health Sciences, Washington, DC

GINA ZINI, MD, PhD
Professor of Hematology and Director of Transfusion Center and Cord Blood Bank, Policlinico Agostino Gemelli, Catholic University of Sacred Heart, Rome, Italy

Contents

Modern automated hematology instruments use either optical methods (light scatter), impedance-based methods based on the Coulter principle (changes in electrical current induced by blood cells flowing through an electrically charged opening), or a combination of both optical and impedance-based methods. Progressive improvement in these instruments has allowed the enumeration and evaluation of blood cells with great accuracy, precision, and speed at very low cost. Future directions of hematology instrumentation include the addition of new parameters and the development of point-of-care instrumentation. In the future, in-vivo analysis of blood cells may allow noninvasive and near-continuous measurements.

Modern hematology laboratories use automated hematology analyzers to perform cell counts. These instruments provide accurate, precise, low-cost differential counts with fast turnaround times. Technologies commonly used include electrical impedance, radiofrequency conductivity, laser light scattering, and cytochemistry. This article reviews the principles of these methodologies and possible sources of error, provides guidance for selecting flagging criteria, and discusses novel, clinically relevant white blood cell parameters provided by new instruments, including immature granulocyte count and granularity index.

Cytomorphological examination of aspirate smears remains the basic method to diagnose hematologic disorders and to evaluate treatment-related changes. Last-generation hematological analyzers can count, besides cells normally circulating in peripheral blood, some types of immature and abnormal cells, such as erythroblasts and immature granulocytes. The complex nature of bone marrow fluid, however, has prevented until now the routine utilization of blood cell counters in this area. Recent studies have shown the possibility of using bone marrow fluid as a substitute for peripheral blood for clinical tests in particular situations and for repetitive cytologic examinations in specific clinical and research fields.

Digital Image Analysis of Blood Cells

Lydie Da Costa

Rapid and accurate counts of red blood cells (RBCs), nucleated RBCs, platelets, and white blood cells (WBCs) (total and differential WBCs) are important requirements for a hematology laboratory. The detection of abnormal blood cell populations and the recognition of pathologic distributions of leukocytes are also of clinical importance. Manual microscopy counts are still required when a sample is flagged by the hematology analyzer and are still the reference method for WBC differential counts. Automated microscopy analyzers can provide accurate WBC differential counts, which may replace manual microscopy, but should not replace the eye of the cytologist.

Platelets: The Few, the Young, and the Active

Carol D'Souza, Carol Briggs, and Samuel J. Machin

Many modern automated cell counters in high-volume clinical hematology laboratories use new, improved technologies for routine platelet analysis. The latest progress includes the use of state-of-the art information technology, specific fluorescent dyes, and monoclonal antibodies to obtain more reliable platelet counts. This information allows the accurate and precise enumeration of platelets even in thrombocytopenic patients and the reporting of novel platelet parameters. In the near future, digital image analysis may permit even better platelet analysis.

Clinical Utility of Reticulocyte Parameters

Elisa Piva, Carlo Brugnara, Federica Spolaore, and Mario Plebani

The reticulocyte count reflects the erythropoietic activity of bone marrow and is thus useful in both diagnosing anemias and monitoring bone marrow response to therapy. Automated flow-cytometric analysis has led to a significant advance in reticulocyte counting, by simultaneously providing additional parameters and indices such as the reticulocyte immature reticulocyte fraction (IRF), the reticulocyte volume, and the hemoglobin content and concentration. IRF has been proposed as an early marker of engraftment. Reticulocyte hemoglobin content is useful in assessing the functional iron available for erythropoiesis, and reticulocyte volume is a useful indicator when monitoring the therapeutic response of anemias.

Hematology Analyzers: Special Considerations for Pediatric Patients

Edward C.C. Wong

Development of hematology analyzers has been predicated on the use of adult blood specimens without consideration for the unique morphologic and cellular content seen in pediatric patient populations. Because both dramatic qualitative and quantitative cellular changes occur in red and white blood cells and platelets from birth to early adulthood, development of pediatric reference intervals is necessary. Because testing is often performed on a small volume of blood, laboratories are required to develop unique approaches in specimen handling and analysis. Many newer instruments offer alternative cellular analysis allowing for unique insights into the hematopoietic response in disease and nondisease states.

CLINICS IN LABORATORY MEDICINE

Preface

Automated Hematology Analyzers: State of the Art

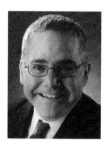
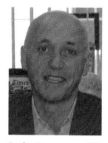

Alexander Kratz, MD, PhD, MPH

Carlo Brugnara, MD

Editors

The invention of the Coulter counter by Wallace H. Coulter in 1953 revolutionized laboratory hematology. It allowed the fast, precise, and accurate enumeration and sizing of the basic cellular elements of the blood. Over the last sixty years, countless additions and enhancements of automated cell counters have made the complete blood count one of the most frequently ordered, most quickly available, and nevertheless cheap laboratory tests. All this occurred while the quality of the results continuously improved and many additional parameters were provided by the newer instruments. This issue of *Clinics in Laboratory Medicine* describes these dramatic advancements.

The issue contains fourteen articles by an international team of leaders in Laboratory Hematology, covering the latest developments and future directions in the field of automated cell counters. After a summary of the history and future of automated cell counters, four contributions focus on red cells, platelets, white cells, and reticulocytes; they describe both well-established applications and novel parameters. Two additional articles are exclusively dedicated to summaries of the most novel parameters and of digital image analysis, among the most exciting new areas within laboratory hematology. Articles on quality control and standardization of cell counters provide readers with an overview of the latest efforts to assure that results are as consistent as possible across different instruments and platforms. Specific applications of automated cell counters are covered in articles on pediatrics, urgent care, body fluid analysis, the assessment of iron deficiency in blood donors, and the integration of blood and bone marrow analysis.

We thank all the authors for their truly outstanding contributions, and we are indebted to them for their willingness to meet our tight deadlines. We express our gratitude to the staff of Elsevier for keeping us on schedule and enabling us to create what

Clin Lab Med 35 (2015) xiii–xiv
http://dx.doi.org/10.1016/j.cll.2014.11.004
labmed.theclinics.com
0272-2712/15/$ – see front matter © 2015 Elsevier Inc. All rights reserved.

we hope will be a significant contribution to laboratory hematology. Most importantly, we thank our families for their support and encouragement in this endeavor.

Alexander Kratz, MD, PhD, MPH
Columbia University College of Physicians and Surgeons
Core Laboratory and Point of Care Testing Service
Columbia University Medical Center
New York Presbyterian Hospital
622 West 168th Street, PH3-303
New York, NY 10032, USA

Carlo Brugnara, MD
Harvard Medical School
Department of Laboratory Medicine
Boston Children's Hospital
300 Longwood Avenue, BA 760
Boston, MA 02115, USA

E-mail addresses:
ak2651@cumc.columbia.edu (A. Kratz)
Carlo.Brugnara@childrens.harvard.edu (C. Brugnara)

Development, History, and Future of Automated Cell Counters

Ralph Green, MD, PhD, FRCPath[a],*, Sebastian Wachsmann-Hogiu, PhD[b]

KEYWORDS

- Automated cell counter • Hematology • Blood • Hemoglobin
- Electrical impedance counting • Flow cytometry • Point of Care • Light scattering

KEY POINTS

- The invention of the microscope allowed the differentiation and counting of blood cells.
- Automated blood cell counters have greatly improved the speed and accuracy of cellular blood analysis, using optical light scattering or changes in electrical current induced by blood cells flowing through an electrically charged small opening.
- Novel methods under development include the addition of new parameters to the complete blood count and white cell differential and the development of smaller, portable instrumentation and of devices that allow in-vivo analysis of blood cells.

> "...for the blood is the life"
> —Deuteronomy 12:23

INTRODUCTION

Even in antiquity, blood was recognized as a singular bodily fluid that was the essence of life, possessing mysterious properties that provided sustenance for human survival. The unraveling of those mysterious properties only became possible once blood could first be characterized according to the appearance and number of its particulate components. Those critical steps comprised, in the first instance, the development of microscopy, enabling the visualization of component blood cells, and subsequently advances made possible through the techniques to measure physical properties of the formed elements of the blood as well as the electronic means of capturing this information.

[a] Department of Pathology and Laboratory Medicine, UC Davis Medical Diagnostics, University of California, Davis Health System, 4400 V Street, PATH Building, Sacramento, CA 95817, USA;
[b] Department of Pathology and Laboratory Medicine, Center for Biophotonics, University of California, 2700 Stockton Boulevard, Sacramento, CA 95817, USA
* Corresponding author.
E-mail address: ralph.green@ucdmc.ucdavis.edu

Clin Lab Med 35 (2015) 1–10
http://dx.doi.org/10.1016/j.cll.2014.11.003   labmed.theclinics.com
0272-2712/15/$ – see front matter © 2015 Elsevier Inc. All rights reserved.

Abbreviations	
CBC	Complete blood count
FOV	Field of view
RBC	Red blood cell
SRS	Stimulated Raman scattering
WBC	White blood cell

The development of the optical microscope made it possible to visualize individual human and plant cells, as well as bacteria. Even the simplest microscope developed by van Leeuwenhoek more than 300 years ago allowed the observation that blood is composed of small red globules, and their size was eventually determined. Progressive developments in optical microscopy followed during the next 2 centuries, such as the addition of an eyepiece to form a compound microscope and improved optics, including objective lenses comprising several lenses to correct for distortions. The application of dyes by Paul Ehrlich in the late 1870s allowed, for the first time, differentiation between different white cell types.[1,2] By then, it was evident that the number of blood cells changes in many diseases and it therefore became clear that it was important to more accurately quantify cell number by doing a blood count. Laborious manual measurements were introduced in which measured volumes of blood were placed on a calibrated slide chamber and cells were counted one by one, the total number being calculated from the known volume and geometry of the chamber. Although still in practice today because of its simplicity, manual counting of cells is prone to large errors and is both time consuming and labor intensive. Automated methods for counting blood cells became a necessity, and engineers began to work together with hematologists to find solutions to this problem. Over the ensuing decades, flow-based cytometers using light, impedance measurements, or both, were developed. These devices provided a large number of parameters related to enumerating and identifying blood elements, including erythrocytes (red blood cells [RBCs]), leukocytes (white blood cells [WBCs]), and thrombocytes (platelets), and differentiating the various leukocyte subtypes. In addition, with the recognition that qualitative differences in the appearance of red cells relating to their size, shape, and degree of hemoglobinization connoted certain types of anemia, the ability to simultaneously and independently measure hemoglobin concentration and hematocrit (or packed cell volume), together with the red cell count, provided Maxwell Wintrobe[3–5] with the tools to promulgate a set of red cell indices that included the mean corpuscular volume, mean corpuscular hemoglobin, and mean corpuscular hemoglobin concentration. This development allowed the morphologic classification of anemias into subtypes according to whether microcytic, normocytic, or macrocytic; and hypochromic, normochromic, or even hyperchromic according to degree of hemoglobinization. Later, it also became possible to quantify the size distribution of red cell populations, expressed as the red blood cell distribution width, thus enabling a further distinction into homogeneous and heterogeneous categories within each morphologic subtype.[6]

UTILITY OF A BLOOD COUNT

Of all the tissues in the body, the blood in circulation is the easiest and least invasive to sample. As such, a blood count represents a biopsy obtained through a simple venipuncture. A complete blood count (CBC) is therefore one of the most commonly used clinical laboratory tests. It provides a rapid and cost-effective assessment of various modalities of a patient's state of health as well as important clues to the

possible presence of disease. A CBC provides information about the cellular components of the blood: RBCs, WBCs, and platelets. CBC data include not only information about the numbers of the 3 basic cell types but also provide information about
the size, shape, and degree of hemoglobinization of the RBCs as well as the
morphologically identifiable types of WBCs; the so-called WBC differential. The
CBC provides clinicians with important information relevant to a patient's state of
health and possible type of underlying disease; these data, along with clinical and
other laboratory data, are often critical in constructing a differential diagnosis for a
patient as well as for monitoring the progression of a disease and its responsiveness
to treatment. At its most rudimentary level, the CBC gives information about low
RBC levels (anemia), high RBC levels (erythrocytosis), low WBC levels (leukopenia),
high WBC levels (leukocytosis), low platelet levels (thrombocytopenia), and high
platelet levels (thrombocytosis). In addition, data on low and high absolute numbers
of the different leukocyte types provide a wealth of information regarding the likely
type and cause of underlying disease, whether infectious, inflammatory, neoplastic,
or other. The blood cell count can therefore be an important first indicator of disease
for many illnesses and is therefore a pivotal starting point in forming a clinical diagnosis, screening for changes in patient health, and for monitoring of disease
progression or treatment. For example, in leukocyte disorders, the number of leukocytes reported and leukocyte differential can assist in assessing infections as well as
in evaluating for hematologic malignancies (leukemias). Given this wealth of information that comes from what is essentially a single laboratory test, the move toward
automation of the CBC was inevitable once the technical capabilities related to measurement, recording, reporting, and rapidity of throughput became available. Moreover, continued improvements in the various components of these integral steps of
automated blood counting have led to progressive advances in both the quality and
quantity of information that is obtained from a CBC. Modern blood counting instruments are able to closely simulate the qualitative information obtained through conventional microscopy with quantitative measurements of the numbers, dimensions,
and properties of the cellular components of the blood, providing a composite multiparameter assessment of the state of the tissue that is the circulating blood.

HISTORY AND CURRENT METHODS

Counting of blood cells was one of the first quantitative methods for blood testing, and
for some time has been the most widely used of tests in clinical settings. Initial measurements were based on careful wet sample preparation on a slide chamber, visualization, and manual counting with the aid of an optical microscope. Later techniques
involved flow methods coupled with either impedance measurements or light scat-
tering/fluorescence techniques to automatically enumerate cells one by one. There
has been a more recent resurgence of microscopy-based techniques as a result of
groundbreaking advances in imaging and image processing tools for automated cell
counting (**Table 1**).

Manual Counting Methods

The first blood count is credited to Karl Vierordt[7,8] at the University of Tübingen, who
published his research on the topic in a series of articles in 1852. His method involved
drawing blood into a capillary tube and spreading a known volume onto a slide, followed by microscopic analysis. During the following years, incremental improvements
of this method followed, including better specimen preparation and refinements in the
counting chamber (including the use of elliptically shaped capillary tubes by Malassez[9]

Table 1	
Brief history of early milestones in blood counting methods leading to automation	
Discoverer, Year	**Methodology**
Vierordt,[7,8] 1852	Microscope
Oliver,[11] 1896	Light scattering and absorption measured by eye
Marcandier et al,[12] 1928	Light scattering and absorption measured with a photodetector
Coulter,[17] 1953	Impedance measurement
Fulwyler,[13] 1965	Impedance measurement and electrostatic cell sorting
Dittrich & Göehde,[14] 1968	Fluorescence-based flow cytometry
Julius et al,[15] 1972	Fluorescence-activated cell sorting
George & Groner,[16] 1973	Light scattering in flow cytometry

Data from Refs.[7,8,11–17]

as well as the addition of etched perpendicular grids in the chamber for easier enumeration of cells). These improvements resulted in counts becoming more accurate but still tedious and slow to perform. A description of subsequent modifications was reviewed and published by Gray.[10] Because of its simplicity, this method is still used in low-resource laboratories around the world.

Automated Counting Methods

Toward the end of the nineteenth century, the prototypes of automated blood counters were first developed, with rapid advances made throughout the twentieth century. These instruments performed measurements using either the light scattered and absorbed by blood cells, or changes in the electrical current induced by blood cells flowing through a small, electrically charged opening.

Methods based on optical measurements

In 1896 a new method for blood cell counting was proposed by George Oliver,[11] based on the measurement (by eye) of light loss caused by scattering and absorption in a test tube filled with diluted blood. This method could be considered the forerunner of eventually the automated blood count, and it provided an RBC count without the need for manual counting of individual cells. However, the inability to accurately quantify the light loss as well as problems related to variations in cell size, shape, or hemoglobin content prevented this method from becoming widely used. Nevertheless, during the 1920s, novel developments in photodetectors (made possible by the discovery of the photoelectric effect and the invention of the photodiode) revived interest in using light scattering and absorption for blood cell counting. Marcandier and colleagues[12] showed in 1928 that, by measuring the light transmitted through a solution of diluted blood, a blood count could be derived after properly calibrating the photometer. However, as in the previously described method by Oliver,[11] the count was not accurate if there were variations in cell size, shape, or hemoglobin content. To address these issues, a flow device that isolated cells in small liquid droplets was first developed by Fulwyler[13] in 1965 for the purpose of separating cells based on their size. In 1968, Dittrich and Göhde[14] coupled a laser beam to this flow device and successfully demonstrated fluorescence-based cytometry. Because of the high speed of the flow, in which thousands of cells pass through the laser beam per second, high-throughput cytometry became a reality. This development may be seen as a watershed in the transition from manual to automated blood counting. In the early 1970s, Julius and colleagues[15] demonstrated fluorescence-based cell sorting, which he called fluorescence-activated cell sorting. The use of fluorescence labels enabled the identification, in addition to the separation, of many types of cells and therefore added a new dimension to the blood count. Up to 11 different fluorophores could be used simultaneously, and, through the use of deconvolution algorithms that allow separation of overlapping spectra, the number could be even larger. Light scattering was also implemented in flow cytometers by George and Groner[16] in 1973, allowing the discrimination of different types of WBCs based on their size/scattering properties. In addition, using light scattering measurements at 2 different angles, they were able to obtain measurements of red cell size (low-angle light scatter) and hemoglobin content (higher-angle scatter) after the cells were isovolumetrically sphered.[16]

Methods based on electrical measurements

During the late 1940s, Wallace Coulter was working on a method to assess particulates in paint. Spurred by his experiences in the Navy and witnessing the effects of the atomic bombs dropped at the end of the Second World War, he looked for ways to apply his technique to blood cell counting. In a discovery that came to be known as the Coulter effect, he started to develop a simplified blood cell analysis tool that could be used for rapid screening of blood from large numbers of people. The Coulter effect is based on the phenomena that cells are poor electrical conductors compared with a saline solution and individual particles passing thorough an orifice at the same time as an electric current produce a change (decrease) in the current caused by the particle-induced increase in electrical impedance. Furthermore, the change in impedance (and therefore in the measured current) is proportional to the volume of the particle, which is the foundation for size-based counting and separation. This simple but elegant concept laid the groundwork for subsequent development of modern automated blood cell counters. After Coulter's[17] first patent on this topic in 1953, many subsequent developments followed, including the popular flow cell format, in which the cells are directed through a flow channel or chamber rather than being passed through an aperture. A significant modification to the system was made in 1965 by Fulwyler,[13] who used a Coulter counter to measure cell volume and then partitioned the cells into droplets of the medium. Because the charge of the droplets is related to the cell volume, an electrostatic field applied to the droplets can deflect them into a collection vessel. Cells can thus be sorted and later reused. Like the fluorescence-based approach pioneered by Julius and colleagues,[15] this approach also played an important part in laying the foundation for automated cell-sorting techniques.

The addition of RNA-binding dyes such as acridine orange enabled automated discrimination and enumeration of reticulocytes as a component of the blood count and substantially improved the accuracy, speed, and precision of reticulocyte counting. Another milestone was the addition of precise size discriminators in electrical and light scattering instruments, which revolutionized platelet counting by enabling automation of this previously laborious measurement.

NOVEL METHODS UNDER DEVELOPMENT

Despite the significant improvements in the technologies described earlier, there are still several limitations to current automated blood counters, such as complex and time-consuming sample preparation, limited number of parameters that can be detected, the need for a blood draw, and lack of capability for continuous monitoring. With rapid technological advancements in optics, electronics, and microfluidics, further improvements are now being directed toward (1) the development of novel contrast agents and methods that will allow higher throughput and multiplexing capabilities, as well as adding new parameters to the measurements such as the analysis of subpopulations of blood cells or counting of smaller particles in blood; (2) the development of smaller, portable, automated blood counters; and (3) the development of in-vivo blood counting techniques.

New Contrast Agents and Methods

Current flow-based blood counters can detect up to approximately 13 parameters simultaneously (11 color and 2 scattered light [side and forward scatter])[18] in a high-speed laminar flow (up to 20 m/s), leading to the discrimination of phenotypic subpopulations of cells and a throughput of up to 100,000 cells per second. However, the heterogeneity and complexity of the immune system as reflected in lymphocyte subsets that have clinical diagnostic relevance may require even higher speed and multiplexing capabilities.

This improvement can be achieved by adding new contrast agents, such as quantum dots or rare earth metals that have narrower emission bands, or through the use of intrinsic markers that are easier to multiplex, such as those based on Raman scattering.[19] The main disadvantage of the Raman-based technique is the significantly reduced speed of measurement caused by the low Raman intensity compared with fluorescence or light scattering. To address this issue, molecular markers that can be used in combination with surface enhanced Raman spectroscopy and are capable of multiparameter blood analysis have been developed.[20] Other possibilities include the use of techniques that can provide additional contrast, such as those based on photothermal and photoacoustic measurements. However, increasing the multidimensionality of the information requires novel computational tools to help analyze these complex datasets and reveal new information, such as the identification of diverse populations of cells. Shekhar and colleagues[21] give an example of a tool that enables automated classification of nearly 40 different proteins to recover the large diversity of $CD8^+$ T cells. In addition, with the recent interest in cellular exosomes, the ability of flow cytometers to measure particles significantly smaller than 1 µm is currently being explored.

Because thousands of blood counts are performed each day in conventional large clinical laboratories, the development and improvement of machine-aided flagging algorithms is also a necessity, because they help reduce the number of false-positives and false-negatives by triggering morphologic review by an expert.

The Need for Portability

Current automated blood counting systems are large devices, the use of which is generally restricted to centralized laboratories. However, the need for delivery of improved but less expensive health care has posed newer challenges to scientists and engineers for the development of automated blood counters that are portable and can be used, for example, in doctor's offices, in disaster areas, in low-resource or remote areas, for monitoring astronauts in space, or even for home testing. The many developments over the past 20 years in microfluidics, optics, electronics, computers, and integration and miniaturization of devices based on such principles are bringing that goal ever closer. Sample preparation has been simplified by the use of microfluidic devices that require much smaller volumes of blood to perform a blood count. Although miniaturized optical components allow the development of smaller devices, faster electronic detectors help increase the throughput of such measurements. In addition, the analysis of recorded data is now aided by computers that can help improve the accuracy of the counts by using better statistical analysis or pattern recognition algorithms.

Miniaturization of flow-based cytometers

Several research groups recently reported the development of miniature flow devices. Such examples include on-chip impedance spectroscopy for a WBC differential count that has a 95% correlation against a commercial flow-based optical/Coulter counter,[22] or fluorescence-based measurements within a sheathless microflow device for a 4-part leukocyte differential count.[23]

The resurgence of image-based blood counters

Before the development of flow-based techniques, blood counting was performed by hand, with technicians examining cells under a microscope using a hemocytometer. The procedure was extremely laborious and it often required hours to generate a blood count. Despite this, image-based counting has some advantages, such as easier sample preparation and handling, and the ability to provide morphologic information that can be useful for the classification of immature and abnormal cells. In addition, imaging systems can be significantly smaller, more portable, and more robust than flow systems. For that reason, there has been a revival of image-based counters, particularly spurred by the development of high-quality, inexpensive camera sensors and of complex, robust image analysis algorithms. Ceelie and colleagues[24] recently examined the performance of 2 state-of-the-art automated image-based instruments and concluded that their accuracy in providing morphologic classification of RBCs and WBCs depends on the type of pathologic changes in the blood sample. One main drawback of image-based blood counters is the limited field of view (FOV), which depends on the magnification and is usually in the range of hundreds of micrometers. For accurate and fast measurements of WBCs and rare cells, the examination of larger areas is needed. Although scanning and tiling together multiple images is possible, a significant advance has been made by the development of a lens-free, in-line holographic imaging technique that uses partially coherent light to record the shadow of cells on an imaging sensor. Cell information can be extracted through the recovery of the phase information of each cell for very large FOVs, limited only by the size of the imaging chip. RBC, WBC (with granulocyte, monocyte, and lymphocyte differential), and hemoglobin concentrations could be measured in this way.[25] More recently, an automated image-based blood counting method that includes RBCs, WBCs with 3-part differential, and platelets has been reported. This method uses a simple sample preparation (that includes WBC and platelet staining) and automated image analysis for performing a blood count on very small volumes of blood and can be adapted to portable devices.[26]

In-vivo Automated Blood Count

Despite the advantages of automated ex-vivo blood counting, the ability to perform an automated in-vivo blood count is appealing because of the potential for noninvasive and near-continuous measurements. Other advantages include that no sample preparation is needed and sampling of larger volumes of blood is possible such that the detection of rare abnormal cells might become feasible.

The blood cells naturally flow through blood vessels, and therefore an adaptation of flow devices first comes to mind. However, there are many challenges that prevent a simple adaptation of the ex-vivo technology to in-vivo measurements. First, the flow is significantly slower ($\sim$0.002 m/s in microvessels and $\sim$0.2 m/s in large vessels, compared with ~10 m/s in flow cytometers) in humans, which would make the measurements significantly slower. Second, poor in-vivo optical conditions require the development of novel contrast mechanisms. Third, the speed of cells is constantly changing, which makes quantitative measurements difficult. An excellent review of in-vivo blood measurements has been published by Tuchin and colleagues[27] and it describes recent efforts to apply optical (absorption, fluorescence, elastic scattering, inelastic scattering [Raman]) as well as ultrasonographic, photothermal, and photoacoustic methods for this purpose. Other potential contrast methods are those that allow deeper penetration of light in the tissue. Examples include optical coherence tomography, nonlinear microscopies such as second harmonic generation, multiphoton fluorescence excitation microscopy, coherent anti-Stokes Raman scattering, and stimulated Raman scattering (SRS). As an example, SRS has been used for in-vivo label-free visualization of RBCs flowing through a capillary.[28]

FUTURE

The difficulty in predicting what the future holds for blood cell counting is best exemplified by considering how difficult it would have been to predict the current situation 50 years ago. However, there will be the dichotomy of building better blood counters for improved diagnostics versus smaller, more portable, or even wearable and implantable in-vivo devices that can provide certain parameters that may be useful as early indicators for changes in disease status and more elaborate tests.

Better, more accurate, and more comprehensive instruments will include more parameters in the blood count, such as the detection of rare-event blood cells, microvesicles, and exosomes, or subpopulations of cells with particular phenotypes that may be of significant clinical value. Measurement of dynamic functional changes in circulating cells is another possibility. Being able to provide multiplexed chemical information will also be important additions to future blood counting devices. Higher throughputs will also likely be the focus of future instruments, and could be achieved by developing new multimodal methodologies based on existing technologies or through the application of newer contrast technologies.

Smaller, portable devices that could do a blood count at the point of care and devices designed for in-vivo measurements will benefit from the use of high-resolution cameras and high-speed transmittance digital microscopy. In this way, cells can be examined under native conditions within the circulation through the use of photoacoustic detection, opening up new possibilities for assessment of cell-cell interactions, detection of circulating tumor cells, in-vivo cell deformability in diseases like sickle cell anemia and other intrinsic cell membrane disorders, and visualization of platelets during thrombus formation.[27]

Ten or more years into the future, automated blood counting instruments are likely to be significantly different from what they are today. Whether any of the directions predicted in this article will come into being is unknown at this time. The opportunity to contemplate this question is one that scientists are free to engage in. It is from such exercises that past developments stemmed and are likely to arise in the future.

REFERENCES

1. Ehrlich P. Beitrag zur Kenntnis der Anilinfaerbungen und ihrer Verwendung in der mikroskopischen Technik. Arch Mikr Anat 1877;13:263–77.
2. Ehrlich P. Methodologische Beitraege zur Physiologie und Pathologie der verschiedenen Formen der Leukocyten. Z Klin Med 1879–1880;1:553–60.
3. Wintrobe MM. A simple and accurate hematocrit. J Lab Clin Med 1929;15:287–9.

4. Wintrobe MM. Macroscopic examination of the blood. Am J Med Sci 1933;185:58–73.
5. Wintrobe MM. Anemia classification and treatment on the basis of differences in the average volume and hemoglobin content of the red corpuscles. Arch Intern Med 1934;54:256–80.
6. Bessman D. What's an RDW? Am J Clin Pathol 1981;76(2):242–3.
7. Vierordt K. Neue Methode der quantitativen Mikroskopischen Analyse des Blutes. Arch F Physiol Heilk 1852;26:9.
8. Vierordt K. Zaehlungen der Blutkoerperchen des Menschen. Arch F Physiol Heilk 1852;26:327.
9. Malassez LC. De la numeration des globules rouges du sang. C R Acad Sci Paris 1872;75:1528.
10. Gray H. Cell-counting technic: a study of priority. Am J Med Sci 1921;162:526–57.
11. Oliver G. A contribution to the study of the blood and the circulation. Lancet 1896; 1:1699.
12. Marcandier M, Bideau L, Dubreuil Y. Applications de la photometrie a la numeration des hemities. C R Soc Biol Paris 1928;99:741.
13. Fulwyler MJ. Electronic separation of biological cells by volume. Science 1965; 150(698):910–1.
14. Dittrich W, Göhde W. Flow-through chamber for photometers to measure and count particles in a dispersion medium. 1968 Patent DE 1815352.
15. Julius MH, Masuda T, Herzenberg LA. Demonstration that antigen-binding cells are precursors of antibody-producing cells after purification with a fluorescence-activated cell sorter. Proc Natl Acad Sci U S A 1972;69(7):1934–8.
16. George W, Groner W. Method and apparatus for analysis of leukocytes using light scattered by each leukocyte at absorbing and non-absorbing wavelength. 1973; US Patent 3781112 A.
17. Coulter WH. Means for counting particles suspended in a fluid. 1953; US Patent #2,656,508.
18. De Rosa SC, Herzenberg LA, Herzenberg LA, et al. 11-color, 13-parameter flow cytometry: identification of human naive T cells by phenotype, function, and T-cell receptor diversity. Nat Med 2001;7(2):245–8.
19. Lau AY, Lee LP, Chan JW. An integrated optofluidic platform for Raman-activated cell sorting. Lab Chip 2008;8(7):1116–20.
20. Watson DA, Brown LO, Gaskill DF, et al. A flow cytometer for the measurement of Raman spectra. Cytometry A 2008;73(2):119–28.
21. Shekhar K, Brodin P, Davis MM, et al. Automatic classification of cellular expression by nonlinear stochastic embedding (ACCENSE). Proc Natl Acad Sci U S A 2014;111(1):202–7.
22. Holmes D, Pettigrew D, Reccius CH, et al. Leukocyte analysis and differentiation using high speed microfluidic single cell impedance cytometry. Lab Chip 2009; 9(20):2881–9.
23. Shi W, Guo L, Kasdan H, et al. Four-part leukocyte differential count based on sheathless microflow cytometer and fluorescent dye assay. Lab Chip 2013; 13(7):1257–65.
24. Ceelie H, Dinkelaar RB, van Gelder W. Examination of peripheral blood films using automated microscopy; evaluation of Diffmaster Octavia and Cellavision DM96. J Clin Pathol 2007;60(1):72–9.
25. Seo S, Isikman SO, Sencan I, et al. High-throughput lens-free blood analysis on a chip. Anal Chem 2010;82(11):4621–7.
26. Smith ZJ, Gao T, Chu K, et al. Single-step preparation and image-based counting of minute volumes of human blood. Lab Chip 2014;14(16):3029–36.

27. Tuchin VV, Tárnok A, Zharov VP. In vivo flow cytometry: a horizon of opportunities. Cytometry A 2011;79(10):737–45.
28. Saar BG, Freudiger CW, Reichman J, et al. Video-rate molecular imaging in vivo with stimulated Raman scattering. Science 2010;330(6009):1368–70.

White Blood Cell Counts
Reference Methodology

Devon S. Chabot-Richards, MD*, Tracy I. George, MD

KEYWORDS

- Automated hematology analyzer • Methodology • Leukocyte
- White blood cell count • Differential count • Laboratory instrumentation

KEY POINTS

- Numerous technologies are used to generate the white blood cell (WBC) differential including electrical impedance, radiofrequency (RF) conductivity, light scatter, cytochemistry, fluorescent labeling, monoclonal antibodies, and automated differential cell counters.
- Most current analyzers report at least a 5-part WBC differential including neutrophils, monocytes, lymphocytes, eosinophils, and basophils.
- It is important to recognize common sources of error in the automated differential, including low cell count, nucleated red blood cells (nRBCs), platelet clumps, and clotted specimens; basophil counts in particular are prone to error.
- Hematology analyzers generate flags on specimens with abnormalities requiring further investigation; these flags are based on criteria, which must be validated by individual laboratories.
- Depending on the specific analyzer, numerous WBC parameters may be reported including nRBC ratio, hematopoietic progenitor cells (HPCs), immature granulocytes (IGs), granularity index, and lymph index.

INTRODUCTION

Historically, WBC counts were performed manually. Skilled technologists are necessary to perform this labor-intensive evaluation. Although manual cell counts are still performed in some situations, modern hematology laboratories use automated hematology analyzers to perform cell counts. These instruments provide accurate, precise, low-cost differential counts with fast turnaround times. Technologies commonly used include electrical impedance volume, RF conductivity, laser light

Disclosures: Sysmex, honorarium (T.I. George); Up To Date, Inc, royalties (T.I. George); Wolters Kluwer/Lippincott Williams & Wilkins, royalties (T.I. George).
Department of Pathology, University of New Mexico, MSC08 4640, 1 University of New Mexico, Albuquerque, NM 87131, USA
* Corresponding author.
E-mail address: Dchabot-richards@salud.unm.edu

Abbreviations	
FITC	Fluorescein isothiocyanate
HPC	Hematopoietic progenitor cell
IG	Immature granulocyte
LUC	Large unstained cells
nRBC	Nucleated red blood cell
PE	Phycoerythrin
PE-Cy5	Phycoerythrin-cyanine 5
RF	Radiofrequency
WBC	White blood cell

scattering, and cytochemistry. In addition to the traditional 5-part differential of neu-trophils, eosinophils, basophils, lymphocytes, and monocytes, with flags for abnormal cells, newer analyzers are better able to quantify abnormal and immature cell types including reactive lymphocytes, IGs, and nRBCs. Some instruments also report a granularity index, indicating toxic granulation of neutrophils. This article reviews the principles of these methodologies and possible sources of error, provides guidance for selecting flagging criteria, and discusses novel, clinically relevant WBC parameters provided by new instruments, including IG count and granularity index and the lymphocyte index.

THE WHITE BLOOD CELL COUNT

WBC count is the number of neutrophils, lymphocytes, monocytes, eosinophils, baso-phils, and immature or atypical cells present in 1 μL of blood. Leukocytosis, or eleva-tion of the WBC, can be seen in a broad range of conditions, including both benign and malignant conditions. Elevation of the WBC requires accurate differential count and morphologic evaluation of the peripheral blood smear along with clinical information to determine the cause.[1,2] Leukopenia, or decrease of the WBC, can also be caused by several conditions and requires accurate differential and morphologic examination to determine which cell line is decreased and to assess whether rare atypical or abnormal cells are present.[3]

METHODS

Historically, the WBC and differential count were determined manually. Cell counts were typically performed using a hemocytometer, a ruled counting chamber. This technique is still routinely used for assessment of cerebrospinal fluid and body fluid specimens and may be available as a backup method or for validating or calibrating automated analyzers. The specimen is diluted in a solution that lyses erythrocytes. The diluted specimen is added to the hemocytometer, a glass slide with ruled chambers of known volume. The technologist then counts the cells on a microscope with a low-power lens. The types of cells are differentiated, and nRBCs are included in the count. The hemocytometer method is prone to error, and skilled technologists are required. Manual differential counts require examination of a stained peripheral blood smear, with enumeration of 100 to 200 WBCs by category. This method is operator dependent and relies on the ability of the technologist to accurately classify cells. In addition, cells may be unequally distributed on the slide. When large cells are pulled to the feather edge of the smear, they may be underrepresented in the area counted by the technologist. There is also an inherent statistical error because the total number of cells analyzed is low.[4]

Automation of the Differential

In the 1970s, attempts to automate the cell differential relied on image analysis. Optical density thresholding was applied to digital images of cells in order to classify the cell types. These instruments were slow, limiting the number of cells counted to 100 to 200, leading to the same statistical imprecision seen in manual counts. Suspect cells required review by technologists for correct identification. These instruments were not cost effective, and development of technologies based on liquid suspensions of cells rather than stained smears became predominant.

Electrical Impedance

The first automated method for counting and differentiating cells using electrical impedance was patented in 1953 by Wallace H. Coulter, an electrical engineer, and his brother Joseph Coulter. The Coulter Corporation rapidly began producing semiautomated instruments for the analysis of peripheral blood specimens.[5] Since then, there have been several refinements and new methods to improve the accuracy of cell counts and differentials and to add additional reporting parameters. Modern analyzers use a combination of multiple techniques for cell counting and differentiation; however, the Coulter principle is still used in some manner by most analyzers.

The Coulter principle relies on electrical impedance to count and sort cells. Cells are nonconductive and produce measurable changes in electrical resistance in a conducting solution. To count and sort white cells, red blood cell lysing agents are added to the sample. Next, the specimen is diluted in an electrolyte solution, such as isotonic saline. This solution is conductive and also preserves cell size and shape. A low-voltage direct current is passed through the liquid. The cell suspension is drawn through an aperture positioned between the 2 electrodes. As cells pass through the aperture, changes in electrical resistance are measured as a voltage pulse. The number of pulses corresponds to the number of cells, and the height of each pulse is proportional to the volume of the cell. The data collected are plotted on a histogram showing the number of cells and their volumes. Thresholds can be set for exclusion of pulses above or below the desired amplitude range (**Fig. 1**).

Early automated instruments generated a 3-part differential based on cell size, because normal samples generally produce 3 distinct peaks on a histogram. The largest size group (>160 fL) includes mature and band neutrophils and eosinophils.

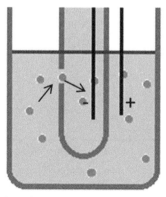

Fig. 1. Schematic diagram of Coulter principle. Cells are suspended in saline and drawn through an aperture, across which a current is flowing. As cells pass through, the current is disrupted, creating a pulse. The pulse amplitude is proportional to the size of the cell.

The intermediate size group (90–160 fL) includes monocytes, immature and mononuclear neutrophils, and eosinophils. The smallest size group (<90 fL) includes lymphocytes and basophils. nRBCs are also included in this group. Abnormal or immature cells and abnormally large populations of eosinophils obscure the distinction between these groups, resulting in inaccurate counts and error flags (**Fig. 2**).

Radiofrequency Conductivity

The principle of RF conductivity can be added to the Coulter principle to give more information about the internal constituents of cells, including nuclear size and density and chemical composition. A high electromagnetic alternating current is generated across the aperture. As cells pass through the aperture, this current penetrates the cell membrane. The resulting pulse amplitude depends on the cell's internal complexity. The electrical impedance and RF conductivity results are combined to classify the cell types. Cells with abnormal localization on the impedance versus RF plot generate flags and require additional review for subclassification.

Light Scattering

Laser light scattering techniques provide information about cell size and structure. These techniques are similar to those used in multiparameter flow cytometry. A flow cell detector is used to analyze light scattering produced as hemodynamically focused blood cells pass through a laser. Recording the number of times the laser is interrupted provides the cell count. The amount and angle of scatter is used to classify cells by size, refractive index, nuclear features, cytoplasmic granularity, and shape of the cell. Multiple angles of scatter are measured. Forward scatter, or 0°, corresponds to cell size. Side scatter of 10° corresponds to internal complexity. A scatter of 90° corresponds to cytoplasmic granularity. Eosinophils show a characteristic depolarized 90° scatter due refraction by their crystalline granules. In addition to classifying the 5 normal subtypes of WBCs, light scatter techniques give characteristic histogram findings for abnormal and immature cells. In addition to light scattering characteristics, WBCs exhibit characteristic autofluorescence when interrogated by the laser, which can further aid in classification (**Fig. 3**).

Cytochemistry

Myeloperoxidase staining can be added to light scattering techniques to provide further information about levels of intracellular peroxidase enzyme. The cells are fixed and stained using a myeloperoxidase substrate. Absorbance of white light by the stained cells is proportional to the intensity of the peroxidase reaction. The

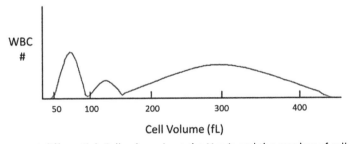

Fig. 2. Three-part differential. Cell volume is on the X-axis and the number of cells is on the Y-axis. The largest cells (>160 fL) include neutrophils and eosinophils. The intermediate cells (90–160 fL) include monocytes, immature neutrophils, and eosinophils. The smallest cells (<90 fL) include lymphocytes and basophils.

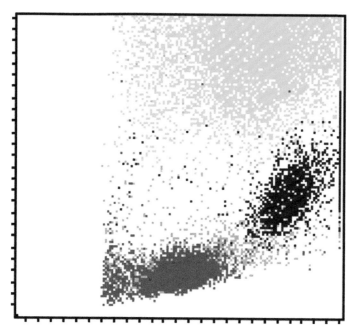

Fig. 3. This scattergram of peripheral blood forward versus side scatter shows 3 separate populations of cells, the lymphocytes (*green*), monocytes (*purple*), and granulocytes (*yellow*).

peroxidase-containing granulocytes, neutrophils, monocytes, and eosinophils give positive results, whereas lymphocytes and basophils give negative results. The cells are further subclassified by size. Large unstained cells (LUCs) may be present; this population includes activated lymphocytes, plasma cells, and blasts.

Fluorescent Labeling

Basic light scattering techniques can be augmented by the use of fluorescent dyes. These dyes stain certain cell structures. As the cells pass through the laser, the dyes emit specific wavelengths of light depending on the fluorochrome, which can be measured. RNA and DNA dyes, such as propidium iodide (PI) or polymethine dyes, are commonly used and can separate nRBCs and reticulocytes from WBCs and also give information about cell viability. PI binds to double-stranded DNA and cannot pass through the membrane of viable cells. If the cells fluoresce with PI, membrane compromise and nonviability are indicated. Cells are separated according to their side scatter and fluorescence emission characteristics to determine the cell type. Polymethine DNA staining is used in conjunction with side scatter characteristics to improve separation of populations of WBCs (**Fig. 4**).

Monoclonal Antibodies

New analyzers offer the use of fluorochrome-conjugated monoclonal antibodies to expand the information given in the cell differential. The Cell-DYN Sapphire (Abbot Diagnostics, Abbot Park, IL, USA), for example, can be used as a 3-color flow cytometer using the fluorescein isothiocyanate, phycoerythrin (PE), and PE-cyanine 5 fluorochromes. The most common panel uses CD3-, CD4-, and CD8-conjugated monoclonal antibodies to specify T-cell subsets and can report CD4 and CD8 cell counts.

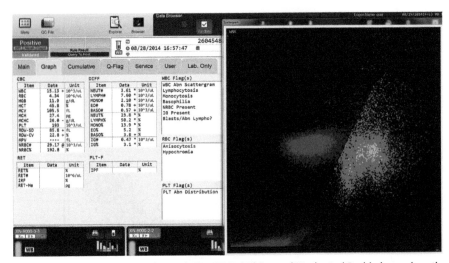

Fig. 4. Sysmex XN-9000 WNR channel. The WNR (White and Nucleated Reds) channel on the Sysmex XN-9000 differentiates cells based on fluorescent intensity and size. The cell membranes are perforated, and the nucleic acids are labeled with a fluorescent marker. The basophil population is yellow, nucleated red blood cells are pink, and other white blood cells are light blue. Debris is dark blue. This sample shows increased nucleated red blood cells.

Automated Differential Cell Counters

In cases in which abnormalities are seen on the automated differential, morphologic review by a trained technologist or pathologist is required for accurate classification. Automated digital image analysis platforms have been developed to facilitate this process. These platforms review stained blood smears and classify WBCs. Images of the cells with the assigned classifications are displayed on a monitor on which a trained technologist can quickly review the cell morphology and confirm or change the classifications. The CellaVision DM9600 automated microscope platforms (CellaVision Inc, Durham, NC, USA) can classify WBCs into 12 different categories: band neutrophils, segmented neutrophils, eosinophils, basophils, monocytes, lymphocytes, promyelocytes, myelocytes, metamyelocytes, blast cells, variant lymphocytes, and plasma cells. The technologist can further subclassify cells into additional categories. Compared with manual methods, these platforms show excellent correlation in normal cases, although accuracy is decreased in the monocyte and basophil categories. In cases with hematologic disease, accurate classification of abnormal cell types is decreased.[6]

Roche Diagnostics (Hoffmann-La Roche, Basel, Switzerland) is currently developing a platform (Cobas m 511 Bloodhound) that uses computer imaging to generate all complete blood cell count (CBC) and differential parameters. This platform generates a 5-part differential using multispectral imaging to classify cells by size, shape, color, and optical density. Abnormal cell types are reviewed by a technologist and assigned to the appropriate categories.

Automated Sampling Modes

Historically, the preparation of samples for analysis required hands-on aliquoting, mixing, and reagent addition by a technologist. Beginning in the 1980s, automated sampling modes were added to analyzers. Samples are aspirated from closed tubes, and mixing and reagent dispension occurs within the analyzer. The instrument includes monitors to evaluate for clots and correct volumes. The addition of barcode readers improves sample identification. Algorithms can be created to initiate additional testing based on initial results, such as the addition of reticulocyte counts in a patient with anemia. Automated slide makers are available that prepare and stain blood smears when laboratory-programmed parameters, such as the presence of abnormal cells, are met. These improvements decrease hands-on time for technologists and improve throughput and efficiency.

SOURCES OF ERROR

There are several common causes of inaccurate automated WBC counts and differentials.[7] Most instruments are sensitive in detecting large populations of abnormal cells; however, when the percentage of abnormal cells drops below 5%, counts may become inaccurate and cells may not be detected. The WBC may be spuriously increased in specimens with increased nRBCs or when many unlysed red blood cells are present. Giant platelets and platelet clumps can also cause an increase in the WBC count, usually classified as a high percentage of lymphocytes. Cryoglobulin and monoclonal protein may also cause a spurious increase because of red blood cell clumping.[8] Most instruments flag the WBC when there is significant interference in the low end of the WBC size region because of these conditions. Apparent decrease in the WBC count may be seen in clotted specimens, when many smudge cells are present, and in patients with uremia.

Abnormalities of WBCs can also cause interference with other CBC parameters. A high WBC can result in a spuriously high red blood cell count and hemoglobin and hematocrit levels. Other red blood cell parameters, including the mean corpuscular volume and mean corpuscular hemoglobin, may also be affected. When WBCs are fragmented or damaged, they may falsely elevate the platelet count.[9]

Depending on the technologies used to generate the differential count, many platforms show lower correlation with manual differentials and increased between-platform variability in the counts of monocytes and basophils in particular. Neutrophil and monocyte counts may be decreased in specimens with delayed processing.[10] Platforms that use the LUC category may include normal monocytes in that group, resulting in a lower monocyte count.[11] Basophil counts performed by automated instruments are notoriously inaccurate.[12] This inaccuracy may be due in part to the low numbers of these cells in normal specimens. Most platforms rely on differential lysing agents to identify basophils, as these cells are resistant to lysis. Abnormal cells may be resistant to lysis and counted in this category. Platforms using light scattering to classify basophils, such as the CELL-DYN Sapphire, require tight gating to exclude lymphocytes from the basophil count and may underestimate the basophil percentage.[13]

REPORTING AND FLAGGING

Several parameters are used to define CBC abnormalities that require further attention, such as morphologic evaluation by a technologist or pathologist. These flags may be instrument or user defined. Most instrument manufacturers recommend thresholds, which must be validated by individual laboratories. Criteria must be selected that minimize the amount of manual blood smear review required while also minimizing the release of erroneous results. Setting the thresholds for flags requires careful consideration of the patient population being tested (**Fig. 5**).[14]

Suspect flags note the presence of abnormal populations of cells that cannot be accurately subclassified, resulting in an inaccurate differential. Common named flags

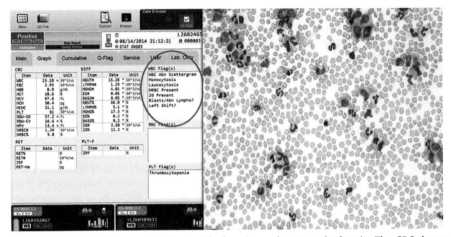

Fig. 5. WBC sample flags on a patient with chronic myelogenous leukemia. The CBC shows leukocytosis with anemia and thrombocytopenia. Immature granulocytes, blasts, and nucleated red blood cells are present on the peripheral smear.

include nRBC, clump (for platelet clumps), blast, IG, bands, left shift, and atypical lymphocyte. Suspect flags may be generated in several situations. nRBCs or platelet clumps or giant platelets may be present in the lowest forward/side scatter region for lymphocytes, resulting in an increased lymphocyte count. This will result in a clump or nRBC flag. Large mononuclear cells may be present at the monocyte/neutrophil interface or may show high 90° light scatter, resulting in a blast flag. Large cells may be seen in the lymphoid region or at the lymphocyte/monocyte interface, giving an atypical lymph or blast flag. The neutrophils may show abnormal forward or side scatter because of the presence of IGs, resulting in an IG or bands flag. When suspect flags are generated, a peripheral blood smear review by a medical technologist or, in certain cases, a pathologist, is required to validate the differential count and further define the abnormality. Studies have demonstrated that although specific flags tend to be poor predictors of the presence of specific abnormalities, the presence of a flag does correlate with the existence of any abnormality. For example, a differential flagged with atypical lymphocyte may show blasts on peripheral blood smear review.[15]

WHITE BLOOD CELL PARAMETERS

Although some small, portable analyzers still report a 3-part WBC differential including small lymphocytes and basophils, intermediate monocytes and mononuclear cells, and large neutrophils and eosinophils, modern analyzers report at least a 5-part differential with neutrophils, monocytes, eosinophils, basophils, and lymphocytes (**Fig. 6**). The monocyte and basophil counts are typically the least accurate and tend to underestimate the actual percentage of cells. Most analyzers also report additional parameters, which can help to identify atypical populations of cells or aid in diagnosis of certain conditions (**Table 1**). Inclusion of these parameters in laboratory algorithms can help to reduce the number of samples requiring manual slide review (**Fig. 6, Table 2**).

Nucleated Red Blood Cells

Enumeration of nRBCs is important because high levels may artificially increase the WBC count. nRBCs are found in the peripheral blood in numerous benign and

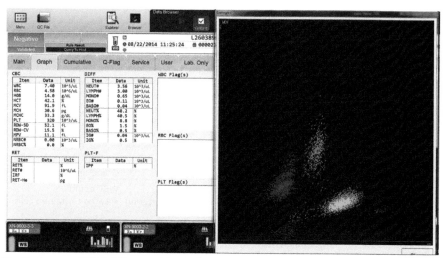

Fig. 6. A normal WBC differential from the Sysmex XN-9000 instrument. The scattergram on the right displays side scatter on the X-axis and side fluorescent intensity on the Y-axis. Monocytes (*green*) show the highest fluorescent intensity, followed by lymphocytes (*pink*), neutrophils and basophils (*light blue*), and eosinophils (*red*). Debris is colored dark blue.

malignant conditions including the neonatal period, with hemolysis, blood loss, sepsis, hematologic malignancy, and bone marrow involvement by other neoplasms. Depending on the technology used, nRBCs may be included in the lymphocyte category or present as a flag for interference in this region. More sophisticated analyzers now report nRBC as a separate category. nRBC can be identified by impedance and light scattering characteristics and high fluorescent intensity. DNA dyes can also be used. nRBCs are reported as a ratio of nRBC to WBC.[16]

Large Unstained Cells

The LUC category includes reactive lymphocytes, plasma cells, blasts, and other abnormal cells. This category is usually defined by light scatter characteristics in conjunction with myeloperoxidase activity and includes cells in the large cell area normally occupied by monocytes and neutrophils that do not exhibit peroxidase activity. In patients with decreased myeloperoxidase activity, the neutrophils will be included in the LUC population. Specimens with LUC counts require manual review of a peripheral blood smear for correct classification of these cells.

Hematopoietic Progenitor Cells

A combination of methods can be used to enumerate the percentage of HPCs. Side scatter and forward scatter characteristics can identify large cells with large nuclei. Differential lysing agents, which lyse mature cells with high membrane lipid content while preserving immature cells, may be used. DNA, RNA, and histone dyes may also be used. In addition to their use in patients with hematologic malignancy and other abnormal states, these counts can potentially be used in stem cell harvesting.[17] Typically, a flow cytometry assay for CD34 is performed to estimate the number of HPCs before leukapheresis for specimen collection. This can be time consuming and requires special equipment and trained personnel. Studies in pediatric populations have shown that the peripheral blood HPC count correlates well with CD34 flow assay, although there seems to be greater variability in adult patients particularly

Table 1
Methodologies and parameters of manufacturer instruments

Manufacturer	Selected Instruments	Methodologies	Parameters
Beckman Coulter (Beckman Coulter, Inc., Brea, CA, USA)	DxH 800 LH780 LH750	Electrical impedance RF conductivity Laser light scattering Flow cytometry	WBC count 5-part differential
Sysmex (Sysmex America, Inc, Lincolnshire, IL, USA)	XE-2100 XE-5000	Electrical impedance RF conductivity Laser light scattering Fluorescence detection	WBC count • Immature granulocytes • Blasts Granularity index
Siemens (Siemens AG, Berlin, Germany)	Advia 2120 Advia 120	Cytochemistry Laser light scattering Fluorescence detection	WBC count • Large unstained cells
Abbott (Abbott Laboratories, North Chicago, IL, USA)	Cell-DYN 4000 Sapphire CD 3500 CD3700	Electrical impedance Fluorescence detection Laser light scattering Monoclonal antibodies	WBC count Leukocyte viability • Blasts • Atypical lymphocytes • Immature granulocytes
Mindray (Mindray Medical International Limited, Shenzhen, China)	BC-6800 BC-5800	Laser light scattering Fluorescence detection	WBC count • Immature granulocytes • High-fluorescence cells[a]
Horiba (Horiba Ltd, Kyoto, Japan)	Pentra DF Nexus	Electrical impedance Light scatter Cytochemistry	WBC count • Atypical lymphocytes • Large immature cells • Immature monocytes • Immature granulocytes • Immature lymphocytes

[a] High-fluorescence cells are blasts and atypical lymphocytes.

at low HPC counts. When the count is greater than 30 HPC/μL, however, the HPC count can be used to justify collection.

Immature Granulocytes

The IG fraction includes promyelocytes, myelocytes, and metamyelocytes. Bands and blasts are not included. These cells are increased in infection, inflammation, malignancy, necrosis, trauma, steroid use, and pregnancy, among other diseases. IG counts are available on many newer instruments and have been suggested as a marker for infection and sepsis. The Sysmex XE-2100 Automated Hematology System (Sysmex America, Inc, Lincolnshire, IL, USA), for example, uses light scattering and fluorescence to identify granulocytes with a larger nuclear volume, consistent with immature cells (**Fig. 7**).[18]

There has been particular interest in using IG counts to discriminate between sepsis and other noninfectious inflammatory conditions, particularly in patients in intensive care units and in pediatric and neonatal patients. Rapid diagnosis of sepsis in these

Table 2
Selected white blood cell parameters and clinical utility

nRBCs	Ratio of nRBCs to WBCs	Diagnosis of anemia, hematologic malignancy, and other disease states
Large unstained cells	Reactive lymphocytes, plasma cells, blasts, other abnormal cells	Diagnosis of hematologic malignancy and other disease states
Hematopoietic progenitor cells	Myeloblasts	Quantification for stem cell harvest, diagnosis of hematologic malignancy and other disease states
Immature granulocytes	Promyelocytes, myelocytes, metamyelocytes	Diagnosis of bacterial infection and sepsis in pediatric and critically ill patients
Granularity index	Degree of neutrophil granulation (hypogranular vs toxic granulation)	Diagnosis of dysplasia, bacterial infection
Lymph index	Reactive lymphocytes	Diagnosis of viral infection

patient groups can be difficult; however, early diagnosis is vital to guide life-saving interventions. Several studies have shown that a significantly increased IG count is specific for infection in patients in intensive care units; however, the sensitivity is lower.[19] Studies attempting to relate IG level to severity of disease and morbidity and mortality have not clearly demonstrated a correlation.[20] The findings are less clear in neonatal populations, however, because healthy neonates have high IG counts.[21] Further characterization of normal IG counts in this age range is required. In addition to infection, this parameter is also being evaluated for a possible role in identifying patients with myelodysplastic syndromes and myocardial infarction, among other conditions.

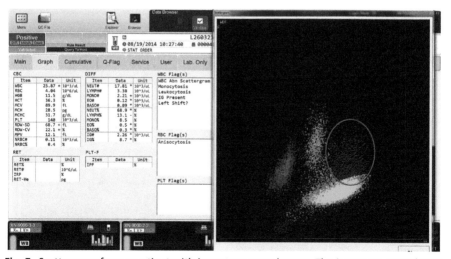

Fig. 7. Scattergram from a patient with immature granulocytes. The immature granulocyte population is dark blue. These cells have higher fluorescent intensity and greater mean volume than the mature granulocytes, shown in light blue.

Granularity Index

In situations in which neutrophil production is stimulated, circulating neutrophils exhibit toxic changes including distinct azurophilic granules in the cytoplasm. Hypogranularity is a dysplastic feature seen in myelodysplastic syndromes and other myeloid malignancies. Morphologic determination of neutrophilic granulation can be highly subjective, particularly in the case of toxic granulation. Using side scatter characteristics, analyzers such as the Sysmex XE-2100 can give a measurement of the granularity of neutrophil cytoplasm. This parameter has been shown to correlate with the grade of toxic granulation or hypogranularity, as determined by morphologic evaluation. Studies have shown that the granularity index increases along with C-reactive protein levels in infection.[22] A low granularity index, particularly in conjunction with other CBC abnormalities such as anemia, platelet distribution width, and standard deviation of red blood cell distribution width, is specific but not sensitive for dysplasia and can help identify specimens for manual slide review.[23] A combination of the granularity index, IG count, and hematopoietic precursor cell count may be even more useful.

Lymph Index

The lymph index relies on impedance, RF, and light scattering to define morphologically distinct populations of lymphocytes. Impedance gives information for cell volume, RF about cytoplasmic chemical composition and nuclear volume, and light scattering about cytoplasmic granularity and nuclear structure. The lymphocyte index is defined as the lymphocyte volume times the lymphocyte volume standard deviation divided by the lymphocyte conductivity. In viral infections, the lymphocyte population shows increased large cells, an increased range of sizes of lymphocytes (lymphocyte volume standard deviation), and decreased conductivity, resulting in an increased lymphocyte index. This may be useful in distinguishing viral from bacterial infection, which is associated with a lower lymphocyte index (**Fig. 8**).[24]

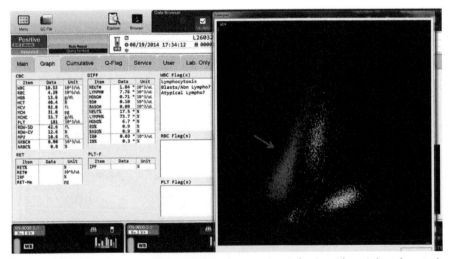

Fig. 8. This report is from a patient with Epstein-Barr virus infection. There is lymphocytosis, and the scattergram shows an abnormal lymphocyte pattern (*pink*) with a greater range of size and fluorescent intensity than the normal pattern.

SUMMARY

Automated hematology analyzers can now use a combination of different technologies to increase the information provided with CBC and differential testing. Understanding the abilities and limits of these instruments is necessary for appropriate triage and reporting of specimens. New parameters can allow for improvement of manual smear review algorithms and aid in diagnosis of benign and malignant conditions.

REFERENCES

1. George TI. Malignant or benign leukocytosis. Hematology Am Soc Hematol Educ Program 2012;2012:475–84.
2. Chabot-Richards DS, George TI. Leukocytosis. Int J Lab Hematol 2014;36(3): 279–88.
3. Valent P. Low blood counts: immune mediated, idiopathic, or myelodysplasia. Hematology Am Soc Hematol Educ Program 2012;2012:485–91.
4. Rümke CL. The imprecision of the ratio of two percentages observed in differential white blood cell counts: a warning. Blood Cells 1985;11(1):137–40.
5. Krause JR. The automated white blood cell differential. A current perspective. Hematol Oncol Clin North Am 1994;8(4):605–16.
6. Cornet E, Perol JP, Troussard X. Performance evaluation and relevance of the CellaVision DM96 system in routine analysis and in patients with malignant hematological diseases. Int J Lab Hematol 2008;30(6):536–42.
7. Cornbleet J. Spurious results from automated hematology cell analyzers. Lab Med 1983;14:509–14.
8. Zandecki M, Genevieve F, Gerard J, et al. Spurious counts and spurious results on haematology analysers: a review. Part II: white blood cells, red blood cells, haemoglobin, red cell indices and reticulocytes. Int J Lab Hematol 2007;29(1):21–41.
9. Zandecki M, Genevieve F, Gerard J, et al. Spurious counts and spurious results on haematology analysers: a review. Part I: platelets. Int J Lab Hematol 2007; 29(1):4–20.
10. Kalpatthi R, Thompson B, Lu M, et al, BABY HUG Investigators. Comparison of hematologic measurements between local and central laboratories: data from the BABY HUG trial. Clin Biochem 2013;46(3):278–81.
11. Grimaldi E, Carandente P, Scopacasa F, et al. Evaluation of the monocyte counting by two automated haematology analysers compared with flow cytometry. Clin Lab Haematol 2005;27(2):91–7.
12. Ducrest S, Meier F, Tschopp C, et al. Flow cytometric analysis of basophil counts in human blood and inaccuracy of hematology analyzers. Allergy 2005;60(11): 1446–50.
13. Amundsen EK, Henriksson CE, Holthe MR, et al. Is the blood basophil count sufficiently precise, accurate, and specific?: three automated hematology instruments and flow cytometry compared. Am J Clin Pathol 2012;137(1):86–92.
14. Barnes PW, McFadden SL, Machin SJ, et al. The international consensus group for hematology review: suggested criteria for action following automated CBC and WBC differential analysis. Lab Hematol 2005;11(2):83–90.
15. Sireci A, Schlaberg R, Kratz A. A method for optimizing and validating institution-specific flagging criteria for automated cell counters. Arch Pathol Lab Med 2010; 134(10):1528–33.
16. Kwon MJ, Nam MH, Kim SH, et al. Evaluation of the nucleated red blood cell count in neonates using the Beckman Coulter UniCel DxH 800 analyzer. Int J Lab Hematol 2011;33(6):620–8.

17. Letestu R, Marzac C, Audat F, et al. Use of hematopoietic progenitor cell count on the Sysmex XE-2100 for peripheral blood stem cell harvest monitoring. Leuk Lymphoma 2007;48(1):89–96.
18. Maenhout TM, Marcelis L. Immature granulocyte count in peripheral blood by the Sysmex haematology XN series compared to microscopic differentiation. J Clin Pathol 2014;67(7):648–50.
19. Nierhaus A, Linssen J, Wichmann D, et al. Use of a weighted, automated analysis of the differential blood count to differentiate sepsis from non-infectious systemic inflammation: the intensive care infection score (ICIS). Inflamm Allergy Drug Targets 2012;11(2):109–15.
20. Nierhaus A, Klatte S, Linssen J, et al. Revisiting the white blood cell count: immature granulocytes count as a diagnostic marker to discriminate between SIRS and sepsis–a prospective, observational study. BMC Immunol 2013;14:8.
21. Cimenti C, Erwa W, Herkner KR, et al. The predictive value of immature granulocyte count and immature myeloid information in the diagnosis of neonatal sepsis. Clin Chem Lab Med 2012;50(8):1429–32.
22. Zimmermann M, Cremer M, Hoffmann C, et al. Granularity Index of the SYSMEX XE-5000 hematology analyzer as a replacement for manual microscopy of toxic granulation neutrophils in patients with inflammatory diseases. Clin Chem Lab Med 2011;49(7):1193–8.
23. Raess PW, van de Geijn GJ, Njo TL, et al. Automated screening for myelodysplastic syndromes through analysis of complete blood count and cell population data parameters. Am J Hematol 2014;89(4):369–74.
24. Zhu Y, Cao X, Tao G, et al. The lymph index: a potential hematological parameter for viral infection. Int J Infect Dis 2013;17(7):e490–3.

Analysis of Bone Marrow Aspiration Fluid Using Automated Blood Cell Counters

CrossMark

Giuseppe d'Onofrio, MD, PhD*, Gina Zini, MD, PhD

KEYWORDS

- Bone marrow analysis • Automated blood cell counters • Reticulocytes
- Flow cytometry • Erythroblast count • Bone marrow aspirate • Toxicologic studies

KEY POINTS

- Automated bone marrow analysis using blood cell counters is not a substitute for microscopic evaluation of bone marrow cytology in aspirate films.
- Potential advantages of automated bone marrow analysis are increased throughput and efficiency, decreased manual labor, reduced costs, increased reproducibility, objectivity of measurements, and less variability due to the individual variation in interpretation and the quality of the smear.
- The main difficulties for bone marrow analysis with blood cell counters are the presence of heterogeneous and immature progenitors, fat droplets, microfibers, and cell aggregates.
- Original information can derive from the comparison of results obtained from the simultaneous analysis of peripheral blood and bone marrow.
- Bone marrow fluid can be used as a substitute for venous blood in emergency situations, at least for the measurement of red cell parameters.
- Automated bone marrow fluid analysis will be useful for repetitive tasks such as toxicologic studies in laboratory animals.

INTRODUCTION

Technology has revolutionized clinical laboratories. Almost all diagnostic tests are currently carried out using highly automated and robotized systems. In hematology, automated blood cell counters were introduced in the 1960s; after half a century of continuous improvements, the latest generation instruments produce in less than a minute dozens of results that are much more precise and accurate than those obtained with the manual techniques formerly in use. The development of increasingly sophisticated methods has transitioned the hematology laboratory from the centrifuge

Disclosure: No conflict of interests.
Research Center for the Development and Clinical Evaluation of Automated Methods in Hematology, Catholic University of Sacred Heart, Largo Agostino Gemelli 8, Rome 00193, Italy
* Corresponding author.
E-mail address: giusdono@gmail.com

Clin Lab Med 35 (2015) 25–42
http://dx.doi.org/10.1016/j.cll.2014.10.001
0272-2712/15/$ – see front matter © 2015 Elsevier Inc. All rights reserved.

labmed.theclinics.com

Abbreviations	
IRF	Immature reticulocyte fraction
LUC	Large unstained cell
MCV	Mean corpuscular volume
NRBC	Nucleated red blood cell
PANDA	Peroxidase activity and nuclear density analysis
PBS	Phosphate-buffered saline
TNCC	Total nucleated cell count
WBC	White blood cell

hematocrit to an in-depth scrutiny of multiple blood cell properties. Any single cell in a peripheral blood sample can now be identified and counted, so that accurate differential leukocyte count, subtle red blood cell features, and even proportions of more or less mature reticulocytes can be measured at a rhythm of hundreds of samples per hour.[1,2] Very few areas still hold out against the technological supremacy; among these, in particular, no significant changes have occurred until now as for bone marrow aspirate. Cytomorphological examination of aspirate smears remains a well-established, basic method to assess the state of hematological cell lineages, to diagnose hematologic disorders, and to evaluate treatment-related changes of the hemopoietic system. Although progress in immunophenotyping techniques using multiangle flow cytometry, together with the recognition of specific genetic and molecular markers, has greatly improved diagnostic sensitivity and accuracy for many hematological conditions, the microscope identification and counting of normal and abnormal cell populations remains an essential tool, and the starting point, for the great majority of hematological diagnoses.[3]

The attempts to obtain a precise quantification of bone marrow cell populations through the utilization of fully automated blood cell counters used in routine hematology laboratories have not been fully successful until now. The complex nature of bone marrow fluid, and the many differences of its composition in comparison to peripheral blood, for which all instruments originally were designed, can justify the present inadequacy of hematological instruments for bone marrow fluid analysis. This article will attempt to summarize the current state of research, the reasons for the presently disappointing results, and opportunities for new forthcoming achievements.

Bone Marrow Fluid

The bone marrow of an adult constitutes 4.7% plus or minus 1.3% of total body weight (equivalent to 1.5–3.7 kg). The red or hemopoietic marrow represents about a quarter of this volume. It is principally located within the central axial skeleton, in the flat bones, and in the epiphyses of the long bones. Its structure consists of a network of trabecular bone lined by endosteum, with multiple cavities rich in sinusoids, reticular stroma, fat cells, and small islands and cords of hemopoietic cells. Although normal peripheral blood only contains 5 classes of mature leukocytes, the bone marrow fluid, aspirated with different techniques, is composed by many different types of cells in different phases of maturation, often aggregated in particles of different size, with fat and fibers.[4,5] The various stages of the granulocyte and erythroid series show a heterogeneous spectrum of sizes and other properties, such as nucleocytoplasmic ratio, cytoplasmic content, and nuclear shapes. Megakaryocytes and other giant cells are dispersed between them. Cellular abnormalities in hematologic disorders, such as myelodysplastic syndromes, leukemia, and myeloproliferative syndromes, produce further changes in the qualitative and quantitative marrow cytology.

Analytical Technologies in Automated Blood Cell Counters

Automated blood cell counters, used in routine hematology laboratories, are dedicated flow cytometers, which use different types of electrical and optical technologies to quantitatively and qualitatively characterize blood cells diluted in a fluid. They have the capability of

- Precisely and accurately counting and sizing all types normal circulating cells (leukocytes, erythrocytes, platelets)
- Flagging the presence of abnormal cells for microscope review (immature granulocytes, blasts, erythroblasts, atypical lymphocytes), with sufficient specificity (to avoid false positives and useless work at the microscope) and specificity (to avoid false negatives and diagnostic errors)

The recent, latest-generation hematological analyzers have improved analytical capabilities, particularly thanks to refined optical, laser, and fluorescence-based detection systems, as much as they can count some types of such abnormal cells, such as erythroblasts and immature granulocytes.[1,2]

Different approaches are being exploited for technologically-assisted analysis of bone marrow aspirates, such as immunophenotype flow cytometry with cell class-specific monoclonal antibodies, and the use of digital virtual bone marrow films with different levels of automated cell identification and counting. These developments, however, are beyond the scope of this article, which is limited to the use of routine blood cell counters for automated bone marrow analysis.

Usefulness of Automated Analysis of Bone Marrow Aspirates

In clinical hematology, as well as in other areas of medicine such as toxicologic research, the demand for bone marrow aspiration testing is continuously increasing, with various indications.[3,4] A few samples are collected from new patients as part of the work-up for possible hematologic disorders. According to World Health Organization (WHO) guidelines, differential counting at the microscope of at least 500 cells for each case by a pathologist is recommended for the diagnosis of hematological diseases.[6] Subtle dysplastic changes; identification of minor populations of atypical cells; evaluation of megakaryocytes and giant cells and architectural and focal abnormalities; and identification of minimal residual disease, all require expert morphologic evaluation on bone marrow aspirates and biopsy sections, in conjunction with flow cytometric immunophenotyping. Most samples, however, are collected for monitoring patients during induction or maintenance chemotherapy, after stem cell transplant or in disease remission; in these samples, which are often hypocellular or normocellular and usually contain only normal cells, an accurate and reproducible quantitative evaluation of the different lineages is more relevant than their fine morphologic evaluation. This is also true for bone marrow analysis in experimental and toxicologic studies in laboratory animals.

Automated bone marrow analysis using blood cell counters cannot supplant microscopic evaluation of bone marrow cytology in aspirate films. When an effective and accurate method is available, however, it will provide ancillary information in a short time, such as a preliminary assessment of sample adequacy in terms of cellularity, representativeness and contamination with peripheral blood, quantitative evaluation of the main cell populations, and even flagging of abnormal samples.

The main potential advantages of the introduction of such methods in the routine practice of hematology, clinical, toxicologic, and research laboratories can be summarized:

- Increased throughput and efficiency
- Decreased manual labor

- Reduced costs
- Increased precision, in terms of improved reproducibility of counting as a result of decreased statistical error allowed by the high number of cells counted
- Objectivity of measurements, based on physical and/or chemical fixed criteria, with disappearance of interobserver differences
- Independence from the competence of the microscopist (although adequate operator training is required for the interpretation of automated results and identification of abnormal cell distributions on the cytograms)
- Analysis of cells in suspension, and consequently lack of dependency on of the quality of smears and absence of artifacts related to irregular cell distribution on the films
- Possible original information from the comparison of results obtained from the simultaneous analysis of peripheral blood and bone marrow

None of these targets is fully accomplished at the present time, despite many attempts and significant technological improvements. Several manufacturers have realized and introduced original methods for the analysis of body fluids different from blood, such as cerebrospinal fluid. None of them, however, has introduced a specific software development or a dedicated analytical channel devoted to the analysis of bone marrow fluid.

DIFFICULTIES IN CELL COUNTING IN BONE MARROW FLUID

The main difficulty for the analysis of bone marrow aspirates using routine automated blood cell counting obviously derives from the previously described complexity of cell compositions. Automated blood cell counters have inherent limitations of their analytical performance when faced with such heterogeneity, so that the separation of the numerous cell types and precursors cannot be sufficiently accurate. Many cells in bone marrow do not normally circulate in peripheral blood, such as erythroblasts, granulocyte precursors, plasma cells, and macrophages. The main cell populations are formed by a continuum of maturing elements, which, while simultaneously proliferating and increasing their number, progressively change their shape, size, and internal composition, until they reach the final stage of their mature progeny ready to be released into peripheral blood. A decrease in size with nuclear chromatin condensation is typical for the majority of bone marrow cell lineages (with the exception of megakaryocytes, which on the other hand cannot be counted owing to their large size). Another problem for accurate cell identification is the presence in the bone marrow aspirate fluid of many different cell types with similar characteristics of size, nucleocytoplasmic ratio, and internal structure, such as mature erythroblasts, lymphocytes, lymphoblasts, monocytes, and some types of blasts (**Fig. 1**). In addition, serious noncell-related interferences have to be considered, depending on the viscous quality of the fluid, which contains solid particles, with irregular cell distribution and aggregation, microfibers, and fat droplets.

Erythroblasts and Other Immature Cells

One of the main difficulties that blood cell counters historically had to face with bone marrow fluid was the failure to count erythroblasts, which are not included within the 5 normal circulating leukocyte classes and, if present, can cause inaccurate differential counts on peripheral blood samples. Generally speaking, with many analyzers the most mature (orthochromatic) erythroblasts are lysed within the analytical channels, and their small pyknotic nuclei are partly lost within debris and background noise and partly admixed within the small lymphocyte clusters, obscuring the

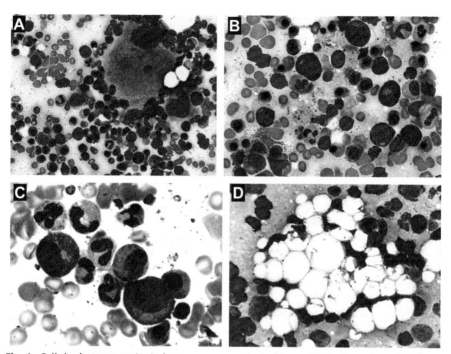

Fig. 1. Cellular heterogeneity in bone marrow aspirate films, with limits and possible interferences for the analysis of bone marrow fluid with automated blood cell counters. (*A*) Area of rich cellularity, crowded with hematopoietic precursors characterized by heterogeneous size and maturity. A giant megakaryocyte and a large promegakaryocyte would escape automated identification because of their large size. Orthochromatic and polychromatophilic erythroblasts are close in size and shape to small lymphocytes. (*B*) The larger, intensely basophilic erythroblasts cannot be identified by the blood cell counters and are usually counted as large lymphocytes, similar to the large plasma cell visible in the middle of the right section of the image. In the upper center, a macrophage nucleus and its cytoplasmic extensions full of cellular debris that can easily interfere with automated analysis. (*C*) The wide spectrum of different sizes, nucleo-cytoplasmic ratio, nuclear shapes, and granular cytoplasmic content in bone marrow cells represent a serious obstacle for the analytical technologies developed for the analysis of peripheral blood cells. (*D*) Fat droplets originating from adipocytes cause serious interferences when bone marrow fluid is analyzed with automated blood cell counters.

noise/lymphocyte separation. The intermediate, polychromatophilic, and basophilic erythroblasts are counted as lymphocytes or large lymphocytes, while the most immature proerythroblast are variously classified as atypical lymphocytes, monocytes, or blasts.

This difficulty is currently well overtaken by 2 analytical methods that use fluorescent nucleic acid stains, such as propidium iodide or another proprietary fluorochrome, and directly count the fluorescent nuclei of partially lysed erythroblasts within a specific analytical channel (like in the Sysmex XE series (Sysmex Corporation, Kobe, Japan), **Fig. 2**A) or in a multiangle leukocyte detection system (like in the Abbott Cell-Dyn/Sapphire series (Abbott Laboratories, Abbott Park, IL USA), see **Fig. 2**B). These methods have shown acceptable performance with bone marrow aspirates. Other instruments apply indirect techniques based on the measurement of cell size and internal content to separate erythroblasts from the other cell types (see **Fig. 2**C, D): similar

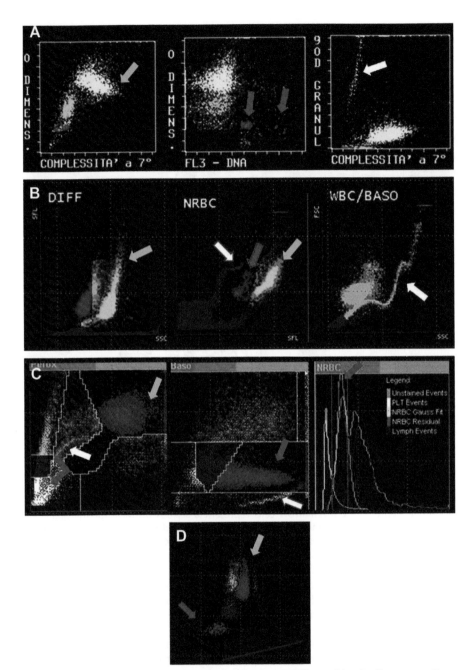

Fig. 2. Scattergrams of bone marrow aspirate fluid with different blood cell counters. Green arrows: immature granulocytes; red arrows: erythroblasts; white arrows: fat droplets. (A) Abbott Cell-Dyn 4000 (fluorescence, impedance, depolarized light). (B) Sysmex XE-2100 (fluorescence, impedance, radiofrequency). (C) Siemens ADVIA 120 (automated cytochemistry). (D) Beckman-Coulter LH750 (VCS technology).

approaches, although acceptably effective in flagging and even measuring the presence of circulating erythroblasts in peripheral blood samples, have not been studied for quantitative bone marrow analysis.

Some instruments can also differentiate and count immature granulocytes in peripheral blood differential count. A partial count of immature granulocytes is possible, for instance, with Sysmex instruments in the immature myeloid information (IMI) channel, which exploits their partial resistance to a surfactant used in that channel. The capability of effectively separating the different granulocyte stages of maturation is still to be reached, so that immature granulocytes are more realistically added to the neutrophilic count when bone marrow is analyzed. Results obtained with the count of blast cells, usually available in automated blood cell counters at least as a research tool or option, will be described.

Large Cells, Cell Particles, and Clusters

A technical limit of automated blood cell counters is the limited volumetric range for cell measurements. Bone marrow cellularity includes large cells present in small numbers, the most important of which are megakaryocytes; their presence, number, disposition, and morphologic characteristics escape any possible automated recognition. Similarly, identification of other large and rare cells that are easily recognizable at the microscope, such as osteoblasts and osteoclasts, plasma cells or mast cells, or normal, reactive or neoplastic groups or clumps of cells (lymphocytes, macrophages, mast cells, erythroid islands, metastases), is impossible. Moreover, maturing cells of the hematopoietic lineages may be unevenly distributed and tightly crowded within bone marrow particles.

Lipid Droplets

Another important limiting factor that caused years of unsuccessful attempts in analysis of bone marrow fluid with automated blood cell counters is the unavoidable presence of fat droplets. Lipid interference is caused by the refractive index of lipid droplets, which have a unique light absorbance and very different sizes along a continuum, thus producing typical thin, curved sigmoid distributions of signals (see **Fig. 1**D). In Sysmex instruments' scattergrams, the fat interference has the distinct appearance of trails, which are sigmoid on the white blood cell (WBC)/Baso and nucleated red blood cell (NRBC) scattergrams, and linear on the IMI scattergram.[7] The linear sigmoid aspect of the fat droplets is also observed in other instruments based on optical cell analysis, like the Siemens Advia and Abbott Cell-Dyn models. Such variable contamination by fat particles is characteristic of the aspirated marrow and can result in overestimation of marrow total nucleated cell count (TNCC) by automated analyzers. The interference is less important in instruments that only utilize the impedance method, such as the former Coulter analyzers.[8]

The lipid nature of such sigmoid clusters has been demonstrated by their disappearance when bone marrow aspirates were cytocentrifuged and plasma was removed and replaced with saline or other isotonic fluids.[9,10] Attempts to eliminate the fat droplets by consecutive wash cycles with BPS, however, did not result in a consistent and complete removal of interferences.[11] Using a Cobas-Helios hematology analyzer, Bentley also tried to exclude signals produced by fat particles by manual adjustment of the threshold lines for each sample analyzed.[9] An effective solution was obtained with a software improvement in the Abbott Cell-Dyn 4000, in which fat particles, originally classified as eosinophils because of their capability to depolarize beams of polarized light, were effectively excluded from the remaining cell clusters and from the TNCC using an adjusted thresholding algorithm.[12]

Impossibility to Store Anticoagulated Specimen

Some authors, in the area of animal experimental research and toxicologic studies, where automated bone marrow analysis could theoretically replace cytomorphological analysis, have claimed as a problem the inability to archive and store fluid bone marrow samples.[13] Therefore, cytocentrifuged or smeared preparation should be prepared and kept available.

TECHNICAL ISSUES: SHOULD BONE MARROW FLUID BE PRETREATED?

Many different approaches have been described and tested in the relatively few papers available in the literature on the analysis of bone marrow aspirates with automated blood cell counters. All authors generally agree that bone marrow samples should be analyzed no later than 6 to 8 hours after collection, even if some have used much older refrigerated samples.[14] Some relatively complex techniques of preanalytical sample preparation have been explored with the aim of removing fat, microfibers, and solid particle. In his early, relatively unsuccessful attempt, for instance, Bentley[9] used cleaned specimens, obtained by diluting 100 µL of bone marrow fluid with 10 mL of NaCl saline buffered with boric acid, centrifuging it, removing the supernatant, and adding 1 mL of saline to the remaining pellet.

Anticoagulation

Bone marrow is a viscous fluid that rapidly undergoes coagulation with platelet aggregation and fibrin formation after aspiration. The use of an anticoagulant is thus mandatory to keep it in a liquid state. Most authors have used the K2 or K3- EDTA in blood tubes of the same type of those used for peripheral blood cell count; others have used lithium heparin.[11,14] The current authors have repeatedly reported acceptable results even with such simple undiluted anticoagulated samples without further pretreatment but using the resistant blood cell mode of the Cell-Dyn 4000 that allows more complete red blood cell lysis, without any occurrence of clotting or clogging in the in the analytical device (eg, aspiration needle, tubing, or flow cell).[7,12,15]

Dilution

Cellular bone marrow can have a high cell concentration, which can prevent accurate measurements because of coincidence error; the Sysmex XE-series instruments do not even report numerical results with hypercellular samples.[16] The effects of dilution can be corrected by applying the ratio of the hemoglobin value of the original liquid specimen against that of a diluted solution to the measurement results.[17] Different researchers have used several approaches to deal with this preanalytical passage:

- A simple twofold dilution in phosphate-buffered saline (PBS) (0.5 + 0.5 mL) in addition to K2-EDTA[18]
- Larger dilutions (10-fold) with normal saline[19]
- Dilution with RPMI medium of the same lithium–heparin samples used for flow-cytometric analysis[14]

Improvement in linearity range with new instruments, however, could reduce the need for a dilution step.

Filtration

This method of sample preparation was applied by a few researchers with the aim of removing solid particles with a simple passage through sterile gauze, or filtration through 100 µm pore filters or 53 µm pore sized nylon mesh.[10,19]

Washing

Some authors tested native samples versus 2 consecutive wash cycles with PBS in order to eliminate interference by microfibers and fat droplets and could not find significant differences between the 2 methods.[11]

Homogenization and Disaggregation

With the aim of disrupting bone marrow particles and obtaining truly representative cell suspension, a rather sophisticated washing, disaggregation, and dilution technique was developed by Criswell and colleagues.[13] They flushed isolated femurs of rats with fetal bovine serum and thoroughly mixed the suspension with pipettes; the resulting cell suspension was treated with inversions and centrifugation, supernatant decantation, pellet resuspension and dilution in 10 mL of PBS.

Shibata and colleagues[17] compared 3 different pretreatment methods; the best results were obtained when cleaned specimens were used. Mori and colleagues[10] used an experimental modification of the XE-2100 consisting of a special bone marrow measurement mode; samples were manually pretreated (anticoagulated with heparin, diluted with RPMI medium, and filtered with 100 μm pore filters); for the measurement of myeloid cells, lysing reagent and polymethine dye were added and incubated at 33°C. Mature granulocytes were stained, while immature granulocytes and myeloblasts, resistant to the lytic action of the reagent, were not stained; pretreated samples were finally directly injected into the optical detector without automatic addition of other reagents.

It is therefore evident that there is a lack of even the minimal attempt to standardize preanalytical steps of bone marrow automated analysis. Together with the difference in each manufacturer's methodological approaches, this is a main obstacle hampering a possible routine implementation.

RESULTS OF PUBLISHED STUDIES

Results of some early studies on the possible use of routine blood cell counters for bone marrow analysis were described as limited and not compatible with a possible routine application, as a consequence of the combination of the previously mentioned methodological difficulties.[9,20,21]

An early clinical application was aimed at exploiting the blast flagging capability for the detection of residual disease in leukemic patients.[22] The modern era of this type of study could start when new methodologies, based on the use of fluorescent nucleic acid dyes, were introduced in the second half of the 1990s. The first instrument capable of counting erythroblast and remove the fat interference was the Cell-Dyn 4000.[23,24] Another valid erythroblast count, associated with an original count of immature granulocytes, became available a few years later, with the Sysmex XE-2100 series of instruments.[25,26] The following sections will summarize the results that several groups reported in published scientific papers on bone marrow analysis with different types of automated blood cell counters.

Nucleated Cell Count as an Indicator of Bone Marrow Cellularity

The bone marrow TNCC is a good indicator of marrow cellularity. This is an area in which automated bone marrow analysis could provide reliable and useful information. The microscope assessment of cellularity on aspirate films, in effect, is limited to a general estimate and to a careful consideration of the quality and adequacy of the aspirate material, in terms of suitability of the films for morphologic analysis. Such evaluation, which is subjective and difficult, does not provide a numerical estimate of cellularity (that is reserved for histologic sections), but only a semiquantitative description (normal; slightly, moderately, or markedly reduced; slightly, moderately, or markedly increased). The availability of a precise, objective, and accurate quantitative count of bone marrow cells is thus useful for diagnostic purposes. Erythroblasts, or NRBCs are usually not included by automated blood cell counters within the WBC count in peripheral blood samples, so that the TNCC of the bone marrow must be calculated as the sum of the different populations (TNCC = NRBC + WBC). In peripheral blood, instruments that do not possess a specific (fluorescent) method to count erythroblasts tend to over-estimate total WBC count and use software adaptation to exclude erythroblast signals. In bone marrow, they tend more often to underestimated TNCC because of the partial disruption of the more mature erythroblast membrane caused by lytic reagent.

The reproducibility of TNCC obtained with the Sysmex XE-2100, evaluated by means of multiple duplicate analysis, has been found to be satisfactory.[7] However, for a high proportion of samples with elevated TNCC (57/264), no results were re-ported by the instrument; dilution with PBS to counts less than 20 to 30 $\times$ 10^9/L reduced the number of rejections. Some authors have compared the automated TNCC with the morphologic assessment of cellularity. Using the Abbott Cell-Dyn 4000, the current authors found good agreement between automated TNCC and 5 morphologic classes corresponding to increasing levels of cellularity.[12] In poorly cellular samples (classes 1 and 2), TNCC was always less than 15 $\times$ 10^9/L; in samples with rich cellularity (classes 4 and 5), TNCC was always more than that value, and often much higher than that. This good level of correlation of TNCC with semiquanti-tative cellularity evaluation was then confirmed using as reference microscopy on bi-opsy sections.[27] Good results were also obtained by comparing microscope assessment with TNCC obtained with Sysmex instrument,[11] Coulter Gen-S[19] (Beck-man Coulter Inc., Brea, CA USA) and VCS technology (Beckman Coulter Inc., Brea, CA USA),[28,29] and Advia (Siemens AG, Munich, Germany).[30] In an experimental context, Criswell and colleagues[31] recently demonstrated that with the veterinary version of the XE-2200i V, TNCC alone provided an immediate and improved assess-ment of potential treatment-related variations in bone marrow cellularity in preclinical rodent studies compared with histologic evaluation alone.

The excellent agreement between TNCC and true bone marrow cellularity has been confirmed by studies of the correlation between automated TNCC and microscope count using Burker-type chambers after sample manual dilution with Türk fluid.[10,17,18]

Differential Bone Marrow Cell Count—Comparison with Microscope

Analytical performance of the hematology analyzers, in general, is inadequate in discriminating the single maturational stages among the heterogeneous multitude of blood cell precursors, so that a true automated bone marrow cell differential count is impossible to obtain. Studies attempting to identify specific bone marrow cell pop-ulations have been published only by groups working with instruments capable of erythroblast count using fluorescent stains. In general, they showed good or accept-able correlations for the main cell lineages, with some specific biases confirmed by the majority of authors. No studies have been published with the latest-generation instru-ments produced by the same or by other manufacturers.

In the first assessment of a full automated bone marrow cell differential count in comparison with traditional morphologic bone marrow differential, the authors found that the relative proportions of the main cell populations were well correlated with morphology, with coefficients of correlation of r = 0.883 for granulocytes and 0.692 for erythroblasts (in resistant red blood cell [RBC] mode to obtain complete erythro-cyte lysis).[12] However, the authors observed a bias of the erythroblast's automated percentage toward slightly lower values than those obtained at the microscope. With the Abbott technology, a lytic reagent selectively damages the erythroblast's membrane to permit propidium iodide binding to the intact nucleus; at least part of the lower automated erythroblast percentage is probably due to some resistance of the most immature proerythroblasts and basophilic erythroblasts to such permeabilizing action.

The good correlation and the instrument's tendency to underestimate the erythroblast count when compared to the microscope have subsequently been confirmed with different preanalytical approaches using the Cell-Dyn 4000,[14,27] and the Sysmex XE-2100.[7,17] Sysmex counts showed an acceptable correlation between automation and the microscope for lymphocytes (however influenced by plasmacytes when present) and eosinophils, and a good correlation for neutrophils (bands + neutrophils), as well as for the automated immature granulocyte count versus microscope myeloblasts plus promyelocytes; monocyte and basophil counts were overestimated because of the interference by fat droplets.[11] Like with the Cell-Dyn 4000, erythroblast counts obtained with the Sysmex showed a poor correlation with microscopy (r = 0.51). Mori and colleagues[10] have found high correlations of their modified XE-2100 counts with immunophenotypic flow cytometric determinations of monocytes, granulocytes, and erythroblasts (r = 0.96), as well as with manual microscope differential count.

Most authors have reported acceptable correlations between the automated and the microscope M:E ratio. Automated M:E ratios, however, were generally slightly higher, as a consequence of the generally underestimated erythroblast count.[18]

Bone Marrow Blasts: Automated Count, Sensitivity, and Specificity

As in peripheral blood, the capability of an automated cell counter to identify and flag the presence of increased percentages of marrow blasts is crucial for the diagnosis and follow-up of patients with acute leukemia and myelodysplastic syndromes. Thus it is also among the most important characteristics to be assessed before considering a routine utilization. In a preliminary study carried out with the Bayer H1 hematology system, based on automated cytochemistry, the blast flag, indicating an instrument count above 5%, was useful for the assessment of bone marrow remission status of patients treated for acute leukemia, with a sensitivity of 82% and a specificity of 90%.[22] With the new Cell-Dyn 4000 technology, permitting direct erythroblast counting and the exclusion of lipid droplets, the authors subsequently showed that the instrument blast cell count (not reportable, but available as research data) had a relatively low correlation with the microscopic blast cell count, and a clear trend toward underestimation.[12] On the other hand, the efficacy of the instrument blast flag for identifying samples with more than 5% blasts in the bone marrow was higher, without false negatives in 20 samples with more than 5% of blasts (100% sensitivity) and with 1 single true false positive result out of 64 negative samples (98.5% specificity). The same instrument could even count a wide range of blasts (1%–64%), with a good correlation for a mixed population of blasts/monocytes, and a sensitivity of 89% and specificity of 98% for blastic marrow with more than 5% blasts, but also for granulocytic hyperplasia, lymphocyte predominance and non diagnostic samples.[14] Cell-Dyn 4000 automated blast cell counts above 3% and presence of blast flag showed a good agreement with increased blast percentages in bone marrow in another study,[18] while the concordance was apparently not as good in 2 studies that correlated blast counts at the microscope with the Sysmex XE-2100 IMI blast percentage.[10,17]

In a recent study, some automated blood count parameters provided by the Siemens Advia 120 analyzer have been measured in bone marrow samples for discriminating patients of acute promyelocytic leukemia.[32] Not unexpectedly, these authors found that the percentage of large unstained cells (large cells devoid of mye-loperoxidase, or LUCs) was particularly low in this group of patients whose blasts are typically rich in peroxidase, compared with other types of myeloid leukemias; more-over, a high LUC value was associated with the increased risk of adverse outcomes and worse survival.

SCATTERGRAMS AND DISTRIBUTION PATTERNS: QUALITATIVE INFORMATION

Besides studies on quantitative measurements and comparison with microscopy and other methodologies, several studies have exploited qualitative aspects of cellular automated analysis, trying to identify diagnostic patterns even with instruments not provided with direct counting capability for erythroblasts and other immature cells.

In a clinical setting, utilization of hematology analyzers for samples suspicious for leukemia can provide hematologists with a rapid and reliable preliminary assessment before microscopic evaluation. Using peripheral blood samples, almost all the different types of blood cell analyzers have been studied to exploit their analytical technologies (eg, impedance, radio frequency, light scatter at different angles, light absorption, fluorescence, and myeloperoxidase content) to identify specific distribu-tions of leukemic cells in terms of size, granularity, nuclear structure, internal compo-sition, and enzyme content. The different types of leukemias exhibit different distribution patterns on instrument scattergrams on the basis of these cell properties. Analyzers based on automated cytochemistry can even provide a clinically useful pre-microscope leukemia classification on the basis of the distribution patterns of the different types of leukemic cell clusters.[33]

Bone marrow scattergram observation provides an immediate general perception of overall sample quality and characteristics, with several possibilities:

- Normal composition with a clear representation of the main cell classes, with var-iable presence of fat
- Samples with erythroid or granulocytic hyperplasia are easily appreciated
- Hypocellular samples are characterized by decreased cell numbers with frequent increase in lipid particles
- Presence of blasts of different types, both myeloid and lymphoid, possibly form-ing clusters in a specific plot area indicative of the leukemia subtype

Automated blood cell counters can be used to evaluate distribution patterns of leukemic cell clusters in bone marrow aspirates samples. It is thus possible to obtain a rapid assessment of overall cellularity, as well as of excessive proportion of blasts or other abnormal populations of cells.[7,15,34] Distinct nucleated cell scattergram patterns were observed with bone marrow samples by several authors.[11,14] Algorithms have been proposed to discriminate between bone marrow samples that can and cannot be evaluated.[16]

Among the many technologies available, the Siemens Advia analytical technologies for the identification of leukocytes frequently provide on the cytogram's specific cellular distributions, which can represent a basis for a type of classification, designated by the acronym PANDA from the initials of the 2 methods used (peroxidase activity and nu-clear density analysis). The analysis of the nuclear density in the basophil/nuclear den-sity channel highlights the presence of blast cells with immature, uncondensed chromatin. The peroxidase channel, on the other hand, allows one to assess the type of blast cell and its degree of differentiation. Peroxidase is a faithful marker of the gran-ulocytic nature of a population and provides valuable information on the maturation characteristics, so that it is possible to recognize certain consistent, reproducible, graphical conformations. Such graphical information constitute a very informative, rapidly available, diagnostic ensemble, which guides and directs the microscopic morphologic analysis, orienting the examination immediately toward the differentiation and degree of maturation of the pathologic cells.[35,36] The PANDA scheme has been evaluated and scientifically confirmed, with good results for both sensitivity and specificity.[37,38] Although originally devised with peripheral blood samples, several studies have shown that this morphologic approach is quite reproducible and equally effective, with bone marrow aspirates both in human and in veterinary pathology.[30,32,39]

BONE MARROW AND PERIPHERAL BLOOD

The possibility of obtaining quick cell counts in marrow samples can represent a source of new information. Interesting data come from the comparison of results obtained from the simultaneous analysis of peripheral blood and bone marrow. The composition in red blood cells of bone marrow and peripheral blood, in particular, is almost the same from both a quantitative and a qualitative point of view.[15] In 91 patients, mean hemoglobin concentration was 9.9 g/dL in the bone marrow aspirate fluid and 10.7 in peripheral blood, with a high correlation ($r^2 = 0.848$); mean corpuscular volume (MCV) was 89.4 and 90.7 fL, respectively ($r^2 = 0.978$). Holdrinet and colleagues[40] showed the similarity of hemoglobin concentration in bone marrow and peripheral blood, using ^{51}Cr-labeled autologous erythrocytes and ^{125}I-labeled albumin; in their study, 97%±4.2% of the hemoglobin content of bone marrow samples was of peripheral blood origin. These findings seem to suggest that most mature red blood cells in the bone marrow samples derive from diluting peripheral blood. On the other hand, TNCC is normally higher in the bone marrow fluid than the WBC count in the peripheral blood, with a gradient that increases with increasing TNCC. This probably reflects the existence of a bone marrow barrier, which prevents the delivery of immature cells into circulating blood. In the authors' study, bone marrow and peripheral blood platelets were correlated below 100×10^9/L, while at normal and higher values there was a trend toward lower platelet counts in bone marrow, with a gradient that rises with increasing counts.[15] Thus probably all platelets in marrow derive from diluting blood, and there could exist an inverse barrier that prevents re-entry of platelets when the platelet count is high.

Bone Marrow Fluid as a Substitute of Peripheral Blood for Laboratory Tests

On the basis of the similarity of blood count parameters between bone marrow and circulating blood, several studies have evaluated the possibility of using anticoagulated samples of bone marrow aspirate (intraosseous blood) as an alternative source of blood for the complete blood cell count and serum biochemical tests, both in human and veterinary pathology.[41–43] Interesting results have been obtained in emergency conditions, where bone marrow analysis could represent an alternative to peripheral blood when venous access could not be established in other vascular sites. In agreement with the authors' findings previously described for adults, in pediatric patients, bone marrow hemoglobin was highly predictive for peripheral blood hemoglobin concentration (<6% difference), while leukocyte counts were usually higher, and platelet counts were usually lower in bone marrow.[44]

Reticulocytes in Bone Marrow and Peripheral Blood

Many authors, using fluorescence flow cytometry and automated blood cell counters, have shown that reticulocyte percentages and absolute counts in bone marrow and peripheral blood are highly correlated; however reticulocytes, as well as the immature reticulocyte fraction (IRF), are consistently higher in bone marrow compared with peripheral blood.[12,15,45,46] Choi and colleagues,[47] for instance, found in healthy subjects mean reticulocyte percentages of 2.0 plus or minus 1.2 standard deviations (SD) in bone marrow versus 1.6 plus or minus 0.8 SD in peripheral blood: cases in which the marrow reticulocyte count was over ten times higher than the peripheral blood rate were observed in myelodysplastic syndromes and megaloblastic anemia. The marked difference in reticulocyte and IRF percentage in patients with ineffective erythropoiesis suggests that the newly generated reticulocytes in bone marrow are incapable of maturing and being released in these cases; an increased marrow-to-blood reticulocyte ratio has been proposed as a useful indicator for the diagnosis of myelodysplastic syndromes.[47,48] The authors have also observed high marrow-to-blood reticulocyte ratio during the follow-up of hemopoietic stem cell transplantation, as a transitory phenomenon likely related to rapid and massive erythroid regeneration.[15] The absence of the normal bone marrow-to-blood gradient in reticulocyte percentage can be ascribed to differences in dilution of the marrow fluid by peripheral blood; the ratio, in fact, increases proportionally with TNCC, so that a value below 1.2 can represent an indicator of excessive contamination of bone marrow aspirates by circulating blood.[15]

ANIMAL HEMATOLOGY: A BREAKTHROUGH IN THE AUTOMATED MARROW ANALYSIS

Bone marrow evaluation is an important step for laboratories working in research and drug development and safety, to test and understand the potential toxicity of new products on the hematopoietic system. Pharmaceutical companies devote considerable personnel and financial resources into bone marrow analysis, which remains a standard requirement to assess treatment-related effects among large animal groups, and to determine potential primary hematotoxicity of new compounds through characterization of changes in bone marrow cellularity, or selective increases or damage of specific cell populations, such as eosinophils.

Two recently published studies on high-throughput automated bone marrow in rats reported interesting applications of blood cell counters in this area. Using the well-established hematology analyzer Sysmex XT-2100iV equipped with species-specific veterinary software, and optimized bone marrow cell-specific gating with defined purified cell populations, these authors found that TNCC alone provided an immediate and improved assessment of potential treatment-related bone marrow cellularity in preclinical studies compared with histologic evaluation.[13] Automated evaluation of the M:E ratio was also useful to refine the overall interpretation of treatment-related bone marrow effects. The original method was tested in healthy control rats, but also in animals with typical treatment related changes, such as erythroid hypoplasia due to cyclophosphamide treatment and erythroid hyperplasia due to erythropoietin treatment and repeat phlebotomies.[31] After a relatively sophisticated procedure of sample preparation, with washing and dilution to dissociate the bone marrow aggregates, the instrument counts were obtained using special gating standards within the Sysmex cytogram; they resulted accurate for TNCC and myeloid cells. Because this instrument does not include any technology for erythroblast identification and counting, a side step of immunologic microbead separation for lymphocytes was added to avoid underestimation of lymphocytes and overestimation of erythroid precursors as a consequence of the similar size and structure characteristics of the 2 cell populations. According to these researchers, the Sysmex XT-2100iV is capable of performing reliable, reproducible, and high-quality bone marrow analysis in rodents when coupled with magnetic bead isolation, purification, and sequestration of bone marrow lymphoid cells. The authors also recommend that smears or cytocentrifuged preparations of bone marrow cell suspensions should always be collected in case cellular morphologic evaluation is necessary, and that automated quantitative bone marrow analysis should always be conducted in conjunction with a histopathological review.

In another recent study, the Advia hematology analyzer was used in healthy dogs as well as in dogs with leukemia and other hematological disorders. The automated TNCC correlated significantly with the microscope evaluation of cellularity on bone marrow films; a good agreement was also found for eosinophils, neutrophils, and the sum of lymphocytes plus erythroblasts.[30] Interestingly, the authors were able to observe distinct and consistent alterations in the Advia cytogram cell distribution patterns in dogs with acute leukemia, similar to those extensively described in people, confirming that the PANDA category system has a potential for analysis of bone marrow fluid.

SUMMARY

In conclusion, the analysis of bone marrow aspirates using automated blood cell counters is not yet satisfactory. Acceptable results are obtained with some analyzers in normal samples for granulocytes, erythroblasts, lymphocytes, and blasts. Each method has typical pros and cons. Among the systems for which literature references are available, the Abbott technique is perhaps the most efficient without need of difficult sample preparation; the problem of lipid interference has been solved thanks to the unique capability of fat droplets to depolarize polarized light. For some instruments sample dilution is still necessary, and the problem of lipid interference has not completely been solved. Other systems do not have a direct quantitative method for erythroblasts counting, but are quite efficient in the premicroscopic classification of the leukemic cell population, both in peripheral blood and in the bone marrow aspirate fluid.

The advent of an effective automated bone marrow analysis would be useful to reduce the repetitive tasks, such as the repeated evaluations of hundreds of cells at the microscope in many samples every day, such as happens in research and pharmacologic industry.[49] Other limitations of the automated approach, such as the lack of the potential for the assessment of subtle morphologic changes (eg, abnormal granulation or inclusions, presence of Auer rods, intra- or extracellular parasites) will be much more difficult to overcome. Cytologic review will thus remain critical whenever a complete classification of all cell types or lineage maturation is required, such as for the assessment of morphologic changes in any lineage, the confirmation of suspect megaloblastic changes, or the evaluation of treatment-related effects.

REFERENCES

1. Buttarello M, Plebani M. Automated blood cell counts: state of the art. Am J Clin Pathol 2008;130:104–16.
2. Briggs C. Quality counts: new parameters in blood cell counting. Int J Lab Hematol 2009;31:277–97.
3. Lee SH, Erber WN, Porwit A, et al. International Council for Standardization in Hematology. ICSH guidelines for the standardization of bone marrow specimens and reports. Int J Lab Hematol 2008;30:349–64.
4. Bain BJ. Bone marrow aspiration. J Clin Pathol 2001;54:657–63.
5. Malempati S, Joshi S, Lai S, et al. Videos in clinical medicine. Bone marrow aspiration and biopsy. N Engl J Med 2009;361:e28.

6. Swerdlow SH, Campo E, Harris NL, et al. WHO classification of tumours of hae-matopoietic and lymphoid tissues. 4th edition. Lyon (France): IARC Press; 2008.
7. Zini G, Mistretta G, Giordano G, et al. Automated analysis of bone marrow fluid with the Sysmex XE-2100 blood cell counter. Infus Ther Transfus Med 2001;28: 277–9. Available at: http://www.karger.com/Journal/Issue/228382. Accessed October 21, 2014.
8. Lesesve JF, Goupil JJ, Larger V, et al. Artefactuqal elevation of the automated white cell count in the context of a bone marrow aspirate analysis. Clin Lab Hae-matol 2000;22:57.
9. Bentley SA, Taylor MA, Killian DE, et al. Correction of bone marrow nucleated cell counts for the presence of fat particles. Am J Clin Pathol 1995;104:60–4.
10. Mori Y, Mizukami T, Hamaguchi Y, et al. Automation of bone marrow aspirate examination using the XE-2100 automated hematology analyzer. Cytometry B Clin Cytom 2004;58:25–31.
11. Goossens W, Brusselmans C, Boeckx N. Preliminary data on the feasibility of bone marrow screening on the Sysmex XE-2100 automated hematology analyzer. Sysmex J Int 2001;11:70–3. Available at: http://scientific.sysmex.co.jp/en/. Ac-cessed October 1, 2014.
12. d'Onofrio G, Zini G, Tommasi M, et al. Quasntitative bone marrow analysis using the Abbott Cell-Dyn 4000 hematology analyzer. Lab Hematol 1997;3:146–53.
13. Criswell KA, Bock JH, Wildeboer SE, et al. Validation of Sysmex XT-2000iV gener-ated quantitative bone marrow differential counts in untreated Wistar rats. Vet Clin Pathol 2014;43:125–36.
14. Fan G, Alvares C, Ismail S, et al. Quantitative and qualitative bone marrow analysis using the Abbott Cell-Dyn 4000 hematology analyzer. Lab Hematol 1999;5:45–51.
15. d'Onofrio G, Zini G, Tommasi M, et al. Automated analysis of bone marrow: routine implementation and differenced from peripheral blood. Lab Hematol 1998;4:71–9.
16. Zini G. Automated bone marrow analysis: dream or reality? Sysmex J Int 2005;15: 15–20. Available at: http://scientific.sysmex.co.jp/en/. Accessed October 1, 2014.
17. Shibata H, Yamane T, Yamamura R, et al. Automatic analysis of normal bone marrow blood cells using the XE-2100 automated hematology analyzer. J Clin Lab Anal 2003;17:12–7.
18. Yamamura R, Yamane T, Hino M, et al. Automated bone marrow analysis using the CD4000 automated haematology analyser. J Autom Methods Manag Chem 2000;22:89–92.
19. Kim M, Kim J, Lim J, et al. Use of an automated hematology analyzer and flow cytometry to assess bone marrow cellularity and differential cell count. Ann Clin Lab Sci 2004;34:307–13.
20. Tatsumi J, Tatsumi Y, Tatsumi N. Counting and differential of bone marrow cells by an electronic method. Am J Clin Pathol 1986;86:50–4.
21. Yokomatsu Y, Tsuda I, Furota A, et al. Reassessment for reference values for total nucleated cell count and myeloid/erythroid ratio of human bone marrow aspirate. Osaka City Med J 1993;39:93–119.
22. den Ottolander GJ, Baelde HA, Huibregtsen L, et al. The H1 automated differen-tial counter in determination of bone marrow remission in acute leukemia. Am J Clin Pathol 1995;103:492–5.
23. Kim YR, Yee M, Metha S, et al. Simultaneous differentiation and quantitation of erythroblasts and white blood cells on a high throughput clinical haematology analyser. Clin Lab Haematol 1998;20:21–9.

24. d'Onofrio G, Zini M, Tommasi M, et al. Integration of fluorescence and hemocytometry in the Cell-Dyn 4000: reticulocytes, nucleated red blood cells, and white blood cell viability studies. Lab Hematol 1996;2:131–9.
25. de Keijzer MH, van der Meer W. Automated counting of nucleated red blood cells in blood samples of newborns. Clin Lab Haematol 2002;24:343–5.
26. Briggs C, Harrison P, Grant D, et al. New quantitative parameters on a recently introduced automated blood cell counter—the XE 2100. Clin Lab Haematol 2000;22:345–50.
27. Sakamoto C, Yamane T, Ohta K, et al. Automated enumeration of cellular composition in bone marrow aspirate with the Cell-Dyn 4000 automated hematology analyzer. Acta Haematol 1999;101:130–4.
28. Lima M, Simon R, Justiça B. Utility of VCS—hematology instruments in bone marrow aspirate analysis. Blood 1993;82(Suppl 1). poster 2154.
29. Varo MJ, Fuertes MA, Escolar JD, et al. Contribution of VCS technology (volume, conductivity and laser light scatter) to the study of bone marrow cellular populations. Blood 1999;94(Suppl 1). poster 5136.
30. Tan E, Abrams-Ogg AC, Defarges A, et al. Automated analysis of bone marrow aspirates from dogs with haematological disorders. J Comp Pathol 2014;151:67–79.
31. Criswell KA, Bock JH, Wildeboer SE, et al. Comparison of the Sysmex XT-2000iV and microscopic bone marrow differential counts in Wistar rats treated with cyclophosphamide, erythropoietin, or serial phlebotomy. Vet Clin Pathol 2014;43:137–53.
32. Jang MJ, Choi HW, Lee SY. Application of bone marrow samples for discrimination of acute promyelocytic leukemia from other types of acute leukemia using the routine automated hematology analyzer. Int J Lab Hematol 2014. [Epub ahead of print].
33. d'Onofrio G, Mango G. Automated cytochemistry in acute leukemias. A new approach to the FAB classification based on cell distribution pattern. Acta Haematol 1984;72:221–30.
34. Schumacher HR. Bone marrow evaluation by Cell-Dyn 4000 system. In: Schumacher HR, editor. Acute leukemias: difficult, controversial and automated analysis. Philadelphia: Williams and Wilkins; 1998. p. 225.
35. d'Onofrio G. PANDA-Innovative classification of haematopoietic malignancies. Bloodline 2001;1:3–6.
36. d'Onofrio G, Zini G. Morphology of blood disorders. 2nd edition. London: Wiley-Blackwell; 2014.
37. Gibbs GJ. Peroxidase activity and nuclear density analysis (PANDA) in the diagnosis of haematological malignancy. Br J Biomed Sci 2005;62:142–4.
38. Maule WJ. Peroxidase activity and nuclear density analysis (PANDA) in the diagnosis of acute promyelocytic leukaemia. Med Technol SA 2012;26:28–32.
39. d'Onofrio G, Zini G. Automated cytochemistry of acute promyelocytic leukemia: there's more than numbers. Int J Lab Hematol 2014. [Epub ahead of print].
40. Holdrinet RS, von Egmond J, Wessels JM, et al. A method for quantification of peripheral blood admixture in bone marrow aspirates. Exp Hematol 1980;8:103–7.
41. Orlowski JP, Porembka DT, Gallagher JM, et al. The bone marrow as a source of laboratory studies. Ann Emerg Med 1989;18:1348–51.
42. Grisham J, Hastings C. Bone marrow aspirate as an accessible and reliable source for critical laboratory studies. Ann Emerg Med 1991;20:1121–4.
43. Greco SC, Talcott MR, LaRegina MC, et al. Use of intraosseous blood for repeated hematologic and biochemical analyses in healthy pigs. Am J Vet Res 2001;62:43–7.

44. Ummenhofer W, Frei FJ, Urwyler A, et al. Are laboratory values in bone marrow aspirate predictable for venous blood in paediatric patients? Resuscitation 1994;27:123–8.

45. Kageoka T. Reticulocyte as indication of the erythroid hematopoiesis: reticulocyte fractions in peripheral blood and bone marrow. Rinsho Byori 2001;49:485–9.

46. Shibata H, Yamane T, Hirose A, et al. Automated analysis of bone marrow reticulocytes using the XE-2100 automated hematology analyzer. Acta Haematol 2004;111:237–8.

47. Choi JW, Pai SH, Choe HW. Significance of the ration of reticulocyte subpopulations in bone marrow and peripheral blood from patients with myelodysplastic syndromes. Ann Hematol 2003;82:259–61.

48. Hirose A, Yamane T, Shibata H, et al. Automated analyzer evaluation of reticulocytes in bone marrow and peripheral blood of hematologic disorders. Acta Haematol 2005;114:141–5.

49. Von Beust B. Automated bone marrowanalysis in rats– a change in paradigm in toxicologic clinical pathology? Vet Clin Pathol 2014;43:121–2.

Red Blood Cell Population Dynamics

John M. Higgins, MD[a,b,*]

KEYWORDS

- Red blood cell population dynamics • Single-RBC measurements
- Mathematical modeling • RBC life span • RBC turnover • Diagnostic applications
- Predictive medicine • Personalized medicine

KEY POINTS

- Traditional complete blood count (CBC) indices (eg, hematocrit level, hemoglobin level, mean corpuscular volume) provide a snapshot of the current state of the hematologic system.
- The hematologic system is constantly changing, with about 2 million red blood cells (RBCs) per second entering the circulation from the bone marrow and about the same number being cleared per second.
- Modern hematology analyzers are sophisticated instruments, measuring single-cell characteristics at high resolution and with high throughput.
- These measured distributions of single-cell characteristics can be combined with our knowledge of physiology to make inferences about RBC population dynamics and to quantify physiologic dynamics, like how quickly new RBCs are being produced, how quickly a typical RBC's volume is changing as it matures during its ~110-day life span in the circulation, and how quickly RBCs are being cleared and recycled.
- Information on physiologic dynamics will reveal new details of physiologic mechanisms and offer new diagnostic opportunities for existing CBC measurements.

INTRODUCTION

The purpose of clinical hematology analyzers is to characterize the health of the patient's hematologic system. These instruments have also supported significant advances in our basic understanding of human physiology. The practical characterization of health by a hematology analyzer is limited both by technical challenges preventing more accurate measurements and by gaps in our understanding of pathophysiology, which compromise our ability to translate measurements into clinical

Disclosure: The author was supported by an NIH Director's New Innovator Award DP2DK098087.
[a] Department of Pathology and Center for Systems Biology, Massachusetts General Hospital, 185 Cambridge Street, Boston, MA 02114, USA; [b] Department of Systems Biology, Harvard Medical School, Boston, MA 02115, USA
* Department of Pathology and Center for Systems Biology, Massachusetts General Hospital, 185 Cambridge Street, Boston, MA 02114.
E-mail address: higgins.john@mgh.harvard.edu

Abbreviations	
CBC	Complete blood count
Hb	Mass of hemoglobin in a single RBC
HCT	Hematocrit
HGB	Mass of hemoglobin per unit volume blood
MCH	Mean corpuscular hemoglobin
MCHC	Mean corpuscular hemoglobin concentration
MCV	Mean corpuscular volume
RBC	Red blood cell count
RDW	Red cell distribution width

action. The modern hematology analyzer represents a great advance in technical capabilities, providing high-throughput and high-resolution measurements of single red blood cell (RBC) characteristics for tens of thousands of cells.[1]

Quantifying Red Cell Dynamics Would Complement the Static Complete Blood Count

The traditional complete blood count (CBC) indices derived from these sophisticated measurements provide a detailed assessment of the current state of a patient's hematologic system: assessment of the total oxygen carrying capacity by the hematocrit (HCT) or hemoglobin (HGB) levels, measurement of the RBC mean corpuscular volume (MCV), mean corpuscular Hb (MCH), mean corpuscular Hb concentration (MCHC), and an assessment of the current magnitude of variation in volume from 1 RBC to the next (red cell distribution width [RDW]). This multivariate characterization of the current state of the hematologic system is relevant to the screening, diagnosis, and monitoring of almost all diseases. However, the circulating RBC population is constantly changing, with about 2,000,000 new RBCs entering from the bone marrow every second and about the same number being cleared and recycled. Knowledge of the rates of change in the circulating RBC population would provide complementary information on the patient's hematologic system, supporting more accurate inference of the prior states of the hematologic system and its likely future states.

Reticulocyte Counts Provide a Glimpse of Value of Red Cell Dynamics

Automated reticulocyte counts demonstrate the clinical usefulness of an assessment of dynamic aspects of the hematologic system.[2,3] The automated reticulocyte count enables estimation of the rate of RBC production, and that estimate can help distinguish between anemias with different cause, for instance, distinguishing those resulting from productive deficits from those resulting from hemolysis or other destructive processes.

Current clinical use of the automated reticulocyte count also provides an example of the added value obtained by combining high-resolution measurements with quantitative models of physiology. In particular, more subtle diagnostic distinctions and prognostications can be made by combining this new quantification of a physiologic process (ie, the reticulocyte count) with traditional CBC indices like HCT or HGB, which assess the size of the current circulating RBC population. Based on our knowledge of physiologic homeostatic mechanisms, we expect a mild anemia to trigger a compensatory increase in reticulocyte production, and we would expect a more significant anemia to trigger a more significant increase in reticulocyte production. The reticulocyte count enables us to determine not only whether reticulocyte production is qualitatively increased in the presence of anemia but also whether the magnitude of increase in production is appropriate. Calculations such as the corrected reticulocyte count are examples of mechanistic model-based inference from clinical laboratory measurements. Using our model of the quantitative physiologic relationship between RBC production rate and anemia, the magnitude of a reticulocyte count can be compared with the magnitude of the anemia and an assessment can be made as to whether the patient's physiologic systems are responding in a healthy fashion. It is thus possible to identify situations that might qualitatively seem to be healthy. For instance, if there is a decreased HCT or HGB level, and the reticulocyte count is increased, the qualitative assessment would be that the patient's response was appropriate and that the anemia was not caused by a deficit in production. The corrected reticulocyte count or the reticulocyte production index are model-based calculations, which provide a more nuanced assessment of erythropoietic output and enable more precise diagnostic interpretations.[4,5] Although the automated reticulocyte count represents a significant technical advance, with proven clinical value, the measurement itself is imprecise, with repeat measurements of the same blood sample varying by more than 10%, and repeat measurements in the same healthy person varying by as much as 30%.[6,7] The fact that such a crude estimate of RBC production rate is so useful underscores the potential clinical value of other, even crude, assessments of RBC population dynamics.

Estimating Red Cell Maturation and Clearance Rates Requires Modeling

The reticulocyte count provides an assessment of the RBC production rate, but there are no corresponding ways to assess the rate of RBC maturation that occurs during an RBC's ~110-day life span in the circulation, nor is there a way to assess the rate of RBC clearance. Other clinical laboratory measurements such as bilirubin and haptoglobin provide some vague information on RBC turnover, but they are of limited value. RBC turnover is difficult to study.[8–10] Methods have been developed and usually involve labeling, reinfusion, and serial sampling of blood. Other techniques using exhaled carbon monoxide are desirable, in that they are less invasive and do not require weeks of preparation and multiple blood samples, but they have other limitations, including poor precision. A better understanding of RBC life span variation and control may suggest better markers of RBC age, which would enable easier determination of RBC age. In the meantime, mathematical models can be used to provide an initial estimate of RBC maturation and turnover. Without a model of RBC aging, RBC clearance cannot be measured noninvasively. Single RBCs would have to be tracked over many weeks up to the time of clearance and beyond, something which is not currently feasible. Estimates of RBC maturation and clearance therefore require modeling but, like automated reticulocyte counts, are likely, even if crude, to provide new insights into physiology[11] and new diagnostic applications.[12]

Modern hematology analyzers provide sophisticated and high-throughput data sets, which present a great opportunity to improve characterization of hematologic health dramatically. In particular, these high-resolution population measurements provide sufficient data to support inferences about RBC population dynamics: how quickly RBC characteristics are changing in the circulating population, and how much those rates vary from 1 RBC to the next and for 1 RBC over time. There are many measurable characteristics of RBCs, and many of them change over time. A study of RBC population dynamics may thus focus on many different cellular characteristics and how they change over time. RBC volume and RBC Hb content are 2 characteristics of known clinical importance, which can be measured accurately and with high throughput. The population dynamics of RBC volume and RBC Hb content, and the rate of clearance of RBCs, are therefore the focus of the rest of this article, in which:

- Current understanding of RBC dynamics from basic scientific studies is summarized
- A conceptual model of RBC population dynamics is synthesized, and a method to infer RBC population dynamics from hematology analyzer measurements is described
- Current and future opportunities for measuring dynamic features of blood cell populations and their potential applications are reviewed

BASIC SCIENTIFIC STUDIES SHOW ASPECTS OF RED BLOOD CELL POPULATION DYNAMICS

The RBC population is in constant flux. About 2 million cells enter the bloodstream from the bone marrow of a typical healthy human adult every second, with about the same number being cleared. The typical RBC circulates for 100 to 120 days, before being recycled and replaced. Basic science studies have shown that many characteristics change during the life span of the RBCs in the peripheral circulation[13]: volume decreases by about 20%,[14–16] Hb mass decreases by about 15%,[14,15] surface area is reduced, surface/volume ratio increases, microvesicles form and are shed, phosphatidyl-serine symmetry changes, and more. Many more changes occur to individual RBCs in specific contexts, and the physiologic basis and implications are not understood for most of them.

Single-RBC measurements of volume provide richer information on in vivo hematologic processes than just the population averages. The combination of automated reticulocyte identification with these single-cell measurements provides this level of detail in an age-stratified way. Some clinical instruments, including the Siemens Advia 120, 2120, and 2120i (Siemens Healthcare Diagnostics, Tarrytown, NY), and the Abbott Cell-DYN Sapphire (Abbott Laboratories, Santa Clara, CA), provide simultaneous measurement of single-RBC volume, single-RBC Hb concentration, and a reticulocyte dye concentration. These measurements provide high-resolution multidimensional characterization (volume, Hb concentration, reticulocyte status) of the full circulating RBC population and the reticulocyte population. Signatures of the in vivo single-RBC dynamics can be seen in the nature and magnitude of variation in each quantity, for instance the single-RBC volume distribution as shown in **Fig. 1** represents the net effects of these processes on the volumes of all circulating RBCs.

Empirical Studies of In Vivo Volume Dynamics

Young RBCs have long been known to be larger than mature or senescent cells. With the advent of automated reticulocyte counts,[2,3,13] it became possible to quantify the volume differences between young RBCs and those that are more mature. There are many open questions regarding the molecular or cellular processes that regulate these changes in volume, but with high resolution measurement of RBC volume distributions, the changes can be quantified and hypotheses tested regarding mechanisms.

Initial volume changes are fast

Several studies have found that the rate of volume change for young RBCs is rapid, with at least half of the total volume change of the RBCs likely occurring during the first week in the circulation.[15,17,18]

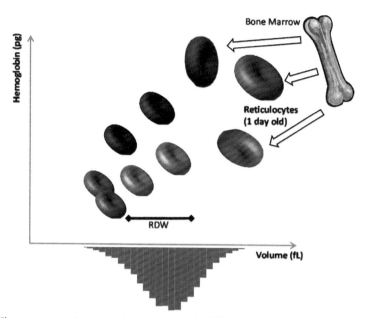

Fig. 1. Changes occurring over the course of the life span of an RBC in the circulation. Single-RBC changes in volume and HGB content integrate over the population and over time to determine the variance in volume and Hb content measured in a CBC. Reticulocytes exit from the bone marrow (*top right*). Their volume and Hb content decline over the course of their ~110-day life span. The single-RBC dynamic processes combine to generate the distributions in volume (RDW) and Hb content, which can be measured by some modern hematology analyzers.

Subsequent volume changes are slow

Experimental studies have also found that the size of each RBC continues to decrease, albeit more slowly, after this first rapid phase occurring early in the lifetime of the RBC in the circulation.[14,16]

Empirical Studies of In Vivo Hemoglobin Content Dynamics

Some modern hematology analyzers measure single-RBC Hb concentration simultaneously with single-RBC volume.[1] Although Hb concentration is the characteristic directly reported by these instruments it is conceptually simpler to work with single-RBC Hb mass or content instead of Hb concentration because simultaneous changes in RBC volume complicate the interpretation. By multiplying the single-RBC Hb concentration by the volume measurement of the same RBC, it is straightforward to derive the Hb mass, with the caveat that Hb mass is derived from two instrument-reported values and may be less accurate than each reported value individually and may also be biased by any correlation in the errors of the 2 values.

The RBC mass is largely determined by the Hb mass, and the RBC density is therefore largely determined by the Hb concentration. It has been challenging to identify physiologic markers of RBC age, and some initial studies suggested that RBC density increased monotonically with age, but because of the strong correlation between RBC density and Hb concentration, this assumption implies that RBC Hb concentration increased monotonically with age. More detailed studies in recent years have resolved some of this confusion and present a picture of Hb content dynamics that is qualitatively similar to that for single-RBC volume.[14]

Initial hemoglobin changes are more significant

RBC density, and thus RBC Hb concentration, seem to increase during the first week or so after a reticulocyte has entered the circulation.[14] Because RBC volume is decreasing during this time as well, a net increase in Hb concentration requires that the Hb content must not decrease as much.[15]

Subsequent hemoglobin changes are less pronounced

Inferences about subsequent changes in RBC Hb content can be made from measurements of RBC volume and Hb concentration. After the first week or so in circulation, RBC density and Hb concentration do not change markedly.[14,16,19] Recent independent measurements with extremely high precision support the conclusion that there is little variation in RBC density across the entire cell population, which represents cells of all ages.[19]

Overall, it seems that for a single reticulocyte entering the peripheral circulation from the bone marrow, the volume changes by about 10% in the first week or so, and the Hb content decreases by about 7%. The volume and Hb content of the single cell then continue to decrease more slowly over the remaining ~3 months of the life span of the RBC, with the total reductions after the first week being comparable to those occurring during the first week, but at slower rates. These volume and Hb content changes are regulated such that there is little variation in the single-RBC Hb concentration from 1 cell to the next.

QUANTIFICATION OF RED BLOOD CELL POPULATION DYNAMICS IN THE CLINICAL LABORATORY

A conceptual and mathematical model can be derived for RBC volume and Hb dynamics from these basic science studies. The model can then be combined with the high-resolution measurements available on some modern hematology analyzers to quantify RBC population dynamics for individual patients. **Fig. 2** shows the volume and Hb distributions measured for an individual healthy patient on an Abbott Cell-DYN Sapphire analyzer. These high-resolution data sets provide additional information on the dynamic processes controlling reticulocyte and RBC maturation. One can begin with the empirical observations described earlier and combine them with these high-resolution data sets to constrain the range of models of RBC dynamics sufficiently that these dynamics can be quantified for individual patients.

Deriving a Model of Red Blood Cell Population Dynamics from Basic Science and Hematology Analyzer Data

The volume of a single RBC changes during its time in the circulation, and the Hb content changes as well. There is strong evidence suggesting that these rates of change are initially relatively fast and subsequently relatively slow. These empirical findings from basic science studies provide constraints on the poorly understood processes responsible for RBC maturation in the peripheral circulation, allowing exclusion of several possible explanations and a focus on a more quantitative description of these processes, even in the absence of any detailed molecular characterization. For instance, **Fig. 3** shows the maturation of a single reticulocyte based on these basic science studies. A model of RBC population dynamics would describe the path through the volume-Hb plane that a young reticulocyte is most likely to take during its lifetime.

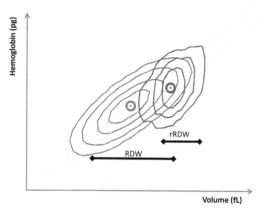

Fig. 2. Single-RBC (*red*) and single-reticulocyte (*blue*) volume and Hb mass distributions. The red contours show the probability density for volume and Hb in the total RBC population of a healthy adult. The red circle shows the MCV, MCH position. The RDW bar shows the extent of the coefficient of variation in volume. There is a thin gray line connecting the MCV, MCH point (*red circle*) to the origin and representing the MCHC. Red contours enclose 90%, 75%, 50%, and 25% percent of cells close to the mean. The blue contours show the same probability density for reticulocytes, with the mean volume and Hb content (rMCV, rMCH) shown as a blue circle. The rRDW bar shows the extent of the coefficient of variation in volume. There is a thin gray line connecting the rMCV, rMCH point to the origin, which represents the average reticulocyte Hb concentration (rMCHC). Blue contours enclose 75%, 50%, and 25% of cells.

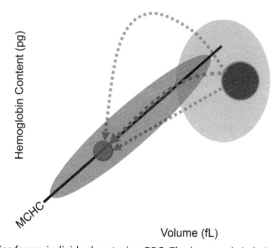

Fig. 3. Trajectories for an individual maturing RBC. The large red circle in the top right represents a reticulocyte sampled from the reticulocyte volume–Hb content distribution (*light blue oval*). The smaller red circle represents a typical mature RBC sampled from the RBC volume–Hb content distribution (*red oval*). The green dashed lines represent 3 hypothetical trajectories. The top trajectory requires an increase in single-RBC Hb content, and any model requiring that sort of trajectory can be excluded based on basic science knowledge. The bottom straight line trajectory can be excluded, because it passes through a space in the plane not covered by either the RBC distribution (*red oval*) or the reticulocyte distribution (*blue oval*). Empirical measurements show that no RBCs of any age are found in these regions, and models requiring this sort of trajectory can be excluded. The middle trajectory is most consistent with basic science findings and hematology instrument measurements.

There are an infinite number of possible trajectories, but many of them can be excluded, because they contradict the empirical results described earlier. For instance, the top trajectory in **Fig. 3** requires an initial increase in the Hb content of the RBC, which is contradicted by basic science studies and available empirical data. Any model of RBC population dynamics that requires such a trajectory can thus be excluded. Using the high-resolution data from the hematology analyzer in **Fig. 2**, the bottom trajectory in **Fig. 3** can also be excluded, because there are no cells in a region of the plane through which many reticulocytes would have to pass according to models requiring this sort of trajectory. The middle trajectory is therefore the most plausible.

To paraphrase the statistician George Box, all mathematical models are wrong, but some are useful. Any model of RBC volume and Hb dynamics is therefore expected to be wrong in some ways, but if it captures enough of the major features of the underlying pathophysiologic processes, the estimates it provides of these true physiologic processes are good enough to be useful in helping us understand dynamic aspects of physiology and useful in complementing traditional diagnostic methods as will be discussed below.

An Example Model of Red Blood Cell Population Dynamics

The range of possible models is strongly constrained by basic scientific studies, some of which were reviewed earlier, and by high-resolution hematology analyzer measurements, such as those shown in **Fig. 2**, but it is still possible to propose different models that are consistent with these studies and data. Informed guesses must then be made, which will certainly not be entirely accurate, but the model can then be tested with new data, its predictions compared, and we can decide if we feel confident that the model is sufficiently accurate to be useful. At least 1 published model has satisfied this sort of validation, and its basic features and assumptions are reviewed, as shown in **Fig. 4**[12]:

- Single-RBC volume and Hb content decrease rapidly until the Hb concentration of the RBC approaches the population mean (MCHC).
- Single-RBC volume and Hb then decrease steadily and more slowly.
- There are small fluctuations in the rates of change in volume and Hb content for individual cells.
- The probability of clearance for a particular RBC can be approximated as a threshold function of its volume and Hb content.

The model describes the rate of volume change for a particular RBC as a function of its current volume and current Hb content.[12] The function has a mathematical form which reflects the 2 phases of volume reduction found by the basic science studies described earlier. The first phase of volume reduction involves faster rates of change and lasts until the Hb concentration of the RBC is close to the population mean (MCHC). The second phase of volume reduction then occurs more slowly. The model includes patient-specific parameters, allowing estimation of rates of volume reduction personalized for each patient, with β_v governing the fast phase of volume change and α governing the slow phase. The model also includes parameters for the Hb dynamics, both the fast (β_h) and slow phases (α), as well as the magnitude of the fluctuations in volume reduction (D_v) and Hb reduction (D_h), and a parameter for the threshold function (v_c) used to approximate the clearance process (**Fig. 5**).

This model then allows these parameters to be quantified for individual patients, yielding estimates of the rates of different dynamic physiologic processes related to RBC rates and clearance. This novel dynamic information provides new insight into physiology, with potential clinical diagnostic applications.

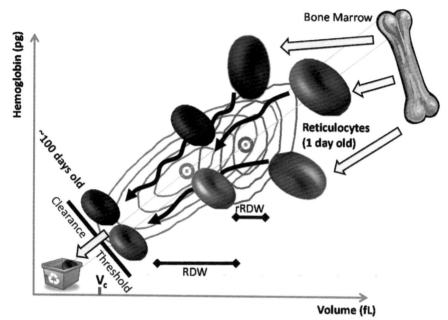

Fig. 4. An example model of RBC population dynamics. Reticulocytes enter from the bone marrow. Their volume and Hb content decrease rapidly at first toward the population mean (gray line through the red circle marking the MCV and MCH). The volume and Hb content of a single RBC continue to decrease with small fluctuations until the cell is cleared and re-cycled, with the probability of clearance approximated by a threshold function of the volume and Hb level of the RBC. A cell with Hb concentration equal to the MCHC is most likely to be cleared when its volume reaches v_c. Cells with higher or lower Hb concentrations are more likely to be cleared at lower or higher volumes, as shown by the clearance threshold line.

APPLICATIONS OF RED BLOOD CELL POPULATION DYNAMICS AND FUTURE DIRECTIONS: TOWARD A MORE COMPLETE BLOOD COUNT

The value of high-resolution data from the modern clinical hematology analyzer derives from the physiologic insights it enables and from the diagnostic applications it supports. The example model described earlier provides an unusual opportunity to compare RBC clearance rates in patients by measuring CBCs and reticulocyte counts. This exercise has suggested, among other things, that the RBC clearance process is tightly regulated and may be modulated in pathologic situations.

Red Blood Cell Clearance Is Tightly Regulated

One of the goals of modeling RBC population dynamics is to generate new insight into basic physiology. RBC clearance processes are difficult to study, and we are only now beginning to understand the magnitude of variation in the RBC clearance process among healthy individuals.[8,9] The clearance rate can be estimated using the model described earlier and shows a coefficient of variation (1.1%) in a healthy population, suggesting that the clearance rate is more tightly controlled than any of the traditional CBC indices (**Fig. 6**). The model itself, as described in Ref.[12] yielded consistent estimates with a range of functional forms for the volume and Hb dynamics. All of the specific equations were deduced from the same set of empirical constraints, and it is reassuring when the quantitative predictions they enable,

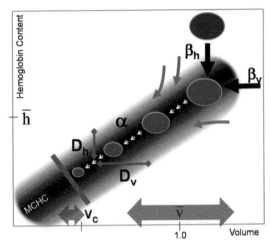

Fig. 5. A model of RBC volume and Hb dynamics. Reticulocytes enter from the bone marrow (*top right*). Their volume and Hb content decrease rapidly at first toward the population mean (*center of thick black line* designated as MCHC), with β_v quantifying the rate of volume change and β_h quantifying the rate of Hb change. The volume and Hb content of a single RBC continue to decrease (α) with small fluctuations (D_v and D_h), until the cell is cleared and recycled, with the probability of clearance approximated by a threshold function of the volume and Hb of the RBC. A cell with Hb concentration equal to the MCHC is most likely to be cleared when its volume reaches v_c. Cells with higher or lower Hb concentrations are more likely to be cleared at lower or higher volumes, as shown by the red clearance threshold line. The thick red horizontal arrows show the coefficient of variation in the v_c and the MCV. There is less variation in the estimated clearance threshold.

such as tight regulation of the clearance process, are robust to the specific functional form. The legitimacy of the estimate of RBC clearance rate rests not on whether the single-RBC Hb and volume dynamics are assumed to be exponential or linear with respect to the current volume or Hb level of an RBC but instead rests only on the knowledge that there is an initial fast phase of volume and Hb reduction followed by a subsequent slow phase, and that the speed of the fast phase is correlated with the difference between the current Hb concentration of the RBC and that of some population-wide target. This enhanced understanding of basic physiology can then be used to improve our understanding of pathologic situations such as iron deficiency anemia.

Red Blood Cell Clearance Seems to be Delayed in States of Red Blood Cell Production Deficits

Having developed and validated this model, it can be used to estimate the RBC clearance rate for patients and compare their estimated clearance rates with those from healthy individuals to understand any effect these diseases may have on the clearance rate or any adaptive response of the clearance rate to these diseases. Iron deficiency is a common condition compromising erythropoiesis. Iron deficiency anemia is associated with a decreased MCV and often an increased RDW. Modeling of the RBC population dynamics in individuals with mild iron deficiency anemia (**Fig. 7**) shows that their clearance threshold has been decreased. Because the clearance threshold is expressed as a fraction of the MCV, this decrease in clearance threshold occurs above and beyond the well-known decrease in MCV.

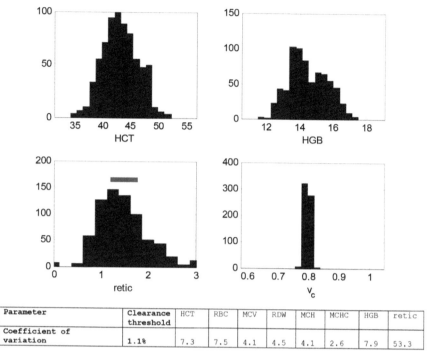

Parameter	Clearance threshold	HCT	RBC	MCV	RDW	MCH	MCHC	HGB	retic
Coefficient of variation	1.1%	7.3	7.5	4.1	4.5	4.1	2.6	7.9	53.3

Fig. 6. Variation in traditional and dynamic CBC indices. The estimated clearance threshold (v_c) has a smaller coefficient of variation in 700 healthy individuals than any of the other traditional CBC indices or the reticulocyte count. The clearance threshold therefore has the potential to be a specific marker of disease, because any variation would be easily distinguishable from the narrow normal range.

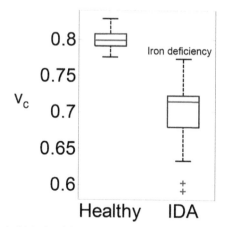

Fig. 7. Clearance threshold in healthy individuals and those with iron deficiency anemia (IDA). The clearance threshold is expressed as a fraction of the MCV, with v_c equal to the volume at which an RBC with an Hb concentration equal to the population mean MCHC would be most likely to be cleared. Healthy individuals have a v_c tightly clustered around 80% of the MCV. Individuals with IDA have a significantly lower v_c. These individuals with IDA had v_cs in the normal range before the development of IDA, and a decreased v_c may therefore serve as an early warning sign for impending IDA.

A delay in RBC clearance transiently increases the circulating mass of RBCs. Given that iron deficiency anemia involves a decrease in erythropoietic output, this model-derived observation of delayed clearance suggests a mechanism: perhaps RBC production decreases slightly as a result of an incipient iron deficiency, and this decreased production triggers compensatory delay in clearance to maintain circulating red cell mass. This hypothesis is shown in **Fig. 8.**

Dynamic modeling of red cell populations in patients with iron deficiency anemia thus suggests that the RBC clearance threshold is decreased, perhaps as compensation for diminished output in the face of decreased iron stores. The lowered clearance threshold maintains circulating RBC mass, confounding the diagnosis of the anemia based on decreasing HCT or HGB levels. By using a model of RBC population dynamics, it might be possible to identify the clearance delay directly and predict the anemia before it appears.

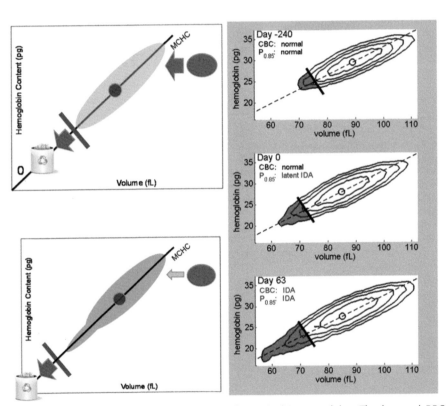

Fig. 8. Hypothesized homeostatic mechanism for RBC clearance delay. The lowered RBC clearance threshold found in patients with decreased erythropoiesis is typical of iron deficiency anemia and suggests that the clearance delay may serve as a temporary compensatory response to decreased RBC production, maintaining RBC mass in the face of decreased production. Left-hand panels show a schematic of the mechanism. Right-hand panels show support for this idea provided by CBC results for an individual when healthy (*top right*), with frank iron deficiency anemia (*bottom right*), and a latent anemia state 2 months before the anemia, when the evidence of clearance delay is shown by the increasing fraction of the RBCs appearing lower than the 85th percentile (*red shaded regions* in each right-hand panel) along the MCHC line.

Delayed Clearance Predicts Iron Deficiency Anemia

A goal of modeling RBC population dynamics is the discovery of novel diagnostic approaches. The model discussed earlier suggests that (1) RBC clearance is tightly regulated in healthy people, (2) it is delayed in the early phases of iron deficiency before anemia has developed, and (3) the clearance rate can be estimated as a threshold function (v_c). It may then be possible to develop an early warning biomarker for iron deficiency anemia by measuring v_c or some other estimate of RBC clearance. Previous studies[12] have found that it is possible to identify cases of iron deficiency anemia in people with normal CBCs using this approach up to 90 days before anemia is discovered, with sensitivity greater than 50% and specificity greater than 90%. Because these people all have normal CBCs, sensitivity of detection using traditional CBC indices alone is 0%.[12] This high sensitivity and specificity for iron deficiency anemia suggest that the timescale for homeostatic response to iron deficient states is sufficiently long (multiple months) that this approach may provide an opportunity to improve screening programs for iron deficiency in adults at risk of gastrointestinal malignancy and in young children at risk of cognitive deficits from nutritional deficiency.

Future Directions

The example model presented in this article characterizes RBC population dynamics using 6 parameters, which describe patient-specific estimates of the fast and slow phases of volume and Hb reduction, the magnitude of their fluctuations, and the clearance rate as estimated by a threshold function. The model allows estimation of these dynamic parameters for individual patients using existing CBC and reticulocyte measurements, thereby providing several new insights into RBC physiology. This article focuses on just one of these insights, namely the tight regulation of RBC clearance rate and its modulation in iron deficiency anemia. The other model parameters provide additional insights into RBC physiology, which complement existing knowledge and present additional opportunities for diagnostic applications. Other models of RBC population dynamics, particularly those that are more accurate because they integrate new understanding, will provide additional and more powerful insights.

Modern hematology analyzers provide high-resolution and high-throughput characterization not just of RBC populations but also of white blood cell lineages and platelets. The characterization of white blood cell lineages and subtypes has become particularly sophisticated in recent years. Models of the population dynamics of these other cell types will likely show important details of physiology, with even greater diagnostic possibilities.

The power of dynamic population models of RBCs depends on the richness of the measurements made by the hematology analyzer. The combined optical measurement of RBC volume and Hb level developed a few decades ago was an important technological step.[1] It is concerning that the availability of instruments with this enhanced technical sophistication may be decreasing as clinical laboratories prioritize features such as automation over the richness of the measurements. This sort of regressive step in terms of technical capability in the clinical laboratory is worrisome for the future role of the clinical laboratory in diagnostic medicine. Almost every other area of medical care has embraced the potential of large data sets to inform personalized and precision medicine. Many hospital departments are collecting vast databases of high-resolution measurements: genetic, proteomic, metabolomic, transcriptomic, cytometric, and more. The current diagnostic purpose of these data sets is not always clear but their future value is unquestioned. If the clinical laboratory does not provide high-resolution CBC data to enable the sort of modeling and analysis described in this article, then other hospital departments will do so. In that case, as large data sets and the expertise to transform them into clinically actionable information become driving forces in modern health care, the clinical laboratory will play a smaller and smaller role. As others have noted,[20] the clinical laboratory currently has the expertise and infrastructure to take a leading role, transforming the recent technical advances in molecular and cellular measurement into clinically actionable information.

ACKNOWLEDGMENT

The author thanks Roy Malka for helpful discussions and comments on the manuscript.

REFERENCES

1. Mohandas N, Kim YR, Tycko DH, et al. Accurate and independent measurement of volume and hemoglobin concentration of individual red-cells by laser-light scattering. Blood 1986;68:506–13.
2. Donofrio G, Chirillo R, Zini G, et al. Simultaneous measurement of reticulocyte and red blood cell indices in healthy subjects and patients with microcytic and macrocytic anemia. Blood 1995;85:818–23.
3. Donofrio G, Zini G, Tommasi M, et al. Automated measurement of total and immature reticulocytes, nucleated red blood cells and apoptotic cells in peripheral blood and bone marrow. Blood 1996;88:3182.
4. Liesveld JL, Rowe JM, Lichtman MA. Variability of the erythropoietic response in autoimmune hemolytic anemia–analysis of 109 cases. Blood 1987;69:820–6.
5. Bain BJ. Leukaemia diagnosis. 3rd edition. Malden (MA): Blackwell; 2003.
6. Piva E, Brugnara C, Chiandetti L, et al. Automated reticulocyte counting: state of the art and clinical applications in the evaluation of erythropoiesis. Clin Chem Lab Med 2010;48:1369–80.
7. Van den Bossche J, Devreese K, Malfait R, et al. Comparison of the reticulocyte mode of the Abx Pentra 120 Retic, Coulter (R) General-S (TM), Sysmex (R) SE 9500, Abbott CD 4000 and Bayer Advia (R) 120 haematology analysers in a simultaneous evaluation. Clin Lab Haematol 2001;23:355–60.
8. Franco RS. The measurement and importance of red cell survival. Am J Hematol 2009;84:109–14.
9. Mock DM, Widness JA, Veng-Pedersen P, et al. Measurement of posttransfusion red cell survival with the biotin label. Transfus Med Rev 2014;28:114–25.
10. Malka R, Delgado FF, Manalis SR, et al. In vivo volume and hemoglobin dynamics of human red blood cells. PLoS Comput Biol 2014;10(10):e1003839.
11. Golub MS, Hogrefe CE, Malka R, et al. Developmental plasticity of red blood cell homeostasis. Am J Hematol 2014;89(5):459–66.
12. Higgins JM, Mahadevan L. Physiological and pathological population dynamics of circulating human red blood cells. Proc Natl Acad Sci U S A 2010;107: 20587–92.
13. Bosch FH, Werre JM, Roerdinkholder-Stoelwinder B, et al. Characteristics of red blood cell populations fractionated with a combination of counterflow centrifugation and Percoll separation. Blood 1992;79:254–60.
14. Franco RS, Puchulu-Campanella ME, Barber LA, et al. Changes in the properties of normal human red blood cells during in vivo aging. Am J Hematol 2013;88:44–51.

15. Willekens FL, Roerdinkholder-Stoelwinder B, Groenen-Dopp YA, et al. Hemoglobin loss from erythrocytes in vivo results from spleen-facilitated vesiculation. Blood 2003;101:747–51.

16. Waugh RE, Narla M, Jackson CW, et al. Rheologic properties of senescent erythrocytes–loss of surface area and volume with red blood cell age. Blood 1992;79: 1351–8.

17. Gifford SC, Derganc J, Shevkoplyas SS, et al. A detailed study of time-dependent changes in human red blood cells: from reticulocyte maturation to erythrocyte senescence. Br J Haematol 2006;135:395–404.

18. Willekens FL, Werre JM, Groenen-Dop YA, et al. Erythrocyte vesiculation: a self-protective mechanism? Br J Haematol 2008;141:549–56.

19. Grover WH, Bryan AK, Diez-Silva M, et al. Measuring single-cell density. Proc Natl Acad Sci U S A 2011;108:10992–6.

20. Louis DN, Gerber GK, Baron JM, et al. Computational pathology: an emerging definition. Arch Pathol Lab Med 2014;138(9):1133–8.

Quality Control of Automated Cell Counters

George S. Cembrowski, MD, PhD[a],*, Gwen Clarke, MD, FRCPC[b]

KEYWORDS

- Quality control • External quality assessment • Hematology • Delta checks
- Biologic variation • Average of patients • Critical values

KEY POINTS

- Hematology quality control should be simplified.
- The use of averages of red blood cell indices for quality control is outmoded and should be replaced with truncated patient averages of all directly measured parameters.
- Patient specimens that have critical concentrations do not need to be repeated in an attempt to improve their accuracy.

QUALITY CONTROL AND EXTERNAL QUALITY ASSESSMENT

Quality control refers to a laboratory's internal assessment of analytical quality. This assessment is accomplished by the regular measurement of quality control (reference) samples. In laboratory hematology, the manufacturer of the laboratory's hematology instrument generally supplies two or three levels of quality control material every 30 to 90 days. The manufacturer's targets for limits of acceptability are generally too broad to be used as quality control limits. With each new lot of control, the hematology laboratory must revalidate or revise its own limits of quality control acceptability to the new control mean ± a multiple of the usual standard deviation. The laboratory's repeated measurements of the quality control (reference) samples by the same analyzer permits the assessment of instrument precision. External quality control (external quality assurance [EQA]), or proficiency testing, allows for the assessment of instrument accuracy and is demonstrated by the laboratory's analyzer/reagent combination producing results that are close to the proficiency provider's target values. Specimens sent to laboratories for EQA are generally acquired by subscription and arrive at the laboratory at bimonthly or longer intervals. Results are generated and

Disclosure: G.S. Cembrowski is the principal of the company Laboratory Concision.
[a] Laboratory Medicine and Pathology, 4B1.24 Mackenzie Health Sciences Centre, University of Alberta Hospital, 8440-112 Street, Edmonton, AB T6G 2B7, Canada; [b] Canadian Blood Services, Medical Office 8249 -114th Street, Edmonton, AB T6G 2R8, Canada
* Corresponding author.
E-mail address: george.cembrowski@albertahealthservices.ca

Abbreviations

CBC	Complete blood count
EQA	External quality assurance
Hct	Hematocrit
Hgb	Hemoglobin
MCH	Mean corpuscular hemoglobin
MCHC	Mean corpuscular hemoglobin concentration
MCV	Mean corpuscular volume
RBC	Red blood cell

---

returned to the proficiency testing provider where they are collated and compared with the results from other participants using the same analyzer and reagent combination. Results of this comparison should be available once all participants have submitted results, potentially days or weeks following testing. This article focuses on quality control. For more specific reading on hematology and EQA, the reader is directed to the work of Cembrowski.[1]

In the hospital environment, quality control samples are routinely analyzed two or three times per day. Reference laboratories tend to run quality control with batches of patient samples, often being inserted at the beginning and end of the patient run. The quality control results are assessed with one or more quality control rules and are available for subsequent charting and evaluation. A wide assortment of quality control rules (**Table 1**) can be used to interpret the quality control results and classify the analytical run as in control, out of control, or as a warning. Each control rule has a specific error detection capability with some control rules being sensitive to systematic errors (shifts) and others sensitive to increased random error (increased imprecision). Because hematology quality control specimens can control the analysis of 16 or more constituents of the complete blood count (CBC), overly narrow limits (eg, ± 2 SD, ± 2.5 SD, and even ± 3 SD) can result in overly frequent "out of control" misclassifications of in control analytical runs.

Caution

We occasionally encounter hematology laboratories that use previously analyzed patient specimens that are then reanalyzed over the next 4 to 24 hours as a secondary control. We do not advise this practice because these specimens are generally less stable than reference sample quality controls and their target range is poorly defined because it is a product of just one or two assays.

BIOLOGIC VARIATION AND ITS INFLUENCE ON THE SELECTION OF QUALITY CONTROL RULES

Patient-related preanalytical influences can affect almost every quantitative test performed in the clinical laboratory. For example, hematocrit (Hct) is increased with exertion (eg, running up several flights of stairs) or just by drawing the blood specimen while the patient is standing compared with sitting or lying down.[2] To minimize these influences and to obtain the most reproducible and comparable test result, diagnostic blood samples should be collected under standard conditions. Even when these recommendations are strictly followed, patients demonstrate nonanalytical variations in the measured analytes. These "usual" within-subject variations are relatively constant from subject to subject. Measurement of this within-subject biologic variation involves the regular sampling of healthy subjects and rapid stabilization of their plasma.

Table 1 Common quality control rules		
Rule	**Summary**	**Use**
1–2SD	Use as a rejection or warning when one control observation exceeds the ± 2 SD control limits.	Overused. Should only be used with manual assays with low number of analytes/control materials. Usually used as a warning.
1–2.5SD	Reject a run when one control observation exceeds the ± 2.5 SD control limits.	Detects random error and large systematic error.
1–3SD	Reject a run when one control observation exceeds the ± 3 SD control limits.	Detects random error and large systematic error.
1–3.5SD	Reject a run when one control observation exceeds the ± 3.5 SD control limits.	Detects large random and systematic error. Use only with highly precise assays.
1–4SD	Reject a run when one control observation exceeds the ± 4 SD control limits.	Detects large random and systematic error. Use only with highly precise assays.
2–2SD	Reject a run when two consecutive control observations are on the same side of the mean and exceed the − 2 SD or + 2 SD control limits.	Detects systematic error.
4–1SD	Reject a run when four consecutive control observations are on the same side of the mean and exceed either the + 1 SD or − 1 SD control limits.	Detects small systematic error; very few applications.
10x	Reject a run when 10 consecutive control observations are on the same side of the mean.	Detects very small errors; do not use.
R-4SD	Reject a run if the range or difference between the maximum and minimum control observation out of the last four to six control observations exceeds 4 SD.	Detects random errors; use within run.

Eventually, these specimens are analyzed as a batch to minimize between-run variation.

To assess the biologic variation of hematology analytes, where primarily whole blood samples are analyzed, newly drawn samples must be analyzed in a timely manner because of the instability of whole blood.[3] **Table 2** presents a summary of estimates of the within-individual variation of components of the CBC. Thus, for Hct, the median within-individual variation is ± 2.8% (expressed as a Coefficient of Variation [CV]). The implication of this statistic is that approximately 95% of an individual's Hct ranges within the patient's mean Hct ± 2 × 2.8% and roughly 99% of an individual's Hct ranges within the patient's mean Hct ± 3 × 2.8%. To identify a patient whose Hct is significantly different from their initial Hct, the Hct must have increased or decreased more that 8.4% of their initial Hct.

Table 2 demonstrates a wide range of biologic variation for hematology analytes, from less than 1% for mean corpuscular volume (MCV) to 20% for enumeration of the different white cell types. To accurately demonstrate changes in MCV, the measurement technology must be exceedingly precise compared with that of the

Table 2
Estimates on the intrasubject biologic variation (expressed as coefficients of variation [%]) of components of the complete blood count

	Zhang et al,[8] 2013	Lacher et al,[9] 2012	Sennels et al,[10] 2011	Van Wyck et al,[11] 2010	Ricós et al,[12] 2007	Ricós et al,[13] 1999	Jones et al,[14] 1996	Maes et al,[15] 1995	Dot et al,[16] 1992a	Dot et al,[17] 1992b	Fraser et al,[18] 1989	H-log: Winkel et al,[19] 1981	H-trak: Winkel et al,[19] 1981	Stattland et al,[20] 1978	Median
Hematocrit	2.44	2.86	2.83	4		2.8	3.7	4	5		2.6			2.7	2.8
Hemoglobin	2.44	2.81	2.95	4	2.8	2.8	3	3.6	2.8		2.7			2.6	2.8
Mean corpuscular hemoglobin	1.31		0.57			1.6		2	1.3		0.8				1.3
Mean corpuscular hemoglobin concentration	0.82		ND			1.7		1.8	1.6		0.8				1.6
Mean cell volume	1.12	0.34	0.18			1.3	0.5	1.4	1.1		1.1				1.1
Mean platelet volume	2.12	3.18				4.3	3.4	3.4							3.4
Platelets	5.27	8.38	2.72			9.1	5	9.1	7.7		9			6.6	7.7
Red blood count	3.04	2.99	2.75			3.2	3.5	4	3		2.1				3
Red cell distribution width	1.49	1	0.39			3.5	2.9	3.4	1.9						1.9
White blood count		15.11	13.03			10.9	14		13.3	12.4	11.2	14.6		15.7	13.3
Eosinophil, #			27.74			21	20					36.6		26.9	26.9
Eosinophil, %		24.18					20							22.1	22.1
Lymphocyte, #		15.23	18.6			10.4	14			12.3	9.4	16.7	20.4	13.2	14
Lymphocyte, %		15.21					14			3.6	10.7				12.3
Monocyte, #		16.92	11.6			17.8	15				11.7		19	19.3	16.9
Monocyte, %		13.52					13				9.9				13
Neutrophil, #		22.2	14.44			16.1	22			21.9		23.1	23.5	26	22.1
Neutrophil, %		9.43					10			8.6					9.4
Basophil, #											7.2				7.2
Basophil, %							33								33

Data from Cembrowski et al, unpublished data, 2014 and Refs.[8-20]

measurement technology to assess the white count differential. Cotlove and co-workers[4] and Fraser and Petersen[5] have shown that the ratios of the biologic variation to the analytical variation (with both the numerator and denominator expressed as either the standard deviation or CV) indicate the goodness of the measurement technology. With a ratio of 2 (deemed desirable), the inherent analytical variation contributes 12% to the observed variation (biologic plus analytical). If the ratio of the biologic to analytical variation is 4 or more, then the analytical variation contributes less than 3% to the observed variation.

The ratio of the biologic to analytical variation provides the laboratorian a perspective on the adequacy of a test's precision to reliably demonstrate a significant change. Thus, if the analytical variation for a particular Hct assay is 0.8%, the contribution to the biologic variation is almost zero and the physician can use the Hct limits of $\pm$ 8.4% to indicate a definite change in the patient's Hct. For optimal interpretation of laboratory results, it is mandatory that laboratorian use optimally precise analyzers. The optimally precise analyzer also simplifies the practice of quality control.

For too long, hematology laboratories have been using quality control rules that require reanalysis or investigation if the quality control results are outside 2 or 3 SD limits. Typical quality control rules are shown in **Table 1**. More than 25 years ago, we recommended the combination 2–2SD, R-4SD, and 1–3SD control rules for hematology quality control.[6] These control rules when applied simultaneously to 18 or 20 different CBC parameters result in a moderate probability of false rejection (ie, in relatively stable hematology analyzers, they tend to signal out of control situations with ensuing investigations demonstrating no clinically significant error in the patients' results). These false rejections result in needless investigation and reanalysis and delays in patient testing. Many of today's hematology analyzers demonstrate improved imprecision as evidenced by small quality control standard deviations and large ratios of biologic to analytical variation. These analyzers permit quality control rules that are forgiving of small shifts and small increases in random error, errors that are made unimportant or "drowned" out by the biologic variation in the test. Based on the criterion of high ratios of medically allowable error to imprecision (another measure of the goodness of analytical testing), we have recommended the 1-3.5SD rule for almost all of the directly measured analytes of a specific highly precise analyzer.[7] For many hematology analyzers, quality control analysis should simply be an exercise that repeatedly demonstrates quality control acceptability (and thus analyzer stability). For hematology laboratories that continually wrestle with shifts and outliers, it is incumbent on the laboratorian to migrate to more stable (and thus more precise) hematology analyzers.

QUALITY CONTROL USING PATIENT RESULTS

In today's hematology laboratories, quality control analysis is the primary indicator that an analytical process is achieving its quality requirements. Patient results can be used to supplement reference sample quality control in the intervals between quality control analysis, during the transitions to new lots of quality control materials and occasionally in evaluating the interparametric validity of the components of the CBC. Patient data can be evaluated on an individual basis or grouped to provide meaningful information about the analytical run.

CRITICAL VALUES

Critical values are defined as those analytical results that signify a serious physiologic change or diagnostic abnormality and requiring urgent clinical intervention to avert significant patient morbidity. Hematologic examples include very low hemoglobin

(Hgb) concentrations that could lead to decreased tissue oxygenation, and infarction or very low platelet counts, if untreated, could result in spontaneous hemorrhage. An analytical result that meets the predetermined definition of a critical value usually results in urgent communication of the result to a patient care provider. Because these critical results are deemed important, it has been a common, but unjustified practice to repeat the testing of critical results before reporting. In 2007, Munoz[21] found that 68% of 340 US hematology laboratories always repeated the analysis of any specimen with a critical value, with small hospitals and independent laboratories having repeat prevalences of 83% and 100%, respectively.

Critical values, although sometimes at the extreme ends of the analytical range, are no more likely to be incorrect than any other analytical result generated on that analyzer. The scientific literature generally demonstrates that 1% or less of the repeated results are significantly different than the original critical values.[22] A recent College of American Pathologists Q-Probes study documented 17- and 21-minute (90 percentile) delays caused by retesting of critical white blood and platelet counts, respectively.[23] The components of ongoing quality control of each analysis together with a quality system underpinning the preanalytic, analytical, and postanalytical phases of analysis are the most important features of accurate analysis and reporting of results. Repeat analysis is a precision check and current hematology analyzers have excellent precision across the analytical range. Accuracy of a result is best monitored through EQA and site-to-site comparison data (discussed later) and is not served by repeats of critical values.

The medical technologist analyst is strongly motivated to repeat the analysis of the critical value specimen. This tendency may arise from the desire to produce the very best answer for clinician interpretation and action. To assuage the desire for repeat testing, articles such as those of Toll[22] and Lehman[23] should be made available in the hematology laboratory. An effective approach to demonstrate the quality of the initial test result is to simply log and graph the differences between the first and second critical pairs against the average of the pairs. Inspection of such graphs should help in the rewriting of the critical value standard operating procedure.[22]

INTERPARAMETRIC CHECKS

Van Kampen[24] introduced the phrase "interparametric quality control" in the late 1970s in his comparison of the chemistry measurement of bicarbonate to the dissolved blood CO_2 derived from blood gas measurements. Similar arithmetical checks may be done within a group of analytes measured on a single specimen (eg, mean corpuscular Hgb concentration [MCHC]), to determine the acceptability of the constituent measurements. For example, the "times 3" rule defines the expected relationship between the red blood cell count (RBC), the Hgb, and the Hct in Coulter-type analyzers and can be used to confirm the accuracy of RBC results in the presence of interfering substances or following dilution or sample manipulation. This check is often used after correction of the MCHC for lipemia or cold agglutinins to ensure that the corrective action has been successful in providing accurate indices. Hct (expressed as percentage) is roughly 3 times the Hgb (expressed as grams per deciliter) and Hgb (grams per deciliter) is approximately 3 times the red count (expressed simply as the decimal coefficient). Equations 1 and 2 demonstrate the use of these relationships:

$$Hct = 3 \times Hgb, \text{ eg: } 30 \, (\%) = 3 \times 9.9 \, \text{g/dL} \tag{1}$$

$$Hgb = 3 \times RBC, \text{ eg: } 9.9 \, (\text{g/dL}) = 3 \times 3.3 \, (\times 10 \, **12/L) \tag{2}$$

DELTA CHECKS

If a patient's previous results are available during the testing of the patient's next specimen, the Laboratory Information System (LIS) can calculate the difference (Δ) between the current and previous measurements. If the delta exceeds a predetermined limit, the large Δ may indicate an analytical or preanalytical error in the previous or current determination, mix-up of the previous or current specimen, or greater than expected biologic (intraindividual) variation. Before reporting the current result, associated with an out of limit delta check, about 40% of US hematology laboratories consistently repeat the current measurement.[21] Such prospective investigations can prevent the reporting of erroneous results associated with the current determination. Although more efficient, investigations that occur after result reporting can lead to erroneous data being reviewed by the clinical staff. Because of improved instrument reliability and the increasing use of barcode identification of specimens, the prevalence of analytical errors and specimen mix-ups has been decreasing. Large Δ values more often indicate a real change in a patient's test values rather than an error. For this reason, Δ check limits should be considered for review on a per analyte basis whenever a technologist suggests that the Δ check limits are too narrow and are resulting in too frequent investigations. Delta checks for detection of analytical errors are most useful for analytes with the least amount of biologic variability. For example, changes in MCV are often meaningful and may indicate a sample mix-up or preanalytical error (including dilution by an intravenous infusion), whereas changes in Hgb concentration more likely indicate a true change secondary to bleeding or transfusion. For some CBC parameters the timing of the change may also be meaningful. Dramatic short-term changes in MCV or MCHC are unlikely to be biologic changes, whereas short-term changes in platelet count, Hgb, and/or white blood cell count may occur because of physiologic or therapeutic interventions. Significant deltas (Δ) in the stable parameters of community patients over a long period of time are more likely to be clinically meaningful compared with changes in hospitalized patients where much of the variability may relate to the underlying condition or to therapy.

Table 3 summarizes the within-day 99% delta check limits for four Edmonton, Alberta hospitals and selected analytes for a patient's first day of hospitalization gathered over 3 months.[25] For most tests, there is little interhospital variation of the 99% delta check limits. For referral laboratories not testing any hospital patients, the delta check limits would be much narrower.[21]

AVERAGE OF PATIENTS

It has been a half century since Hoffmann and Waid[26] suggested that series of "normal" patient laboratory results could be averaged to demonstrate either no error condition during the analysis (patient average within limits) or the existence of an error situation (patient average outside of limits and presumably caused by an analytical shift with many of the results either increased or decreased). Because laboratory results outside their usual limits tend to be repeated more often than normal results, Hoffmann and Waid recommended that only results within the normal range be averaged.

Many research publications have explored this average of patients procedure. One of the most popular approaches to hematology quality control is Bull's approach (also known as $\overline{X}_b$, pronounced "x bar b"), which uses a unique average of sequential batches of 20 patient red cell indices to demonstrate (in)stability in the red cell associated Coulter measurements.[27] The red cell indices consist of the directly measured MCV; the mean corpuscular Hgb (MCH) calculated from Hgb and RBC count; and

Table 3
Summary of the within-day 99% delta check limits for four Edmonton, Alberta hospitals and selected analytes for a patient's first day of hospitalization, over the course of 3 months

Test	99% Numeric Deltas				99% Percentage Deltas			
	UAH (2 LH-750)	RAH (2 Gen-S)	GNH (Gen-S, HmX)	MH (Gen-S, HmX)	UAH (2 LH-750)	RAH (2 Gen-S)	GNH (Gen-S, HmX)	MH (Gen-S, HmX)
HB, g/L	(−43, 39)	(−42, 39)	(−40, 44)	(−69, 72)	(−35, 49)	(−35, 51)	(−31, 60)	(−45, 86)
HCT, L/L	(−0.12, 0.11)	(−0.12, 0.11)	(−0.12, 0.12)	(−0.12, 0.10)	(−34, 46)	(−34, 48)	(−32, 53)	(−32, 48)
MCH, pg	(−1, 1)	(−1, 1)	(−1, 1)	(−2, 2)	(−5, 5)	(−3, 4)	(−4, 4)	(−6, 7)
MCHC, g/L	(−15, 16)	(−12, 13)	(−16, 15)	(−17, 18)	(−4, 5)	(−3, 4)	(−5, 5)	(−5, 5)
MCV, fL	(−4, 3)	(−2, 3)	(−3, 3)	(−3, 3)	(−4, 4)	(−3, 3)	(−3, 4)	(−3, 3)
NE, 10^9/L	(−31, 36)	(−34, 36)	(−38, 36)	(−31, 29)	(−57, 172)	(−47, 103)	(−47, 108)	(−41, 78)
NEA, 10^9/L	(−11, 11)	(−11, 12)	(−14, 17)	(−13, 14)	(−75, 326)	(−71, 239)	(−68, 450)	(−69, 149)
PLT, 10^9/L	(−161, 144)	(−178, 172)	(−507, 533)	(−125, 113)	(−64, 146)	(−100, 75)	(−87, 123)	(−46, 56)
RBC, 10^12/L	(−1.4, 1.30)	(−1.4, 1.3)	(−1.4, 1.4)	(−1.3, 1.2)	(−36, 50)	(−36, 51)	(−31, 56)	(−34, 46)
RDW	(−1.80, 2.11)	(−1.95, 1.67)	(−1.73, 1.96)	(−1.78, 2.25)	(−9, 12)	(−11, 11)	(−11, 12)	(−10, 13)
WBC, 10^9/L	(−12, 13)	(−12, 11)	(−15, 17)	(−13, 16)	(−61, 172)	(−59, 126)	(−59, 152)	(−55, 126)

Abbreviations: HB, hemoglobin; MCH, mean corpuscular hemoglobin; NE, neutrophils percentage; NEA, neutrophils — absolute; PLT, platelets; RDW, red cell distribution width; WBC, white blood cell.

Adapted from Tran DV, Clarke G, Etches W, et al. Derivation and comparison of complete blood count (CBC) delta check limits for four city hospitals in Edmonton, Canada. Paper presented at: International Society of Laboratory Hematology Symposium. Chicago, May, 2006. Available at: http://www.mylaboratoryquality.com/4cityhospitals1.pdf.

the MCHC derived from Hgb, RBC, and MCV. When a large number of CBCs are measured by a normal functioning Coulter (eg, a few weeks worth or several thousand CBCs), the statistical average of that large number of red cell indices should be very constant. When 20 indices are averaged, intermittent or persistent deviations of X_b can occasionally indicate an analytical shift in one or more of the constituents of MCH or MCHC. Too often, especially with today's highly precise hematology analyzers, these outlying average indices in hospital patients indicate the analysis of nonrandomized selection of patients with a high proportion of abnormal indices including neonates, patients in renal failure, or oncology patients undergoing chemotherapy.

In the 1980s and 1990s, review of control every 20 specimens probably had significant utility. Today many more samples are being analyzed. To decrease the implicit variation of the patient average and to improve its error signaling, it is intuitive to average more specimens. In an evaluation of patient averages, we found that the error-detection capabilities of patient averages depend on multiple factors[28] with the most important being the number of patient results averaged (Np) and the ratio of the standard deviation of the patient population (s_p) to the standard deviation of the analytical method (s_a). Other important factors included the limits for evaluating the mean (control limits), the limits for determining which patient data are averaged (truncation limits), and the magnitude of the population lying outside the truncation limits.

Douville and colleagues[29] have provided a formula for determining the number of patient results that must be averaged to provide the error-detection capabilities of Nc controls.

$$N_p = 2 \times N_c \times \left(s_p^2 / s_a^2 \right)$$

Douville and colleagues recommended that the number of patient samples to be averaged should reflect at least two control specimens.

$$N_p > 4 \times s_p^2 / s_a^2$$

It is important to prevent the averaging of specimens with expected outlying results. In the referral laboratory that analyzes primarily specimens from fairly healthy patients, the occasional incorporation of blood from a patient with renal failure or chemotherapy does not affect the patient mean. To monitor hospital hematology analyzers, either middleware or the analyzer's own software should be programmed to eliminate from averaging patients from specific units (renal failure, oncology) or patients of specific ages (ie, the neonate). Before averaging, to reduce the effect of the more frequent testing of outlying abnormal results, these data can be excluded (truncated) from averaging. In a referral hematology laboratory we used an average of patients system to monitor every test that was reported to the clinician, including platelets, white blood cells, and the differential.

Intermittent shifts in the patient averages can largely be ignored. The troubleshooting of persistently shifted patient averages must incorporate assessment of preanalytical and postanalytical (especially laboratory information) issues. The laboratorian must have an understanding of the clinical reasons for shifts in the patient averages before assuming analytical error and adjusting analyzer parameters. It is not always clear to laboratory staff whether a persistent shift is caused by a subtle patient population shift or an altered analytical process. As such, persistent outlying patient averages should be investigated with careful inspection of the current quality control data followed by analysis of quality control samples.

INTERLABORATORY (PEER) QUALITY CONTROL COMPARISONS

Today, many hematology laboratories function in integrated health care systems and, within that system, tend to run similar analyzers and even identical lots of quality control materials. For these distributed, integrated laboratories, site-to-site comparisons of quality control results provide a combination of the benefits of quality control and external quality assessment. Each quality control measurement can be directly compared with measurements by similar analyzer type within the laboratory system. These peer comparison data are continuously available through user-accessible Internet portals and permits the immediate recognition of out of control, potentially inaccurate results.

Such peer or site-to-site comparison is provided by instrument manufacturers who also provide instrument-specific quality control samples, or through manufacturers of quality control materials. In the latter case the peer comparison scheme must separate the data provided from different analyzer types for comparison. This type of comparison may be a service offered with purchase of a particular hematology analyzer, or may be available as a purchased service together with quality control materials. Internet-connected analyzers using specific quality control materials may allow for upload of results with comparison at user-defined intervals, or in some cases, automatic uploading of results with each run. Manual entry of results to user-accessible web sites is also used in some schemes.

The use of peer comparison data may be helpful in several ways. First, it can confirm precision and ensure that analysis of the same quality control material remains constant over the lifetime of the material. In addition, quality control values that match the results achieved by many other laboratories using the same analyzer type also provide assurance of accuracy. In this case, the mean of many laboratories serves as a surrogate for the most accurate or gold standard result. Peer comparisons therefore provide the precision data traditionally tracked through quality control, and the accuracy data that traditionally was monitored through the EQA process. Within-laboratory precision may result in very "tight" ranges, however, such that apparent deviations actually reflect minimal and unimportant analytical variations. Site-to-site comparisons provide an intermediate range, typically a wider range than parameters established within the laboratory but not as broad as those that accompany purchased quality control reagents. These peer or site-to-site comparison data and ranges may be a useful reference when out-of-control samples are encountered.

Analyzers are calibrated in the process of installation and validation, and following major maintenance. Calibration involves the analysis of calibrators, specimens with assigned values for all analytes, and requires adjustment of instrument-measured parameters to match those of the calibrators. The expected range for each measured parameter of the CBC is often very narrow. Ensuring that one parameter is within the range may result in another CBC parameter veering out of range. This difficulty in calibration is another instance where the peer mean and standard deviation can provide useful guidance on expected results and help determine whether the calibration process has achieved the desirable accuracy.

PORT (MODE TO MODE) COMPARISONS

Port comparisons or mode to mode comparability refers to the comparability of the analytical results when blood (whole blood or quality control material) is aspirated by the hematology analyzer via the primary mode and when the blood is manually aspirated through a separate, secondary port. Mode to mode comparability should be evaluated during the instrument's initial verification evaluation and then at least annually (Clinical Laboratory Standards Institute [H26A] guidelines,[30] CAP hematology and coagulation checklist[31]). The manufacturer's guidelines for monitored parameters (background counts, all reported CBC constituents, and carryover) and tolerance limits should be strictly observed. Although either quality control or whole blood samples can be used to assess mode to mode comparability, we prefer fresh whole blood with an Hgb exceeding 15 g/dL. Repeat sampling of a fresh, whole blood sample on the primary mode for all analyses should be repeated two to three times. **Fig. 1** shows an example of a worksheet used to compile and compare mode to mode means. The

 Alberta Health Services

Covenant Health

Regional Laboratory Services
Hematology
RHEAHF01306MUL
Version: 1.0

Hematology Mode to Mode Correlation Excel Worksheet
Effective Date: March 5, 2014

This document is applicable at site(s):

| CCI | DVH | EEHC | FSH | GNH | LEH | MIS | NEC | RAH | RED | SGH | STO | UAH |

Hematology Mode to Mode Correlation Excel Worksheet

Date:_____

Instrument #1:

	WBC				RBC				HGB				PLT			
Sample	auto mode mean	manual mode mean	DIF	% DIF	auto mode mean	manual mode mean	DIF	% DIF	auto mode mean	manual mode mean	DIF	% DIF	auto mode mean	manual mode mean	DIF	% DIF
1			0.00	#DIV/0!			0.00	#DIV/0!			0.00	#DIV/0!			0.00	#DIV/0!
2			0.00	#DIV/0!			0.00	#DIV/0!			0.00	#DIV/0!			0.00	#DIV/0!
3			0.00	#DIV/0!			0.00	#DIV/0!			0.00	#DIV/0!			0.00	#DIV/0!
Mean			0.00	#DIV/0!			0.00	#DIV/0!			0.00	#DIV/0!			0.00	#DIV/0!

Instrument #2:

	WBC				RBC				HGB				PLT			
Sample	auto mode mean	manual mode mean	DIF	% DIF	auto mode mean	manual mode mean	DIF	% DIF	auto mode mean	manual mode mean	DIF	% DIF	auto mode mean	manual mode mean	DIF	% DIF
1			0.00	#DIV/0!			0.00	#DIV/0!			0.00	#DIV/0!			0.00	#DIV/0!
2			0.00	#DIV/0!			0.00	#DIV/0!			0.00	#DIV/0!			0.00	#DIV/0!
3			0.00	#DIV/0!			0.00	#DIV/0!			0.00	#DIV/0!			0.00	#DIV/0!
Mean			0.00	#DIV/0!			0.00	#DIV/0!			0.00	#DIV/0!			0.00	#DIV/0!

Instrument #3:

	WBC				RBC				HGB				PLT			
Sample	auto mode mean	manual mode mean	DIF	% DIF	auto mode mean	manual mode mean	DIF	% DIF	auto mode mean	manual mode mean	DIF	% DIF	auto mode mean	manual mode mean	DIF	% DIF
1			0.00	#DIV/0!			0.00	#DIV/0!			0.00	#DIV/0!			0.00	#DIV/0!
2			0.00	#DIV/0!			0.00	#DIV/0!			0.00	#DIV/0!			0.00	#DIV/0!
3			0.00	#DIV/0!			0.00	#DIV/0!			0.00	#DIV/0!			0.00	#DIV/0!
Mean			0.00	#DIV/0!			0.00	#DIV/0!			0.00	#DIV/0!			0.00	#DIV/0!

Acceptable Limits:

	DIF		%DIF
WBC	$\pm 0.4 \times 10^9$/L		$\pm 5\%$
RBC	$\pm 0.20 \times 10^{12}$/L	OR*	$\pm 2\%$
HB	± 3 g/L		$\pm 2\%$
PLT	$\pm 20 \times 10^9$/L		$\pm 7\%$

*Whichever is greater

Corrective action for parameters outside of established limits:_____

Performed by_____Date_____

Reviewed by_____Date_____

Fig. 1. Example of a worksheet used to compare mode to mode measurements. (*Courtesy of Alberta Health Services, Edmonton, Alberta, Canada; with permission.*)

mean of these multiple repeats is compared with results from the alternate/manual sampling mode.

REFERENCES

1. Cembrowski GS. Hematology quality practices. In: Kottke-Marchant K, Davis BH, editors. Laboratory hematology practice. Oxford (United Kingdom): Wiley-Blackwell; 2012. p. 686–706.
2. Jacob G, Raj SR, Ketch T, et al. Postural pseudoanemia: posture-dependent change in hematocrit. Mayo Clin Proc 2005;80(5):611–4.
3. Vives-Corrons JL, Briggs C, Simon-Lopez R, et al. Effect of EDTA-anticoagulated whole blood storage on cell morphology examination: a need for standardization. Int J Lab Hematol 2014;36(2):222–6.
4. Cotlove E, Harris EK, Williams GZ. Biological and analytic components of variation in long-term studies of serum constituents in normal subjects III. Physiological and medical implications. Clin Chem 1970;16(12):1028–32.
5. Fraser CG, Petersen PH. Analytical performance characteristics should be judged against objective quality specifications. Clin Chem 1999;45(3):321–3.
6. Cembrowski GS, Carey RN. Laboratory quality management: QC [and] QA. Chicago: ASCP Press; 1989. p. 186–212.
7. Cembrowski GS, Smith B, Tung D. Rationale for using insensitive quality control rules for today's hematology analyzers. Int J Lab Hematol 2010;32(6 Pt 2): 606–15.
8. Zhang P, Tang H, Chen K, et al. Biological variations of hematologic parameters determined by UniCel DxH 800 hematology analyzer. Arch Pathol Lab Med 2013; 137:1106–10.
9. Lacher DA, Barletta J, Hughes JP. Biological variation of hematology tests based on the 1999–2002 National Health and Nutrition Examination Survey. Natl Health Stat Report 2012;54:1–11.
10. Sennels HP, Jorgensen HL, Hansen AS, et al. Diurnal variation of hematology parameters in healthy young males: the bispebjerg study of diurnal variations. Scand J Clin Lab Invest 2011;71:532–41.
11. Van Wyck DB, Alcorn H Jr, Gupta R. Analytical and biological variation in measures of anemia and iron status in patients treated with maintenance hemodialysis. Am J Kidney Dis 2010;56:540–6.
12. Ricós C, Iglesias N, García-Lario JV, et al. Within-subject biological variation in disease: collated data and clinical consequences. Ann Clin Biochem 2007;44: 343–52.
13. Ricós C, Alvarez V, Cava F, et al. Current databases on biological variation: pros, cons and progress. Scand J Clin Lab Invest 1999;59:491–500.
14. Jones AR, Twedt D, Swaim W, et al. Diurnal change of blood count analytes in normal subjects. Am J Clin Pathol 1996;106:723–8.
15. Maes M, Scharpé S, Cooreman W, et al. Components of biological, including seasonal, variation in hematological measurements and plasma fibrinogen concentrations in normal humans. Experientia 1995;51:141–9.
16. Dot D, Miró J, Fuentes-Arderiu X. Within-subject viological variation of hematological quantities and analytical goals. Arch Pathol Lab Med 1992;116:825–6.
17. Dot D, Miró J, Fuentes-Arderiu X. Biological variation of the leukocyte differential count quantities. Scand J Clin Lab Invest 1992;52(7):607–11.
18. Fraser CG, Wilkinson SP, Neville RG, et al. Biologic variation of common hematologic laboratory quantities in the elderly. Am J Clin Pathol 1989;92(4):465–70.

19. Winkel P, Statland BE, Saunders AM, et al. Within-day physiologic variation of leukocyte types in healthy subjects as assayed by two automated leukocyte differential analyzers. Am J Clin Pathol 1981;75:693–700.
20. Statland BE, Winkel P, Harris SC, et al. Evaluation of biologic sources of variation of leukocyte counts and other hematologic quantities using very precise automated analyzers. Am J Clin Pathol 1978;69:48–54.
21. Munoz O. Workload efficiency in the hematology laboratory. Doctoral dissertation. Salt Lake City (UT): The University of Utah; 2008.
22. Toll AD, Liu JM, Gulati G, et al. Does routine repeat testing of critical values offer any advantage over single testing? Arch Pathol Lab Med 2011;135(4):440–4.
23. Lehman CM, Howanitz PJ, Souers R, et al. Utility of repeat testing of critical values: a Q-probes analysis of 86 clinical laboratories. Arch Pathol Lab Med 2014;138(6):788–93.
24. Van Kampen ES. Interparametric quality control in acid base balance. In: Mass AHJ, editor. Blood pH and gases. Utrecht (Netherlands): Utrecht University Press; 1979. p. 49–56.
25. Tran DV, Clarke G, Etches W, et al. Derivation and comparison of complete blood count (CBC) delta check limits for four city hospitals in Edmonton, Canada. Paper presented at: International Society of Laboratory Hematology Symposium. Chicago (IL), May, 2006.
26. Hoffmann RG, Waid ME. The "average of normals" method of quality control. Am J Clin Pathol 1965;43:134.
27. Korpman RA, Bull PS. Letter: the implementation of a robust estimator of the mean for quality control on a programmable calculator or a laboratory computer. Am J Clin Pathol 1976;65(2):252–3.
28. Cembrowski GS, Chandler EP, Westgard JO. Assessment of "average of normals" quality control procedures and guidelines for implementation. Am J Clin Pathol 1984;81(4):492–9.
29. Douville P, Cembrowski GS, Strauss JF. Evaluation of the average of patients: application to endocrine assays. Clin Chim Acta 1987;167(2):173–85.
30. Clinical Laboratory Standards Institute. H26–A2 validation, verification, and quality assurance of automated hematology analyzers; Approved Standard—Second edition. Wayne, PA: Clinical Laboratory Standards Institute; 2010.
31. Alberta Health Services and Covenant Health. Mode to mode hematology correlation excel worksheet. Alberta, Canada: Alberta Health Services; 2014.

Laboratory and Genetic Assessment of Iron Deficiency in Blood Donors

Joseph E. Kiss, MD

KEYWORDS

- Blood donation • Iron deficiency • Ferritin • Soluble transferrin receptor
- Reticulocyte hemoglobin content • Hypochromic mature red blood cells
- Hereditary hemochromatosis (HFE) • TMPRSS6

KEY POINTS

- Iron depletion is common in blood donors, especially women and frequent donors.
- Hemoglobin level is useful to detect anemia but has limited value in assessing blood donor iron status.
- Red blood cell indices, such the percentage of hypochromic mature RBC and reticulocyte hemoglobin content can improve the assessment of iron status over hemoglobin alone.
- Current studies suggest that measurement of ferritin at a level of 26 to 30 ng/mL optimally identifies donors who are iron depleted.
- Genetic assessment of iron pathways may reveal new approaches for selecting individuals who are more or less able to donate blood on a regular basis.

BLOOD DONORS AND IRON DEPLETION

Blood donors and the red blood cells (RBCs) they provide serve as a vital link in the delivery of health care worldwide. More than 9 million volunteer blood donors donate each year in the United States.[1] Nearly 70% are repeat donors, many of whom become iron deficient as a result of regular blood donation.[2,3] Moreover, nearly 7% of presenting donors are deferred from donating because they cannot meet the minimum hemoglobin standard of 12.5 g/dL obtained by finger-stick testing. The US Food and Drug Administration (FDA) defines this as the minimum hemoglobin value in both men and women to determine donor eligibility, but no requirement currently exists for determining iron levels. Low hemoglobin, a late consequence of iron deficiency,

Division of Hematology-Oncology, Department of Medicine, University of Pittsburgh Medical Center, and The Institute for Transfusion Medicine, 3636 Boulevard of The Allies, Pittsburgh, Pittsburgh, PA 15213, USA
E-mail address: jkiss@itxm.org

Clin Lab Med 35 (2015) 73–91
http://dx.doi.org/10.1016/j.cll.2014.10.011
0272-2712/15/$ – see front matter © 2015 Elsevier Inc. All rights reserved.
labmed.theclinics.com

Abbreviations	
AIS	Absent iron stores
AUC	Area under the curve
CHCMm	Cellular hemoglobin concentration of mature RBC
CHr	Reticulocyte hemoglobin content
FDA	Food and Drug Administration
GWAS	Genome-wide association studies
HYPOm	Hypochromic mature red blood cells
HYPOr	Hypochromic reticulocyte red blood cells
IDA	Iron-deficiency anemia
IDE	Iron-deficient erythropoiesis
MCH	Mean corpuscular hemoglobin
MCHC	Mean corpuscular hemoglobin concentration
MCV	Mean corpuscular volume
rHuEpo	recombinant human erythropoietin
R/F ratio	sTfR/ferritin ratio
RBC	Red blood cell
RISE group	Retrovirus Epidemiology and Donor Evaluation Study-II Iron Status Evaluation group
ROC	Receiver operating characteristic
SNP	Single nucleotide polymorphism
sTfR	Serum soluble transferrin receptor
TIBC	Total iron-binding capacity
ZPP	Zinc protoporphyrin

represents the largest category of blood donor deferral and occurs more frequently in women. In addition, women are 3 times more likely to be iron deficient than men.[4] Even in the absence of anemia, iron depletion has been associated with several conditions arising from the key role iron plays in the central nervous system and neuromuscular function,[5] including fatigue,[6] decreased exercise capacity,[7] neurocognitive changes,[8] pica (the compulsive ingestion of non-nutritive substances, such as ice), and restless legs syndrome.[9,10]

Overall, 35% of the blood donor population in the United States is estimated to be iron deficient.[4] The large number of affected blood donors and recognition of the potential health consequences has prompted the main blood banking organization, the American Association of Blood Banks, to recommend that measures be adopted to identify and to prevent iron deficiency in all or in selected high-risk individuals. As a result, blood collection centers worldwide are examining potential strategies to manage donor iron loss, including changes in acceptable hemoglobin level, donation interval, donation frequency, testing of iron status, and iron supplementation. This review considers the relative merits of different laboratory and genetic tests to assess the iron status of blood donors and their suitability as screening tests for blood donation.

BRIEF REVIEW OF IRON PHYSIOLOGY IN MEN AND WOMEN

Iron is an essential element in many physiologic processes. In association with heme, it participates in the reversible binding of oxygen by RBCs and is also a key constituent in the myoglobin of muscle and mitochondrial cytochromes. Nonheme iron plays a key role in the activity of many enzymatic reactions. Iron may also be toxic when present in excess; absorption is tightly regulated because there is no active mechanism for excretion. Dietary iron is absorbed in the proximal small intestine. Iron from animal sources (heme iron) has greater bioavailability (~30% absorbed) than nonheme (ie, plant products) iron (~10% absorbed).[11] Men normally absorb approximately 1 mg/d, equaling basal losses primarily from the gastrointestinal tract. Iron absorption in premenopausal women is greater, approximately 1.3 to 1.5 mg/d, because of additional losses from menstruation. Absorption capacity increases proportionate to the level of iron deficiency (ie, ferritin level) to an average maximum of 4 to 5 mg/d in very active blood donors.[12] The average iron absorption is more in the range of 2 to 3 mg/d.[11] Absorbed iron binds to transferrin and is transported to transferrin receptors located on early erythroid and all other nucleated cells. Iron that is not directly used in physiologic pathways is stored intracellularly as ferritin; small amounts present in blood are in equilibrium with intracellular ferritin, the serum level of which is considered a reliable indicator of available storage iron in the absence of inflammation.

Total body iron content in men averages approximately 50 mg/kg (~3500 mg), whereas in women, who have lower hemoglobin levels and less blood volume in proportion to weight, the average is closer to 35 mg/kg (~2100 mg). Seventy percent to 80% of body iron exists in RBCs in the form of hemoglobin. Cook and colleagues[13] estimated average tissue iron stores of only 776 ± 313 mg in men and 309 ± 346 mg in women. Thus, it should not be surprising that the loss of approximately 230 mg iron with each whole blood donation along with the limited capacity for absorption leads to a high incidence of iron deficiency in regular donors, especially women.

With losses in excess of absorption, iron deficiency occurs progressively, beginning with the gradual loss of storage iron, followed by the development of iron-deficient erythropoiesis (IDE), and culminating in iron-deficiency anemia (IDA).[14] Measurement of hemoglobin is a poor indicator of iron depletion and IDE because anemia occurs as the last stage in this sequence. In the clinical setting, the laboratory evaluation of iron deficiency is usually undertaken in the setting of anemia and begins by examining the complete blood count. Microcytic RBCs (mean corpuscular volume [MCV] <80 fL) and reduced mean cellular hemoglobin (MCH) are often present, and a reticulocyte count is decreased (absolute <50,000/μL). The usual biochemical panel includes a serum iron and a total iron-binding capacity (TIBC). The serum iron level is the least reliable test because it has a diurnal fluctuation and is affected by inflammation and infectious stimuli. The TIBC assesses the iron-binding capacity of the transport protein (transferrin). In IDE, the serum iron is low and the TIBC is high reflecting unsaturated transferrin. The normal saturation of transferrin (serum iron/TIBC) is 20% to 50%, with values less than 15% being characteristic of IDE. Ferritin, a measurement of storage iron, is also commonly performed. In IDE, stores are low; however, ferritin becomes elevated during inflammation because of the release from storage sites (eg, liver) making this test less reliable. A laboratory test that can be used to avoid the confounding effects of inflammation on ferritin is the serum soluble transferrin receptor (sTfR), a transmembrane receptor that is elevated in IDE because of shedding into the blood by iron-depleted erythroid cells.[15] Finally, the gold standard concerning the presence or absence of storage iron is an assessment of a sample of bone marrow stained for the presence of iron (Prussian blue). Examination of bone marrow material solely to assess iron stores is not routinely done because of the discomfort and invasiveness of the procedure.

Molecular defects have been described that impact iron homeostasis. In hereditary hemochromatosis, the protein that normally downregulates iron absorption is defective, leading to excessive accumulation of iron in the body. In addition, a common transferrin polymorphism (G277S mutation) has been elucidated that predisposes individuals to the development of iron deficiency.

TESTS TO IDENTIFY IRON DEPLETION AND IRON-DEFICIENT ERYTHROPOIESIS IN BLOOD DONORS

In one important sense, blood donors are quite different from clinical patients who often have inflammatory, infectious, or neoplastic disorders that alter the diagnostic variables used to define iron deficiency. Serum iron and, to a lesser degree, transferrin levels decrease in response to inflammation; ferritin levels increase, irrespective of iron stores. These alterations describe a clinical state termed *iron-restricted erythropoiesis* in which iron is not depleted per se but is sequestered in storage sites and is also less able to be absorbed, resulting in functional iron deficiency. We now know that the primary regulator of iron homeostasis, hepcidin, mediates this state through inhibition of the transmembrane iron-chaperone receptor, ferroportin.[16,17] Hepcidin is increased in inflammatory states, which leads to iron-restricted erythropoiesis and chronic disease anemia by this and other mechanisms. On the other hand, blood donors behave more like a normal control population. Before they are accepted for donation, they must affirmatively answer several questions regarding their physical well-being (starting with asking, are you feeling well and healthy today?) and must have normal vital signs including body temperature. This screening approach selects against those with inflammatory and or infectious disease. Thus, studies that have evaluated acute phase proteins, such as C-reactive protein, in blood donors have found low levels.[15] As a result, serum ferritin levels in blood donors are less influenced by acute-phase changes and provide a more reliable indication of true iron status than in clinical medicine.

Ferritin has been used alone and in combination with other biochemical tests to assess the iron status in blood donors. In addition, both standard RBC measurements (eg, MCV and mean corpuscular hemoglobin concentration [MCHC]) and more specialized hematology analyzer indices (eg, percent hypochromic mature RBCs [HYPOm] and reticulocyte hemoglobin content [CHr]) have been used. It is important to again emphasize that as a practical matter, hemoglobin is the only point-of-care test currently used to qualify the donor. Therefore, in addition to accurately detecting iron depletion on the current donation it may be important that any proposed test be evaluated in the context of its ability to identify subsequent (ie, next visit) blood donor iron status and/or low hemoglobin deferral.

Serum Iron, Total Iron Binding Capacity, and Percent Transferrin Saturation

Box 1 lists representative iron assays that have been investigated in blood donors. Transferrin is the major iron transport protein in plasma, binding Fe^{3+} ions, and is measured as the TIBC. Normally one-third of the binding sites are occupied (20%–50% saturated, abbreviated as %Sat). The use of %Sat has been limited to historical

---

Box 1
Measurements of iron status in blood donors

- Serum iron/transferrin (% transferrin saturation)
- Ferritin
- sTfR
- sTfR/ferritin ratio
- Zinc (free erythrocyte) protoporphyrin
- RBC indices (% hypochromic RBC and so forth)

studies. It has not been used without other biochemical assays, such as ferritin, because the %Sat level has a relatively low sensitivity in detecting iron depletion.[18] For example, in the study by Simon and colleagues[3] using ferritin 12 ng/mL or less to define iron *depletion*, the overall frequency in repeat blood donors was 8% in men and 23% in women.[3] Iron *deficiency* (as defined by both a low ferritin and transferrin saturation of <16%, the latter indicating decreased iron availability for transport into RBCs) was found in a smaller subset of those with low ferritin, 2% of male and 13% of female donors. Defining iron deficiency is relevant to the diagnosis of clinical anemia and associated symptoms, whereas the identification of iron depletion and the ability to tolerate additional iron loss (and prevention of frank iron deficiency) is a more important goal in the management of blood donors.[19]

Serum (or Plasma) Ferritin

Ferritin can be measured in either serum or plasma (using ethylenediaminetetraacetic acid plasma, ferritin concentration is approximately 5% lower than serum[20]) and is considered to reflect the level of tissue iron stores, at least in blood donors who generally have reduced iron stores compared with epidemiologically normal populations. The level in blood results from equilibration or leakage from cellular or tissue sources. Each nanogram per milliliter of ferritin in blood corresponds to 8 to 10 mg of iron in the storage compartment.[15,21] As mentioned, in contrast to the situation in blood donors, ferritin is an acute-phase protein with variable levels that imperfectly measure iron stores in clinical medicine. The classic cutoff value, 12 ng/mL, was originally based on a US population survey performed before the international standard for ferritin was established in 1985.[22] Since then, it has been adopted as a specific but insensitive indicator of absent iron stores (AIS).[23] Bone marrow analysis for the presence of iron in iron-deficient and replete women revealed that a serum ferritin cutoff of 15 ng/mL correctly classified 98% iron-replete and 75% iron-deficient subjects.[24] A systematic review of high methodologic quality studies (bone marrow iron determined in more than half) found ferritin levels to be superior to several other measurements (MCV, %Sat, zinc protoporphyrin [ZPP]), and ferritin less than 15 ng/mL "confirms the diagnosis" of IDA.[25] Other studies suggest higher levels (22–40 ng/ml) more sensitively reflect depleted iron stores.[14,25,26] Patients with chronic renal disease have shown hematologic responses to intravenous iron at even higher ferritin levels.[18]

In blood donors, the original description by Finch and colleagues[2] used the ferritin assay to show that blood donation was associated with a significant decrease in ferritin levels, which was related to the intensity of blood donation over the previous 4 to 5 years. Studies consistently show the same predictable effect of donation intensity on iron stores (**Fig. 1**).[3,27,28] Simon and colleagues,[3] in an observational study of blood donors, showed the frequency of iron depletion as measured by serum ferritin 12 ng/mL or less was less than 3% in male first-time donors but 12% in female first-time donors, reflecting the impact of menstrual blood loss. Each successive lifetime donation reduced the mean ferritin values, particularly in men, so that both sexes reached apparent iron equilibrium after approximately 5 to 6 lifetime donations. Postmenopausal women had higher ferritin levels than premenopausal women but lower values than male donors. Premenopausal women taking iron supplements had improved iron stores approaching those of male donors. No change in hemoglobin levels was seen with blood donation in this retrospective study.

O'Meara and colleagues[29] conducted a large single-center longitudinal study to determine the value of routine ferritin measurement in blood donors. A total of 160,612 donations in 23,557 donors from 1996 to 2009 were assessed for serum ferritin at each blood donation starting in 2004. Values less than 10 ng/mL were

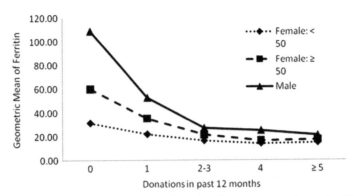

Fig. 1. RISE study: effect of previous RBC donation frequency on plasma ferritin level at enrollment. (*From* Cable RG, Glynn SA, Kiss JE, et al. Iron deficiency in blood donors: analysis of enrollment data from the REDS-II Donor Iron Status Evaluation (RISE) study. Transfusion 2011;51:511–22; with permission.)

identified as iron depleted and resulted in medical counseling by a blood bank physician to assess other potential medical reasons for low iron or to be referred to their physician and to consider steps to improve iron balance, such as decreasing donation frequency and/or taking iron supplements. The major results comparing groups after and before the intervention revealed the following: (1) Hemoglobin levels increased by 0.26 g/dL in women and 0.19 g/dL in men. (2) The prevalence of anemia, defined as hemoglobin less than 12 g/dL (women) or 13 g/dL (men) declined from 3.6% to 2.2% in women and from 0.7% to 0.5% in men. (3) Hemoglobin deferrals (cutoff of <12.3 g/dL for women and <13.3 g/dL for men) also declined, from 2.8% to 1.9% in women. (4) The donor return rate decreased to 60% - 64% (from 72% - 75%), after the institution of ferritin screening. It can be seen from this study that ferritin monitoring has a positive impact on anemia and hemoglobin deferral, although some donors stop donating entirely.

As in clinical studies, it is clear that a ferritin cutoff of 12 ng/mL is a specific indicator of iron depletion in blood donors but also lacks sensitivity.[30] One study found that this cutoff failed to identify iron depletion in more than one-third of cases in blood donors.[31] The investigators found that a higher ferritin level (22 ng/mL) indicated functional iron depletion. These investigations were not based on the gold standard bone marrow iron stains or a hematologic response to iron but relied instead on serum soluble transfer receptor measurements to indicate functional iron deficiency.

Soluble Transferrin Receptor and Soluble Transferrin Receptor/Ferritin Ratio

The sTfR is a truncated form of the transferrin receptor that is shed when early erythroid cells are deprived of iron or if there is increased erythropoietic proliferative activity (eg, hemolytic anemia, thalassemia). Serum levels are also affected by race (~9% higher in African American subjects) and altitude (~9% higher).[15] Until recently, there has been no uniform reference standard. However, there is now agreement on a source standard that promises to enhance the reliability of the assay[31] in combination with ferritin to define IDE as a more sensitive measure of iron status. Increased sTfR levels reflect the functional iron compartment and have been shown to correlate with depleted iron stores in bone marrow preparations.[23] The sTfR levels also show excellent correspondence to oral iron treatment in otherwise healthy anemic women.[14] The transferrin receptor is expressed primarily on the surface of erythroid cells. Reduced iron levels lead to increased TfR synthesis and shedding into circulating blood. Levels greater than the normal reference range (95% confidence interval) have been used to suggest tissue iron deficiency. In addition, ferritin measurements (which reflect storage iron) and sTfR values (which reflect functional iron) have been combined into a ratio, log (sTfR/ferritin), as a derived measurement. Experience to date in blood donors using the 2 inversely related measurements has shown efficacy in assessing iron status.[32-34] An index (sTfR/log ferritin) has been advocated as another way to discriminate IDE from storage iron depletion.[14,23,35]

Using the log (receptor/ferritin [R/F]) ratio, however, carries with it another important advantage because it can be used to assess iron stores quantitatively. Based on the work of Skikne and colleagues[36] and Cook and colleagues,[13] we know there is a log linear relationship between (sTfR/ferritin) and storage iron, as expressed by the following formula:

$$\text{Body iron (mg/kg)} = - [\log (R/F \text{ ratio}) - 2.8229]/0.1207$$

The use of this equation allowed the estimation of the tissue iron stores in men as described earlier as well as the ability to quantify the iron deficit because sTfR continues to increase as ferritin levels reach the lower limit of detection. Body iron can be expressed as the iron surplus in stores or the iron deficit in tissues. In addition, quantifying iron stores in this manner in serial follow-up studies permits an estimation of iron absorption in blood donors.[37]

The US Retrovirus Epidemiology and Donor Evaluation Study-II (REDS-II) Iron Status Evaluation (RISE) group conducted a multicenter, prospective, longitudinal study of iron status in more than 2400 first-time and frequent (men who donated $\geq$3 times per year and women $\geq$2 times per year) blood donors who were followed for 15 to 24 months while continuing to donate.[4,27] Two measures of iron depletion were studied: AIS defined as ferritin 12 ng/mL or less and IDE defined as log (sTfR/ferritin) 2.07 or greater (97.5% of the upper limit of the reference range in first-time iron-replete male donors). In RISE, half of the repeat male donors and two-thirds of the repeat female donors demonstrated evidence of IDE at enrollment (**Table 1**). By the time of the final visit, the first-time donors had developed similar levels of iron depletion as the repeat donors at enrollment and the repeat donors continued to maintain a similar levels of AIS and IDE, highlighting the impact of donation frequency on iron losses. The RISE study identified donation intensity, female sex, and younger age as the most important factors increasing the likelihood of iron deficiency. Donor self-reported iron supplement intake was beneficial. Of the 9.9% of donors deferred for low hemoglobin,

Table 1
Findings from the RISE study: iron status at enrollment and final visit

	Enrollment Visit		Final Visit ($\geq$15 m)	
	IDE (%)	AIS (%)	IDE (%)	AIS (%)
First Time Females	25	6.6	51	20
Repeat Females	67	28	62	27
Frist Time Males	2.5	0	20	8
Repeat Males	49	16	47	18

IDE log (sTfR/ferritin) 2.07 or greater; AIS ferritin 12 ng/mL or less.
Abbreviation: m, months.
Data from Cable RG, Glynn SA, Kiss JE, et al. Iron deficiency in blood donors: the REDS-II Donor Iron Status Evaluation (RISE) study. Transfusion 2012;52:702-11.

77% had evidence of IDE. As expected, female sex was an important predictor of hemoglobin deferral. In addition, interdonation intervals at less than 14 weeks were found to be associated with increased hemoglobin deferral (odds ratio [OR] ~2.0–2.5) and iron deficiency (OR ~3.0–4.4 for ferritin <12 ng/ml).

In the RISE analysis, plasma ferritin was highly correlated with IDE, R^2 −0.96, whereas sTfR was less so: R^2 0.54.[32] Multivariate regression analysis revealed that log (sTfR/ferritin) of 2.07 (97.5% of the upper limit of the reference range) equated to a ferritin level of 26.7 ng/ml, indicating evidence of IDE. Ferritin at this cutoff value had 95.1% sensitivity and 89.6% specificity in detecting IDE. The investigators concluded that this ferritin threshold had optimal sensitivity and specificity to detect early iron depletion in blood donors and that sTfR added little diagnostic information. A ferritin of 26.7 ng/mL is in the range that has been proposed for detection of iron depletion in other studies discussed earlier.[3,11]

Zinc Protoporphyrin

Zinc protoporphyrin (ZPP), also called free erythrocyte protoporphyrin, is measured using a portable hematofluorometer as a point-of-care test using capillary (finger stick) samples. Zinc is chelated by protoporphyrin IX if iron is not available during the last step of porphyrin ring synthesis, resulting in elevated erythrocyte ZPP per mole of heme (ferrous protoporphyrin).[38] The normal reference range (method specific) is less than 60 μmol ZPP per mole of heme. Among conditions that have a low prevalence in blood donors, such as lead intoxication, values are also increased in thalassemia, occurring in as many as 51% of subjects with a beta-thalassemia trait and 20% with an alpha-thalassemia trait.[39] Limited studies in blood donors show early detection of iron deficiency and correlation with hemoglobin deferral. Erythrocyte ZPP was measured in 102 women to evaluate iron deficiency anemia and hemoglobin deferral. Women with increased ZPP values all had low serum ferritin concentrations (≤12 ng/ml). The positive predictive value of an increased ZPP in predicting deferral of the donor after one or 2 donations was 75%, whereas a serum ferritin concentration of 12 ng/ml or less predicted deferral in 26% of the donors.[40] Another group of investigators found in a multivariable analysis that elevated ZPP levels (using venous blood) aided in the prediction of future hemoglobin deferral when added to other variables, including previous hemoglobin value, age, sex, time since previous visit, and total number of blood donations over a 2-year period (OR ~2.0 and 2.2 in men and women, respectively).[41] However, they were unable to validate the model using ZPP in a different donor population in which different hemoglobin eligibility criteria were in place[42] Additional trials using ZPP as a point-of-care screening test for detecting and managing iron deficiency in blood donors are in progress.[43]

Red Blood Cell Indices for Assessment of Functional Iron Status

As discussed previously, the conventional morphologic hallmarks of iron deficiency anemia, low MCV, MCH, and MCHC, occur relatively late in the development of iron depletion. Alexander and colleagues[44] found a significant trend correlating lower MCV and MCH and donation frequency (as a risk factor for low iron) in men and women; however, the strength of the correlation was weak (R^2 only −0.08 to −0.17). Insufficient sensitivity is also a limitation in predicting the likelihood of low hemoglobin deferral. For example, Stern and colleagues[45] found RBC parameters including MCHC less than 330 g/L ($R^2 = 0.12$) and MCV less than 80 fL ($R^2 = 0.00$) to be inferior to hemoglobin ($R^2 = 0.63$) in predicting subsequent hemoglobin deferral. In line with results of other studies, the ferritin level was similarly nonpredictive ($R^2 = 0.07$), highlighting the fact that most iron-depleted donors continue to meet donor eligibility criteria for donating blood despite iron depletion. Their analysis prompted a change in the blood donor management strategy (reported earlier[29]) from the original strategy based on serum ferritin determination in all donations to one focused on annual serum ferritin as a routine check and then only in donors with hemoglobin values within 0.5 g/dL of the hemoglobin deferral threshold in Switzerland (<12.3 g/dL in women and 13.3 g/dL in men).

Technologic advances in the assessment of functional iron status by measuring RBC indices using a next generation of hematology analyzers (ADVIA 120, Siemens Healthcare Diagnostics, Deerfield, IL and Sysmex XE-5000, Kobe, Japan)[46] have also been reported to be useful in monitoring the iron status in blood donors (**Table 2**). In functional iron deficiency, a reduction in hemoglobin content of RBCs results from an imbalance between iron supply and iron requirements of erythropoiesis, which is increased in blood donors. Analysis of the fraction of individual RBCs with deficient hemoglobinization using laser scatter techniques reflects changes in the availability of iron during erythropoiesis, which may be comparable with and possibly better than biochemical markers.[47] CHr reflects iron incorporation to developing reticulocytes (ie, iron availability during formation of reticulocytes that can be detected within the 3-day lifespan of these cells), whereas the proportion of HYPOm is a time-averaged marker of iron availability that is detected within the 3-month lifespan of mature RBCs. These measurements have been likened to monitoring glucose levels and hemoglobin A_{1c} levels in patients with diabetes, respectively.

RED BLOOD CELL INDICES IN CLINICAL POPULATIONS

The RBC indices have been found to be more sensitive indicators of functional iron deficiency than biochemical iron tests in patients with renal failure who are treated with erythroid-stimulating agents, in pregnancy, and in pediatric patients with iron deficiency.[48–52] Adequate iron stores are essential for optimizing the treatment response to rHuEpo. For example, a state of functional iron deficiency as detected by decreased CHr can be induced with rHuEpo administration in normal individuals when ferritin levels are less than 100 ng/mL,[53] and increases in CHr can be observed in response to iron treatment (**Fig. 2**).[54] Functional iron deficiency is frequently seen at even higher ferritin values in patients with renal disease and other patient populations, including malignancy, infection, and in collagen vascular diseases whereby serum

Table 2
RBC indices definitions

Channel	Parameter[a]	Cell Population
Mature: reflects Fe incorporation during 3-mo lifespan of mature RBCs	HYPOm	% Of mature RBC population with HGB <280 g/L
	CHCMm	MCHC in mature cells (g/L)
Reticulocyte: reflects Fe incorporation into 3-d lifespan of reticulocytes	HYPOr	% Of reticulocytes with HGB <280 g/L
	CHr	Cellular Hgb content of reticulocytes (pg)

Abbreviations: CHCMm, hemoglobin content of mature cells; Fe, serum iron; Hgb, hemoglobin; HYPOm, hypochromic mature RBCs; HYPOr, hypochromic reticulocyte RBCs.
[a] ADVIA 120 Hematology Analyzer terminology. Sysmex XE2100 uses similar technology: RET-Y (compares with CHr) and RBC-Y (compares with HYPOm).
Data from ADVIA 120 Hematology system operator's guide: glossary version 1.02.00. Copyright © 1997, 2002 Bayer Corporation.

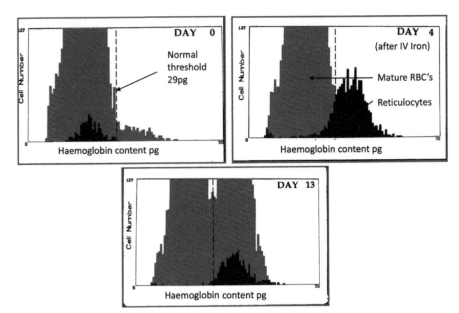

Fig. 2. Response in hemoglobin content of mature red cells (CH, *red*) and of reticulocytes (CHr, (*blue*) to iron dextran in a patient unresponsive to oral iron therapy. Hemoglobin increased concomitantly from 7.8 g/dL at day 0 to 11.2 g/dL at day 13.

ferritin is an acute-phase response protein that is an unreliable indicator of iron stores. Another RBC index marker, the percentage of hypochromic red cells (%HYPO; RBCs with MCHC less than 28 g/dL) has been shown to indicate functional iron lack in dialysis patients and in normal individuals treated with rHuEpo.[53,55] Additionally, HYPOm was found to have a high degree of correlation with sTfR (area under receiver operating characteristic [ROC] curve = 0.98) in female students with iron deficiency anemia, in whom the increased %HYPO returned to normal after oral iron therapy.[48] This finding suggests that measurement of RBC indices may be efficacious for assessing iron depletion in normal otherwise healthy individuals as represented by blood donors.

RED BLOOD CELL INDICES IN BLOOD DONOR POPULATIONS

Because biochemical measures such as sTfR and the hematologic indices CHr and HYPOm reflect iron currently available for erythropoiesis, normal values may be seen in a blood donor with AIS who is maintaining sufficient dietary iron intake. Thus, the potential value of these tests may be in assessing the ability of some donors who continue to successfully donate (without deferral) or in predicting future donor deferrals (at-risk donors). In a study using the ADVIA 120 analyzer in the evaluation of blood donor iron status, Radtke and colleagues[34] found reasonable sensitivity of CHr at the 32-pg cutoff and HYPOm at the 0.3% cutoff individually (57.5% for both measures), and combined (69%) in the identification of IDE, with high specificity (~90%). In a smaller study, Nadarajan and colleagues[33] found 81% sensitivity and 89% specificity for a HYPOm-equivalent parameter, RBC-Y and lower sensitivity, 69%, versus 93% specificity for CHr at the 28-pg cutoff. Both investigators used the log (sTfR/ferritin) ratio as the gold standard to define iron deficiency. These investigators reported greater sensitivity and specificity using serum ferritin over RBC parameters: 88% and 92% at the ferritin cutoff of 20 ng/mL[31] and 100% and 90% (area under the curve [AUC] 0.99) at a cutoff of 15 ng/mL, respectively.[33] However, the analyses were methodologically biased in ascribing these results to ferritin because ferritin was compared with log (sTfR/ferritin) in the ROC analysis.[32] The investigators concluded that despite logistical issues in obtaining RBC indices, they were superior to hemoglobin values in assessing blood donor iron status.

In the multicenter RISE analysis, plasma ferritin and sTfR were compared with RBC indices including CHr and the %HYPO to characterize AIS and IDE in blood donors.[32] The RBC index that performed the best overall was %HYPOm (**Fig. 3**). At a %HYPOm cutoff value of 0.55%, the sensitivity and specificity were 85% and 57% for AIS and 72% and 68% for IDE, respectively. Comparative values for CHr at 32.6 pg (optimized according to ROC curve analysis) were 81% and 49% for AIS and 69% and 53% for IDE, respectively, with poorer results at the conventional cutoff of 28 pg. CHr had lower diagnostic usefulness than HYPOm or several other indices including proportion of reticulocyte hypochromic RBCs (HYPOr) or hemoglobin content of mature cells (CHCMm). The RBC assays were better (greater AUC) at identifying more severe iron depletion (ie, AIS or ferritin less than 12 ng/mL). At 28 pg for CHr, there was extremely poor sensitivity (7%), no better than MCV of 80 fL. In a recent single-center study in blood donors, CHr using a cutoff value of 28 pg was reported to have excellent specificity with slightly higher sensitivity for detection of AIS (defined in their study as sTfR/log ferritin >97.5th percentile, or 1.5): 27.3% (men) and 40.8% (women); however, the investigators also expressed reservations that CHr did not identify a considerable proportion of latent iron-depleted donors.[42]

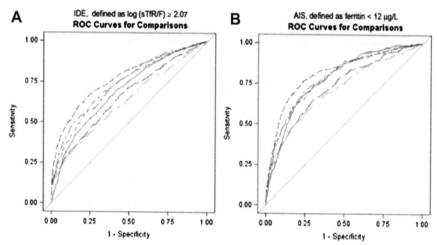

Fig. 3. RBC indices for detection of iron deficiency in RISE donors. ROC curves for hematology indices at enrollment visit. (*A*) IDE, defined as log (sTfR/F) of 2.07 or greater. (———) Hemoglobin (Hb) (0.6951); (– – –) HYPOm (0.7692); (— · —) hemoglobin content of mature cells (CHCMm) (0.7369); (—— ——) CHr (0.6549); (– – – –) reticulocyte hypochromic RBCs (HYPOr) (0.7281); (—— ·) MCV (6257). (*B*) AIS, defined as ferritin less than 12 μg/L. (———) Hb (0.7820); (– – –) HYPOm (0.8177); (— · —) CHCMm (0.7920); (—— ——) CHr (0.7302); (– – · – –) HYPOr (0.7871); (—— ·) MCV (0.7079). (*From* Kiss JE, Steele WR, Wright DJ, et al. NHLBI Retrovirus Epidemiology Donor Study-II [REDS-II]. Laboratory variables for assessing iron deficiency in REDS-II Iron Status Evaluation [RISE] blood donors. Transfusion 2013;53:2766–75; with permission.)

Technical issues affecting some of the measured RBC parameters are critical to the accuracy of RBC index tests. The manufacturer recommends testing within 6 hours because cell swelling may affect the accuracy of some measured parameters, including HYPOm, HYPOr, CHCM, and MCV but not CHr.[32,46] Whether these sample preparation/storage issues affected the reported differences in results between HYPOm and CHr are not clear. Some studies report better results using CHr,[35,56] whereas others report that HYPOm is superior. For example, HYPOm was found to have better sensitivity and specificity than CHr in 2 hemodialysis/erythropoietin treatment trials[57,58] and a study of iron-deficient young women or patients hospitalized with anemia.[50] Mitsuiki and colleagues[59] found that a higher cutoff for CHr, 32 pg, improved the sensitivity and specificity of this test in the diagnosis of iron deficiency. In particular, because of the immediate uptake of iron into developing immature RBCs, reticulocyte variables (CHr, HYPOr) may indicate recent or real-time hematinic therapy; HYPOr and CHr have been shown to have more rapid correction than HYPOm after iron replacement in anemic young women.[46] CHr ranked low as an indicator of AIS and IDE in the RISE study.[32] The RISE investigators theorized that the reticulocyte hemoglobin compartment may be preserved because regular blood donors may be able to compensate as they either consciously or unconsciously consume more iron-rich foods and/or iron supplements leading up to their scheduled donation, thus replenishing the reticulocyte hemoglobin compartment while remaining chronically iron depleted.

In conclusion, the RISE study found that RBC indices had only a modest value in assessing the iron status of blood donors. Although clearly superior to hemoglobin in detecting iron depletion, using HYPOm or CHr detected IDE in about 70% of true-positive donors while falsely classifying approximately 32% (HYPOm) and approximately 47% (CHr). A plasma ferritin value of 26.7 ng/ml (comparable serum level of ~28 ng/ml) provided the simplest and best discriminatory value overall used in conjunction with the 12.5 g/dL capillary hemoglobin standard. It would be advisable that blood centers considering using RBC indices as a screen for iron depletion in blood donors to rigorously validate their results, especially with regard to ROC curve-based threshold values, in comparison to ferritin levels. Future research would benefit greatly from well-designed prospective studies using RBC indices in donor management.

GENETIC ASSESSMENT OF IRON STATUS IN BLOOD DONORS

A growing body of research is beginning to uncover genetic variations involved in iron metabolism and hemoglobin production, many affecting the actions of the central regulator of iron metabolism, hepcidin (**Table 3**). Indeed, a new term has been coined *ironomics* to emphasize the interplay between genomics and iron pathways.[60] Current guidelines that govern blood donation are fairly uniform for all donors despite considerable individual differences in the ability to donate without being deferred for low hemoglobin. For example, there are subsets of very frequent/high-intensity donors that seem to be less susceptible to iron deficiency and hemoglobin deferral. Mast and colleagues[61,62] have characterized a group of female superdonors with 6 donations in the previous 12 months that had less than one-half the odds for low hemoglobin deferral than those with only one donation. Data such as this, at the extremes of donor tolerance of iron losses, suggest there may be individuals that can respond by more efficient dietary iron absorption. At the other end of the spectrum are donors who are deferred after they donate once or only a few times, suggesting a vulnerability to iron loss from blood donation.

Table 3
Genetic alterations and iron status in blood donors

Genetic Polymorphism	Iron Pathway Effect
HFE: C282Y, H63D	Hepcidin regulation (*increased* Fe absorption)
TF G277S	Transferrin mutation (*decreased* iron transport and iron deficiency anemia)
HIF-1α	Erythropoietin and hepcidin regulation (RBC production and iron absorption)
TMPRSS6	Hepcidin regulation (iron absorption)

Genotype Data RISE Study	
HFE Genotype	**TF G277S Genotype**
Wild-type 1568 (64.7%)	Wild-type 2107 (86.9%)
Heterozygous H63D 573 (23.6%)	Heterozygous or homozygous 254 (10.5%)
Heterozygous C282Y 194 (8.0%)	Missing 64 (2.6%)
Homozygous H63D 39 (1.6%)	
Homozygous C282Y 7 (0.3%)	
Double mutation 41 (1.7%)	
Missing 3 (0.1%)	

Abbreviations: Fe, serum iron; HFE, hereditary hemochromatosis; HIF-1α, hypoxia inducible factor 1α; TF, transferrin.

Data from Mast AE, Lee TH, Schlumpf KS, et al, NHLBI Retrovirus Epidemiology Donor Study-II (REDS-II). The impact of HFE mutations on hemoglobin and iron status in individuals undergoing repeated iron loss through blood donation. Br J Haematol 2012;156:388–401.

Hereditary Hemochromatosis Polymorphisms

Hereditary hemochromatosis (HFE) is associated with 2 major polymorphisms affecting the HFE gene, 845 G ->A (C282Y) and 187 C ->G (H63D). Clinical iron overload occurs in individuals who are either homozygous for C282Y or are C282Y/H63D compound heterozygotes[63] who cannot upregulate hepcidin to decrease iron absorption. As a result, individuals with hemochromatosis have inappropriately low hepcidin for the amount of iron stores they possess. It is reasonable to think that individuals with HFE polymorphisms might be ideal blood donors; in fact, the FDA has approved a program that allows them to donate more frequently than regular donors.[64] In a large population survey, Beutler and colleagues[65] found a significantly lower prevalence of iron depletion without anemia (defined as a transferrin saturation of <16%, serum ferritin <21 ng/mL, and hemoglobin concentration ≥12 g/dL) in female C282Y carriers compared with controls: 1.9% versus 4.1% in all women and 4.1% versus 9.2% in women less than 50 years of age. No protective effect of HFE polymorphisms was observed on the frequency of iron deficiency anemia (which affected only 3.3% of women between 25–50 years of age). These results are consistent with a relatively modest effect stemming from defective hepcidin regulatory function as a consequence of HFE mutations, leading to relatively increased iron levels compared with control individuals.

HFE polymorphisms are quite common, being found in approximately 34% (10% C282Y and 24% H63D) of the US Caucasian population.[66] Similar or only slightly higher prevalence rates have been found in blood donors (see **Table 3**), even among high-intensity donors who might be at an advantage to absorb more iron to compensate for the physiologic stress of repeated iron losses and avoid the development of iron deficiency anemia. Could HFE polymorphisms be protective of iron balance and hemoglobin levels in regular blood donors? Mast and colleagues[67] genotyped first-time and repeat blood donors participating in the REDS-III-RISE study, who were assessed for iron and hemoglobin status at each donation up to 24 months. Among first-time donors, the proportion of those without HFE mutations was lower than a large population database reported previously, 66.7% versus 76.0% (P = .0006), suggesting blood donors (or those that volunteer to participate in clinical trials) may be enriched for HFE. There was no difference overall between first-time and repeat donors in HFE at enrollment, except that the frequency of H63D was found to be higher in black repeat donors compared with first-time donors, 15.8% versus 3.8% (P = .01). First-time donors with 2 HFE polymorphisms had significantly higher ferritin, CHr, and hemoglobin levels initially; carriers had slightly higher levels. However, after donating blood a few times the changes in iron and hemoglobin status decreased in parallel to donors who did not have these polymorphisms. Laboratory measures that were found to affect iron and hemoglobin changes longitudinally included ferritin and CHr, which were suggested as better indicators of iron status and ability to donate repeatedly than HFE status. Similar analysis of another genetic polymorphism, the transferrin (G227S) gene, was also performed. This mutation is associated with a reduction in TIBC and predisposes menstruating women to iron deficiency.[68] However, blood donors in the RISE study with this variant gene did not show an increased risk of iron depletion or iron deficiency anemia greater than the controls.[67]

TMPRSS6 and Other Genomic Studies

With the recognition of hepcidin as the central iron regulatory hormone that controls body iron,[69] other molecules involved in the regulation of hepcidin biosynthesis have been identified along with polymorphisms that alter hemoglobin and iron status in recent genome-wide association studies (GWAS).[70] TMPRSS6 is a membrane-associated serine protease that decreases hepcidin biosynthesis. TMPRSS6 knockout mice have iron deficiency and microcytic anemia.[71] Single nucleotide polymorphisms (SNPs) in the TMPRSS6 gene are associated with changes in hemoglobin concentration.[72] One of the SNPs, rs855791, encoding a valine to alanine amino acid change, was strongly associated with hemoglobin levels and changes in MCV; it seems that it affects TMPRSS6-mediated changes in hepcidin expression, thereby influencing iron metabolism.[73] Mast and colleagues[74] analyzed the A736V TMPRSS6 polymorphism and found approximately 40% AA, 40% AV, and 20% VV variants in a random sample. For women, the average hemoglobin was 0.74 and 0.53 g/dL higher in AA (P<.0001) and A/V (P = .0057) than in VV, respectively. This finding correlated with average ferritin, which was 77% and 54% higher in AA (P = .0024) and A/V (P = .022) than in VV donors. The female AA donors maintained 0.35 to 0.50 g/dL significantly higher hemoglobin levels over the course of successive donations. Although preliminary, these investigations have identified the TMPRSS6 genotype as a common polymorphism of iron status that may influence individual responses to blood donation.

There is another example of a high prevalence polymorphic gene that impacts hemoglobin levels and tolerance to repeated blood donation.[75] Hypoxia inducible factor (HIF)-1α is involved in iron homeostasis by increasing erythropoietin and suppressing hepcidin expression in the liver under conditions of hypoxia. Men who were carriers of the HIF-1αPro-582-Ser polymorphism (affecting 25%–30% of reported subjects) were found to have higher hemoglobin and ferritin levels than individuals homozygous for the wild-type allele. In addition, the HIF-1α polymorphism protected blood donors from developing iron deficiency and was shown to reduce low hemoglobin and low ferritin deferrals, allowing more intensive blood donation activity.

These seminal studies using genomic analysis make it likely that there are additional polymorphisms in other iron regulatory proteins that account for either high intensity donation success or vulnerability in becoming anemic and being deferred. Careful comparison with phenotypic data including longitudinal studies using measures of hemoglobin and iron status will need to be performed to determine their overall usefulness. Along these lines, the National Heart, Lung, and Blood Institute–sponsored REDS-III group has initiated a study called RBC-Omics,[75] which will examine the hypothesis that genetic variation underlies the different ability of individuals to repeatedly donate blood without low hemoglobin deferral or to develop adverse consequences associated with iron depletion, including pica (the compulsive eating of non-nutritional substances such as ice) and restless legs syndrome (involuntary spastic leg movements, occurring typically at night), which are reported in 10% to 20% of iron-depleted blood donors. Investigations will include exome sequencing, GWAS analyses, and metabolomic studies. This study and similar studies are expected to impact transfusion medicine by providing genomic markers of a wide range of red cell parameters including hemoglobin production and iron metabolism, ultimately leading to a better understanding of the determinants of pica and restless leg syndrome. Increasingly available genetic information from this study and others may one day allow customized recommendations that enhance donor safety and reduce the adverse effects of those who voluntarily participate in the blood donation experience.

REFERENCES

1. Whitaker BI, Hinkins S. The 2011 National Blood Collection and Utilization Survey Report. The United States department of health and human services. Available at: http://www.hhs.gov/ash/bloodsafety/2011-nbcus.pdf. Accessed December 08, 2014.
2. Finch CA, Cook JD, Labbe RF, et al. Effect of blood donation on iron stores as evaluated by serum ferritin. Blood 1977;50:441–7.
3. Simon TL, Garry PJ, Hooper EM. Iron stores in blood donors. JAMA 1981;245:2038–43.
4. Cable RG, Glynn SA, Kiss JE, et al. Iron deficiency in blood donors: the REDS-II Donor Iron Status Evaluation (RISE) study. Transfusion 2011. http://dx.doi.org/10.1111/j.1537–2995.2011.03401.x.
5. Jahanshad N, Kohannim O, Hibar DP, et al. Brain structure in healthy adults is related to serum transferrin and the H63D polymorphism in the HFE gene. Proc Natl Acad Sci U S A 2012;109:e851–9.
6. Krayenbuehl PA, Battegay E, Breymann C, et al. Intravenous iron for the treatment of fatigue in nonanemic, premenopausal women with low serum ferritin concentration. Blood 2011;118:3222–7.
7. Brownlie T 4th, Utermohlen V, Hinton PS, et al. Tissue iron deficiency without anemia impairs adaptation in endurance capacity after aerobic training in previously untrained women. Am J Clin Nutr 2004;79:437–43.
8. Murray-Kolb LE, Beard JL. Iron treatment normalizes cognitive functioning in young women. Am J Clin Nutr 2007;85(3):778–87.
9. Bryant BJ, Yau YY, Arceo SM, et al. Ascertainment of iron deficiency and depletion in blood donors through screening questions for pica and restless leg syndrome. Transfusion 2013;53:1637–44.
10. Spencer BR, Kleinman S, Wright DJ, et al. Restless legs syndrome, pica, and iron status in blood donors. Transfusion 2013;53(8):1645–52.

11. Hallberg L, Hulten L, Gramatkovski E. Iron absorption from the whole diet in men: how effective is the regulation of iron absorption? Am J Clin Nutr 1997;66:347–56.

12. Garry PJ, Koehler KM, Simon TL. Iron stores and iron absorption: effects of repeated blood donations. Am J Clin Nutr 1995;62:611–20.

13. Cook JD, Flowers CH, Skikne BS. The quantitative assessment of body iron. Blood 2003;101(9):3359–64.

14. Suominen P, Punnonen K, Rajamäki A, et al. Serum transferrin receptor and transferrin receptor ferritin index identify healthy subjects with subclinical iron deficits. Blood 1998;92(8):2934–9.

15. Worwood M. Serum transferrin receptor assays and their application. Ann Clin Biochem 2002;39:221–30.

16. Ganz T, Nemeth E. Regulation of iron acquisition and iron distribution in mammals. Biochim Biophys Acta 2006;1763:690–9.

17. Goodnough LT, Nemeth E, Ganz T. Detection, evaluation, and management of iron-restricted erythropoiesis. Blood 2010;116:4754–61.

18. Thomas DW, Hinchliffe RF, Briggs C, et al, British Committee for Standards in Haematology. Guideline for the laboratory diagnosis of functional iron deficiency. Br J Haematol 2013;161:639–48.

19. Farrugia A. Iron and blood donation - an under-recognized safety issue. Advances in Transfusion Safety – volume IV. Dev Biol 2007;127:137–46.

20. Ferritin [Package Insert]. Advia centaur assay manual. 111353 Rev J, 2005–02. Bayer HealthCare LLC; 1998.

21. Cook JD, Skikne BS. Serum ferritin: a possible model for the assessment of nutrient stores. Am J Clin Nutr 1982;35:S1180–5.

22. Cook JD. Serum ferritin as a measure of iron stores in normal subjects. Am J Clin Nutr 1974;27:681–7.

23. Punnonen K, Irjala K, Rajamaki A. Serum transferrin receptor and its ratio to serum ferritin in the diagnosis of iron-deficiency anemia. Blood 1997;89:1052–7.

24. Hallberg L, Bengtsson C, Lapidus L, et al. Screening for iron deficiency: an analysis based on bone-marrow examinations and serum ferritin determinations in a population sample of women. Br J Haematol 1993;85:787–98.

25. Guyatt GH, Oxman AD, Ali M, et al. Laboratory diagnosis of iron-deficiency anemia: an overview. J Gen Intern Med 1992;7:145–53.

26. Mast AE, Blinder MA, Gronowski AM, et al. Clinical utility of the soluble transferrin receptor and comparison with serum ferritin in several populations. Clin Chem 1998;44(1):45–51.

27. Cable RG, Glynn SA, Kiss JE, et al. Iron deficiency in blood donors: analysis of enrollment data from the REDS-II Donor Iron Status Evaluation (RISE) study. Transfusion 2011;51:511–22.

28. Rosvik AS, Ulvik RJ, Wentzel-Larsen T, et al. The effect of blood donation frequency on iron status. Transfus Apher Sci 2009;41:165–9.

29. O'Meara A, Infanti L, Stebler C, et al. The value of routine ferritin measurement in blood donors. Transfusion 2011;51:2183–8.

30. Punnonen K, Rajamäki A. Evaluation of iron status of Finnish blood donors using serum transferrin receptor. Transfus Med 1999;9:131–4.

31. Thorpe SJ, Heath A, Sharp G, et al. A WHO reference reagent for the Serum Transferrin Receptor (sTfR): international collaborative study to evaluate a recombinant transferrin receptor preparation. Clin Chem Lab Med 2010;48:815–20.

32. Kiss JE, Steele WR, Wright DJ, et al. NHLBI Retrovirus Epidemiology Donor Study-II (REDS-II). Laboratory variables for assessing iron deficiency in REDS-II Iron Status Evaluation (RISE) blood donors. Transfusion 2013;2013(53):2766–75.

33. Nadarajan V, Sthaneshwar P, Eow GI. Use of red blood cell indices for the identification of Iron deficiency among blood donors. Transfus Med 2008;18: 184–9.

34. Radtke H, Meyer T, Kalus U, et al. Rapid identification of iron deficiency in blood donors with red cell indexes provided by Advia 120. Transfusion 2005;45:5–10.

35. Semmelrock MJ, Raggam RB, Amrein K, et al. Reticulocyte hemoglobin content allows early and reliable detection of functional iron deficiency in blood donors. Clin Chim Acta 2011. http://dx.doi.org/10.1016/j.cca.2011.12.006.

36. Skikne BS, Flowers CH, Cook JD. Serum transferrin receptor: a quantitative measure of tissue iron deficiency. Blood 1990;75:1870–6.

37. Kiss JE, Cable RG, Steele WR, et al. Quantification of iron stores and iron absorption in REDS-II iron evaluation study (RISE) donors. Transfusion 2013;53. S47–030G.

38. Labbe RF, Vreman HJ, Stevenson DK. Zinc protoporphyrin: a metabolite with a mission. Clin Chem 1999;45:2060–72.

39. Graham EA, Felgenhauer J, Detter JC, et al. Elevated zinc protoporphyrin associated with thalassemia trait and hemoglobin E. J Pediatr 1996;129:105–10.

40. Harthoorn-Lasthuizen EJ, Lindemans J, Langenhuijsen MM. Zinc protoporphyrin as screening test in female blood donors. Clin Chem 1998;44:800–4.

41. Baart AM, deKort WL, Moons KG, et al. Zinc protoporphyrin levels have -added value in the prediction of low hemoglobin deferral in whole blood donors. Transfusion 2013;53:1661–9.

42. Baart AM, deKort WL, Moons KG, et al. External validation and updating of a Dutch prediction model for low hemoglobin deferral in Irish whole blood donors. Transfusion 2013. http://dx.doi.org/10.1111/trf.12211.

43. Gorlin J. Commentary: iron man pentathlon or "we have met the enemy and they is us!". Transfusion 2014;54:747–9.

44. Alexander HD, Sherlock JP, Bharucha C. Red cell indices as predictors of iron depletion in blood donors. Clin Lab Haematol 2000;22:253–8.

45. Stern M, O'Meara A, Infanti L, et al. Prognostic value of red blood cell parameters and ferritin in predicting deferral due to low hemoglobin in whole blood donors. Ann Hematol 2012;91:775–80. http://dx.doi.org/10.1007/s00277-011-1371-4.

46. Harris N, Kunicka J, Kratz A. The ADVIA 2120 hematology system: flow cytometry-based analysis of blood and body fluids in the routine hematology laboratory. Lab Hematol 2005;11:47–61.

47. Thomas C, Thomas L. Biochemical markers and hematologic indices in the diagnosis of functional iron deficiency. Clin Chem 2002;48:1066–76.

48. Kotisaari S, Romppanen J, Penttilä I, et al. The Advia 120 red blood cell and reticulocyte indices are useful in diagnosis of iron-deficiency anemia. Eur J Haematol 2002;68:150–6.

49. Kotisaari S, Romppanen J, Agren U, et al. Reticulocyte indices rapidly reflect an increase in iron availability for erythropoiesis. Haematologica 2003;88: 1422–3.

50. Ervasti M, Kotisaari S, Heinonen S, et al. Use of advanced red blood cell and reticulocyte indices improves the accuracy in diagnosing iron deficiency in pregnant women at term. Eur J Haematol 2007;79:539–45 [Erratum in: Eur J Haematol 2008;80:92].

51. Buttarello M, Pajola R, Novello E, et al. Diagnosis of iron deficiency in patients undergoing hemodialysis. Am J Clin Pathol 2010;133:949–54.

52. Brugnara C, Zurakowski D, DiCanzio J, et al. Reticulocyte hemoglobin content to diagnose iron deficiency in children. JAMA 1999;281:2225–30.

53. Brugnara C. Iron deficiency and erythropoiesis: new diagnostic approaches. Clin Chem 2003;49(10):1573–8.
54. Brugnara C, Laufer MR, Friedman AJ, et al. Reticulocyte hemoglobin content (CHr): early indicator of iron deficiency and response to therapy. Blood 1994; 83(10):3100–1.
55. Macdougall IC, Cavill I, Hulme B, et al. Detection of functional iron deficiency during erythropoietin treatment: a new approach. BMJ 1992;304:225–6.
56. Mast AE, Blinder MA, Lu Q, et al. Clinical utility of the reticulocyte hemoglobin content in the diagnosis of iron deficiency. Blood 2002;99:1489–91.
57. Bovy C, Gothot A, Delanaye P, et al. Mature erythrocyte parameters as new markers of functional iron deficiency in haemodialysis: sensitivity and specificity. Nephrol Dial Transplant 2007;22:1156–62.
58. Tessitore N, Solero GP, Lippi G, et al. The role of iron status markers in predicting response to intravenous iron in haemodialysis patients on maintenance erythropoietin. Nephrol Dial Transplant 2001;16:1416–23.
59. Mitsuiki K, Harada A, Miyata Y. Assessment of iron deficiency in chronic hemodialysis patients: investigation of cutoff values for reticulocyte hemoglobin content. Clin Exp Nephrol 2003;7:52–7.
60. Waldvogel-Abramovski S, Waeber G, Gassner C, et al. Iron and transfusion medicine. Blood Rev 2014;27:289–95.
61. Mast AE, Foster TM, Pinder HL, et al. Behavioral, biochemical, and genetic analysis of iron metabolism in high-intensity blood donors. Transfusion 2008;48(10): 2197–204.
62. Mast AE, Schlumpf KS, Wright DJ, et al. Demographic correlates of low hemoglobin deferral among prospective whole blood donors. Transfusion 2010. Haematol 1993;85(4):787–98.
63. Feder JN, Gnirke A, Thomas W, et al. A novel MHC class I-like gene is mutated in patients with hereditary haemochromatosis. Nat Genet 1996;13(4):399–408.
64. US Food and Drug Administration Guidance for Industry: variances for blood collection from individuals with hereditary hemochromatosis. Available at: www.fda. gov/.../guidancecomplianceregulatoryinformation/guidances/blood/ucm076719. htm - 48k - 2014-06-05. Accessed December 08, 2014.
65. Beutler E, Felitti V, Gelbart T, et al. Haematological effects of the C282Y HFE mutation in homozygous and heterozygous states among subjects of northern and southern European ancestry. Br J Haematol 2003;120:887–93.
66. Adams PC, Reboussin DM, Barton JC, et al. Hemochromatosis and iron-overload screening in a racially diverse population. N Engl J Med 2005;352(17):1769–78.
67. Mast AE, Lee TH, Schlumpf KS, et al, NHLBI Retrovirus Epidemiology Donor Study-II (RES-II). The impact of *HFE* mutations on hemoglobin and iron status in individuals undergoing repeated iron loss through blood donation. Br J Haematol 2012;156:388–401.
68. Lee PL, Halloran C, Trevino R, et al. Human transferrin G277S mutation for iron deficiency anemia. Br J Haematol 2001;115:329–33.
69. Nemeth E, Ganz T. Regulation of iron metabolism by hepcidin. Annu Rev Nutr 2006;26:323–42.
70. Ganesh SK, Zakai NA, van Rooij FJ, et al. Multiple loci influence erythrocyte phenotypes in the CHARGE Consortium. Nat Genet 2009;41(11):1191–8.
71. Du X, She E, Gelbart T, et al. The serine protease TMPRSS6 is required to sense iron deficiency. Science 2008;320:1088–92.
72. Chambers JC, Zhang W, Li Y, et al. Genome-wide association study identifies variants in TMPRSS6 associated with hemoglobin levels. Nat Genet 2009;41(11):1170–2.

73. Benyamin B, Ferreira MA, Willemsen G, et al. Common variants in TMPRSS6 are associated with iron status and erythrocyte volume. Nat Genet 2009;41(11): 1173–5.
74. Mast AE, Langer JC, Bialkowski W, et al. The TMPRSS6 Ala736 Val polymorphism is associated with decreased hemoglobin and iron status in females undergoing repeated phlebotomy. Available at: https://ash.confex.com/ash/2013/webprogram/Paper58169.html. Accessed December 08, 2014.
75. Kleinman S, Busch MP, Murphy EL, et al. The National Heart, Lung, and Blood Institute Recipient Epidemiology and Donor Evaluation Study (REDS-III): a research program striving to improve blood donor and transfusion recipient outcomes. Transfusion 2014;54(3 Pt 2):942–55. http://dx.doi.org/10.1111/trf.12468.

Body Fluid Cell Counts by Automated Methods

Linda M. Sandhaus, MD, MS

KEYWORDS

- Cell counting • Body fluids • Automated body fluid analysis • Hematology analyzers

KEY POINTS

- The introduction of body fluid modes on automated hematology analyzers is an important advance in automated body fluid analysis.
- The current limits of precision for low white and red blood cell counts pose barriers to wider acceptance of automated cell counts for cerebrospinal fluid.
- Improved analyzer flagging algorithms for abnormal cell distributions in body fluid samples will help define criteria for microscopic review.
- The impact of automated body fluid analysis on laboratory efficiency depends on many factors and will vary among laboratories.

BACKGROUND AND INTRODUCTION: WHY AUTOMATE BODY FLUID CELL COUNTS?

Cellular analysis of body fluids (BFs) is medically important in the diagnosis of infectious and other inflammatory processes, hemorrhage, and malignancies that may involve body cavities and the central nervous system (CNS). Historically, BF cell counts have been done by hemocytometer chamber counts. As with other manual microscopic techniques, this method is subject to high interobserver variability and poor reproducibility. The limitations of manual cell counts and the adaptability of automated hematology analyzers to the cellular analysis of BF specimens has led to greater interest and innovation in automated BF analysis in recent years. Many published studies have demonstrated that a variety of automated analyzers initially developed for blood or urine analysis can provide acceptable alternatives to manual cell counts for most BF sample types. Potential benefits of automation include improvements in accuracy, precision, laboratory efficiency, and cost-effectiveness. This article reviews the current state of automated BF cellular analysis and discusses its advantages, current limitations, and future directions.

Department of Pathology, University Hospitals Case Medical Center, 11100 Euclid Avenue, Cleveland, OH 44106-3205, USA
E-mail address: Linda.Sandhaus@UHhospitals.org

Clin Lab Med 35 (2015) 93–103
http://dx.doi.org/10.1016/j.cll.2014.10.003 labmed.theclinics.com
0272-2712/15/$ – see front matter © 2015 Elsevier Inc. All rights reserved.

Abbreviations	
BF	Body fluid
CBC	Complete blood count
CNS	Central nervous system
CSF	Cerebrospinal fluid
CV	Coefficient of variation
ED	Emergency Department
LOQ	Limit of quantitation
MN	Mononuclear cells
PMN	Neutrophils
QC	Quality control
RBC	Red blood cell
TAT	Turnaround time
TNC	Total nucleated cell count
WBC	White blood cell

AUTOMATED METHODOLOGIES FOR BODY FLUID CELLULAR ANALYSIS

Currently available automated hematology analyzers use different combinations of technologies to quantify and classify the cellular components of blood. These methods include impedance technology, cytochemical reactivity, differential cell lysis, and flow cytometric analysis of light scatter and nuclear fluorescence staining intensity. Most published studies on automated BF analysis have evaluated the performance of hematology analyzers.[1–25] An automated analyzer that was initially developed for urinalysis uses flow through digital imagery and neural network software to quantify and classify cells and other particles, and has also been evaluated for automated BF analysis.[26,27] The aggregate evidence presented in these studies indicates that automated BF analysis has already become a reality in many clinical laboratories.

BFs differ from whole blood in their cellular composition, cellular stability, and matrix effects. The introduction of a BF mode is a major innovation that some manufacturers have incorporated into their hematology analyzers. The purpose of the BF mode is to optimize the analyzer's unique combination of technologies for the analyses of BF samples, taking into account their different cellular composition and matrix effects. It is important for users to understand the technological modifications and software algorithms of the BF mode for the analyzer under evaluation, as these features will determine the capabilities and limitations of the method. For example, a BF mode that has a gating strategy to exclude mesothelial cells from the white blood cell (WBC) count should produce more accurate WBC counts than the complete blood count (CBC) mode. Similarly, an extended counting capability can improve the accuracy for very low cell counts in BF samples by counting a larger volume of fluid than is used for CBC samples. On the other hand, the BF mode WBC differential count might be limited to 2 cell types (neutrophils [PMN] and mononuclear cells [MN]), in contrast to the whole blood differential capabilities of 5 or 6 cell types. **Table 1** lists features that might be present in some BF modes of currently available automated hematology analyzers.

VALIDATION OF AUTOMATED METHODS FOR BODY FLUID CELL COUNTS

Manufacturers are required to provide a statement of intended use, which indicates the types of BFs that have been validated on the analyzer, and the analytical measurement range for each BF type. Laboratories must verify the manufacturer's claims for each type of BF that they plan to run on the analyzer. Analysis of BFs that are not

Table 1	
Features of body fluid modes on some hematology analyzers	
Feature	**Effect**
Short time to transition between modes	Improves turnaround times
No sample dilution requirement	Improves accuracy and efficiency
Reports TNC and WBC	Improves accuracy of WBC
Differential count excludes tissue cells	Improves accuracy of differential counts
Flags samples with abnormal cellular distributions	Improves detection of malignant cells
Reports RBC counts to more significant figures than CBC mode	Improves accuracy for low RBC counts and assessment of traumatic taps
Extended counting for low cell counts	Improves accuracy for low cell counts

Abbreviations: CBC, complete blood count; RBC, red blood cell; TNC, total nucleated cell count; WBC, white blood cell count.

included in the manufacturer's intended use statement are considered laboratory developed tests, and require more extensive validation. Method verification/validation includes determinations of accuracy, precision, sample carry-over, linearity, lower limits of quantitation (analytical sensitivity), analytical specificity, reportable range, and reference intervals (as appropriate) for each BF type. Method validation protocols generally recommend comparison of at least 40 patient samples; however, more samples might be needed to cover the analytical measurement range for a particular BF type. Readers are referred to excellent publications by the Clinical Laboratory Standards Institute and International Council for Standardization in Hematology for detailed explanations of the requirements for validation studies.[28,29] This discussion focuses on a few key aspects of the validation process.

Accuracy

Accuracy is typically evaluated by demonstrating comparability of results obtained by the new method and the reference method using split patient samples. However, this approach is fundamentally flawed for the evaluation of automated BF methods because the new (automated) method is being compared with a reference (manual) method that is very imprecise. Recent College of American Pathologists proficiency surveys for manual BF cell counts have demonstrated coefficients of variation (CVs) of 20% to 40% over the range of WBC and red blood cell (RBC) counts assayed, with the highest CVs being obtained at the lower cell counts.[30] For this reason, the manual method cannot be considered a gold standard in the statistical analysis.

Large CVs for either method will yield lower correlation coefficients in method comparison studies.[31] The measures of comparability that are commonly used in laboratory correlation studies are the Pearson correlation coefficient and ordinary linear regression. These parametric statistical methods are based on assumptions that the data and the error in each method have normal (bell-shaped) distributions. Use of these parametric statistical methods should be discouraged for BF method comparisons, because often the data do not meet these assumptions. Passing-Bablok regression, Deming regression, Spearman correlation, and Bland-Altman difference plots are more appropriate measures of correlation and methodological bias, because these nonparametric statistical methods are not based on assumptions about the distribution of the data or the error in each method. There is no well-defined value for the correlation coefficient that indicates an acceptable correlation, as this depends on how the test will actually be used in clinical practice. Each laboratory must decide if the correlation is satisfactory for their use.

Another challenge in performing correlation studies is that sample integrity deteriorates over time. Therefore, it is important for the split samples to be analyzed in close time proximity to minimize differences caused by cellular degeneration. Assay of commercial control material and recovery of expected values within predefined limits of precision can also be used to assess accuracy. However, commercial control materials can only supplement, not replace patient samples, as they do not have the same matrix effects or other variability that occurs in actual patient samples.

Analysis of the correlation data may indicate statistically significant differences between the 2 methods for some BF types, certain cell types, or a particular range of values. It is important to ask whether these differences are also clinically significant and likely to affect patient care. For example, if the 2 methods produce statistically significant differences in the range of cell counts that are near the upper limit of the existing reference ranges for cerebrospinal fluid (CSF), some samples might be classified as normal by the reference method and abnormal by the automated method. The apparent misclassifications by the automated method could affect patient diagnosis and management.[12]

Limit of Quantitation and Specificity

The limit of quantitation (LOQ) is the lowest cell count that is reliably detected and meets the laboratory's limits of bias and imprecision.[29] Functional detection limit and functional sensitivity are synonymous terms. For practical purposes, LOQ can be defined as the lowest cell count for which the CV does not exceed 20%. Because automated methods analyze a much greater volume of sample than hemocytometers (typically, 85–300 μL compared with 1–3 μL), they can achieve better precision (lower CVs) at lower cell counts. The LOQ will generally be higher than the manufacturer's stated lower limit of linearity, and will also be higher than the limit of detection (analytical sensitivity).[29] Recently published studies on the performance characteristics of some automated analyzers have demonstrated functional sensitivities in the range of 10 to 30 WBCs/μL.[5,10,15,20] The LOQ has the most bearing on automated cellular analysis of CSF because all other BF types generally have cell counts that far exceed the LOQ of the analyzers.

The term analytical specificity has slightly different, but related interpretations in the context of automated BF analysis. One interpretation refers to interfering substances that might cause erroneous cell counts. The manufacturer should identify known substances that might interfere with the analysis, such as high viscosity, crystals in synovial fluids, or microorganisms.[11,32] Analytical specificity can also refer to the false-positive rate (eg, the percentage of samples that would be misclassified as abnormal when the automated cell count exceeds the manually determined reference range).[12] Calculation of the false-positive rate is a useful way to demonstrate the analytical differences between methods that might have clinical implications. However, it has not yet been clearly established whether or to what extent interfering substances may be contributing to higher automated cell counts.

Validation of Automated Methods for Leukocyte Differential Counting

The purpose of WBC differential counts on BFs is to quantify the cell types that are present to provide diagnostically useful information. As previously mentioned, WBC differential cell counts performed in the usual CBC mode of a hematology analyzer will be inaccurate, because mesothelial cells and other tissue cells may be counted as leukocytes and misclassified as neutrophils or monocytes. Therefore, automated

WBC differential counts should only be performed on hematology analyzers that have a dedicated BF mode for this purpose.

Automated differential counts must be validated against manual differential counts, preferably those performed on cytospin smears.[33–35] At present, BF modes offer limited differential counts, consisting of PMN and MN cells. Depending on the analyzer software, other cell types might be included in the PMN and MN categories (eg, eosinophils and basophils might be included in the PMN category and lymphocytes in the MN category). To obtain a valid measure of correlation, these combined cell categories must be taken into account when correlating automated 2-part BF differential counts with the manual differential counts performed on Wright-Giemsa–stained cytospin smears. In addition to the usual limitations of manual differential counts (imprecision, subjectivity), time delays and cytocentrifugation will affect cell recovery and may affect the proportion of cell types that are present in the split samples.[21,36] Recent studies have shown that for BFs with WBC greater than 10 cells/μL, automated 2-part differential counts correlate well with manual differential counts.[3,10,14,15,37] Some of these studies showed an apparent positive bias for PMNs, especially when the WBC is less than 20 cells/μL. A possible explanation is that there is disproportionate loss of the more labile PMNs over time and with cytocentrifugation, which will decrease the proportion of PMNs on the cytospin smear. Different laboratories may reach different conclusions about which BF samples are appropriate for automated differential counts.

Although current technology may be satisfactory for WBC differential counting in some BF samples, microscopic examination is still indicated for the detection of malignant cells. Leukemic blasts, lymphoma cells, and metastatic carcinoma may be present in low numbers in CSF, and even samples with normal cell counts may contain malignant cells. Some recent studies suggest that flags generated by abnormal cell distributions in the BF mode might be useful in screening samples for malignant cells.[21,36,38] Therefore, method validation studies should also include an evaluation of the flagging capabilities of the BF mode. Most laboratory technologists, though skilled in WBC differential counts, have limited training in the detection of non-hematopoietic malignant cells.[39] By contrast, cytopathology laboratories are staffed by cytotechnologists whose primary concern is the detection of malignant cells. However, when malignancy is not clinically suspected and the samples are not submitted to cytopathology, the hematology laboratory may have the first opportunity to detect malignant cells. Therefore, reliable flagging to signify the presence of atypical cells could potentially improve the detection of malignancies in hematology laboratories.

SPECIFIC ISSUES RELATED TO DIFFERENT BODY FLUID TYPES

The different BF types pose different challenges for automated analysis. CSF and synovial fluid are normally present in healthy persons, whereas serous cavity effusions represent pathologic conditions. Therefore, reference ranges are important in the interpretation of CSF and synovial fluid cell counts, but are of less value in the interpretation of pathologic effusions.

Cerebrospinal Fluid

CSF poses the greatest challenges for automated cellular analysis. CSF is examined for a variety of medical indications, and most patient samples are normal. Therefore, method correlation studies tend to be skewed toward extremely low cell counts. Imprecision is higher for both manual and automated methods when cell counts are low. As shown in **Fig. 1**A, a range of automated WBC values may be obtained for

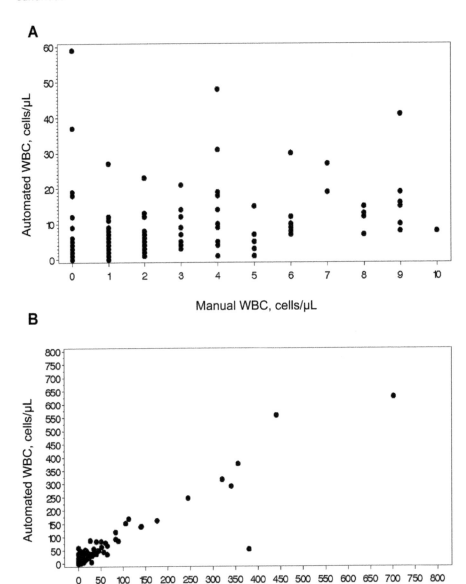

Fig. 1. Manual hemocytometer white blood cell (WBC) counts versus automated WBC counts on 200 clear cerebrospinal fluid samples. (*A*) Expanded scale for manual cell counts ranging from 0 to 10 cells/μL. Spearman correlation coefficient: $\rho = 0.47$. (*B*) Complete data set. Spearman correlation coefficient: $\rho = 0.77$. (*Adapted from* Sandhaus L, Ciarlini P, Kidric D, et al. Automated cerebrospinal fluid cell counts using the Sysmex XE-5000. Am J Clin Pathol 2010;134:736; with permission.)

each increment in the manual cell count. This nonlinear relationship between the 2 sets of values will yield a weak correlation coefficient (Spearman $\rho = 0.47$), even though a strong correlation (Spearman $\rho = 0.77$) may be obtained when the full range of data is included in the analysis (see **Fig. 1**B). The reason for this is that a few samples with high cell counts can exert a disproportionate effect on the correlation coefficient.

Furthermore, as RBCs and WBCs are not normal constituents of CSF, the accepted reference ranges are extremely low and generally exceed the limits for which the analyzers were originally intended. Published reference ranges were established by manual methods and are widely accepted, despite poor documentation of how the reference range studies were done and uncertainty about pediatric reference ranges.[35] As mentioned earlier, several correlation studies with automated analyzers have shown a positive bias in CSF samples when WBC counts are extremely low. The reasons for the observed positive bias by automated methods are not clear, but various explanations have been suggested, including "electronic noise" and inclusion of cellular debris or other particulate debris in the cell counts.[10,15] Therefore, some samples that have normal manual cell counts may appear abnormal by automated methods. For this reason, some investigators have recommended that samples with low cell counts should be excluded from automated analysis,[12] whereas others have suggested that new reference ranges for automated methods may need to be determined.[22] Until the causes of the discordant results are better understood, it remains unclear as to which results are more accurate.

Enumeration of RBCs by automated analyzers poses another set of technical and interpretive difficulties for CSF. RBC counts are useful in the diagnosis of intracranial hemorrhage, and for determining whether a traumatic tap has contaminated the sample with peripheral blood and has potentially introduced blood into the CNS. For an acute intracranial hemorrhage, the RBC count is generally high enough to be enumerated by the analyzer with adequate precision for clinical interpretation. However, most hematology analyzers do not report RBC counts at the low concentrations that might exist with mildly traumatic tap. The clinical significance is that peripheral blood introduced into the sample by a traumatic tap might lead to misinterpretation of the source of the leukocytes, such as neutrophils or leukemic blasts. The traditional approach has been to calculate the ratio of RBC/WBC, with a ratio greater than 500/μL favoring peripheral blood contamination.[35,40,41] However, if the RBC count falls below the lowest reportable value of the analyzer, either no result or a result of zero might be produced. There is no widely accepted agreement on the number of RBCs that signify a traumatic tap. Some pediatric oncology protocols use 10 RBCs/μL as an indicator of peripheral blood contamination,[42–44] although most laboratorians would consider this value to be unrealistically low. Another pediatric study used 1000 cells/μL as the cutoff for traumatic tap and determined that for CSF profiles with RBC counts of less than 10,000 cells/μL, adjustments to the CSF WBC count were not warranted and that blood in the CSF was not sufficient to explain an increased WBC.[45] Establishing criteria for defining traumatic tap by automated RBC counts would help promote clinical acceptance of this methodology, especially among pediatric oncologists, who rely on standardized protocols for defining CNS involvement by leukemia.

Serous Fluids (Pleural, Peritoneal, Pericardial, Peritoneal Lavage, and Dialysate Fluids)

The reporting of cell counts on serous BFs has been inconsistent and confusing. The inconsistency arises from different approaches to the mesothelial cells that are normally present in these fluids and can be numerous. Some laboratories include these cells in their hemocytometer cell counts and report a total nucleated cell count (TNC), whereas others exclude them. Some laboratories include mesothelial cells in the differential count as MNs, whereas others exclude them. There is similar inconsistency in the reporting of macrophages. Automated analyzers with BF modes use gating strategies to exclude tissue cells from the WBC count. The WBC differential count produced by the BF channel will include only those cells that fall within the

WBC clusters. Therefore, automation offers the potential to standardize reporting of serous BF results.

Reference ranges for WBCs or RBCs are generally not reported for pleural, peritoneal, and pericardial fluids, although WBC counts of less than 1000 cells/µL are generally found in transudates while WBC counts greater than 1000 cells/µL are associated with exudates.[35] In continuous ambulatory peritoneal dialysis fluid, a WBC count greater than 100 cells/µL and PMN 50% or greater is considered to indicate peritonitis.[35,46] Spontaneous bacterial peritonitis is suspected when the absolute PMN count is greater than 250 cells/µL.[35,47] RBC counts can be useful in interpreting the results of diagnostic peritoneal lavage in cases of abdominal trauma. The ranges considered clinically significant are well above the lowest values reported by hematology analyzers.

Synovial Fluid

Few studies have evaluated automated methods for cell counting in synovial fluid samples. Cell counts are generally higher, and there is better agreement between WBC and PMN counts when samples are pretreated with hyaluronidase.[11,48] Pretreatment with hyaluronidase might also help prevent clogging of the flow cells in some analyzers. There are no reference ranges for RBCs in synovial fluid, and a WBC count of less than 150 cells/µL is generally considered normal. The potential for interference with automated cell counts by the presence of crystals, fat globules, or microorganisms should be carefully evaluated.

QUALITY CONTROL

Quality control (QC) material should be analyzed in the same manner whereby the BFs will be processed and analyzed. For automated analysis, this means that the QC material must follow the same fluidics pathways and be analyzed with the same software algorithms used for actual BF samples. QC should also include performance of background counts of the fluidic system, and any additional diluents or reagents that are used for BF analysis that are not used in the analysis of blood samples.

LABORATORY EFFICIENCY AND COST-EFFECTIVENESS OF AUTOMATED BODY FLUID ANALYSIS

It is generally assumed that automated methods will improve laboratory turnaround times (TATs) in comparison with labor-intensive manual methods. However, whether faster TATs are achieved in practice depends on the unique combination of variables in each laboratory. Laboratories with high BF test volumes will certainly benefit from automation. One laboratory determined that manual WBC counts took an average of 19.2 minutes, compared with 4.8 minutes for automated WBC count and differential count.[17] Another laboratory achieved a 7.5-fold reduction in TAT for CSF cell counts (635 vs 85 seconds).[25] However, potential time savings may be offset by other rate-limiting laboratory practices. For example, in the author's laboratory the practice of holding automated cell counts until a cytospin smear review was completed caused unacceptable delays in reporting CSF cell counts to the Emergency Department (ED). A decision to report CSF cell counts before cytospin smear review on ED patients significantly reduced TATs. The availability of the analyzer for BF analyses can also cause delays. The time required to change between CBC and BF modes can be up to several minutes. Therefore, efficiency can be improved by minimizing the need to transition between modes. For high-volume laboratories with an automated track, multiple analyzers, and a high BF sample volume, the option to designate one analyzer for BF analysis might improve efficiency without interrupting the CBC workflow.

The potential cost savings with automated BF analysis are largely attributable to reduced labor costs. One study calculated a mean cost of €1.22 for the automated method compared with €6.74 for the manual method, largely attributable to savings in technologist time.[25]

CURRENT CHALLENGES AND FUTURE DIRECTIONS IN AUTOMATED BODY FLUID ANALYSIS

Some hematology analyzer manufacturers have clearly taken the lead in automated BF cellular analysis. This discussion has attempted to highlight both the advantages and the limitations of current automated methodology. The introduction of BF modes offers the potential to improve accuracy and reporting of BF cell counts and differential counts, and to standardize performance, which will make these results more clinically useful. However, there is a need to validate reference ranges for BF cell counts performed by automated methods, especially for CSF. Multi-institutional studies would be helpful to determine whether reference ranges can be standardized across multiple analyzer platforms.

Improvements in BF mode flagging capabilities may lead to improved detection of malignant cells in the hematology laboratory.

REFERENCES

1. Andrews J, Setran E, McDonnel L, et al. An evaluation of the Cell-Dyn 3200 for counting cells in cerebrospinal and other body fluids. Lab Hematol 2005;11: 98–106.
2. Aulesa C, Mainar I, Prieto M, et al. Use of the Advia 120 hematology analyzer in the differential cytologic analysis of biological fluids (cerebrospinal, peritoneal, pleural, pericardial, synovial, and others). Lab Hematol 2003;9:214–24.
3. Aune MW, Sandberg S. Automated counting of white and red blood cells in the cerebrospinal fluid. Clin Lab Haematol 2000;22:203–10.
4. Bellamy GJ, Clark SJ, Simpkin PS, et al. Automated counting of cells in cerebrospinal fluid [letter to the editor]. Clin Lab Haematol 2005;27:353–4.
5. Boer K, Deufel T, Reinhoefer M. Evaluation of the XE-5000 for the automated analysis of blood cells in cerebrospinal fluid. Clin Biochem 2009;42:684–91.
6. Bottini PV, Pompeo DB, Souza MI, et al. Comparison between automated and microscopic analysis in body fluids cytology [letter to the editor]. Int J Lab Hematol 2014. [Epub ahead of print].
7. Brown W, Keeney M, Chin-Yee I, et al. Validation of body fluid analysis on the Coulter LH 750. Lab Hematol 2003;9:155–9.
8. Danise P, Maconi M, Rovetti A, et al. Cell counting of body fluids: comparison between three automated haematology analysers and the manual microscope method. Int J Lab Hematol 2013;35:608–13.
9. De Smet D, Van Moer G, Martens GA, et al. Use of the Cell-Dyn Sapphire hematology analyzer for automated counting of blood cells in body fluids. Am J Clin Pathol 2010;133:291–9.
10. Fleming C, Brouwer R, Lindemans J, et al. Validation of the body fluid module on the new Sysmex XN-1000 for counting blood cells in cerebrospinal fluid and other body fluids. Clin Chem Lab Med 2012;50(10):1791–8.
11. Froom P, Diab A, Barak M. Automated evaluation of synovial and ascetic fluids with the Advia 2120 hematology analyzer. Am J Clin Pathol 2013;140:828–30.

12. Glasser L, Murphy C, Machan J. The clinical reliability of automated cerebrospinal fluid cell counts on the Beckman-Coulter LH750 and Iris iQ200. Am J Clin Pathol 2009;131:58–63.

13. Harris N, Kunicka J, Kratz A. The ADVIA 2120 hematology system: flow cytometry-based analysis of blood and body fluids in the routine hematology laboratory. Lab Hematol 2005;11:47–61.

14. Hoffman JJ, Janssen WC. Automated counting of cells in cerebrospinal fluid using the CellDyn-4000 haematology analyzer. Clin Chem Lab Med 2002;40:1168–73.

15. de Jonge R, Brouwer R, de Graaf M, et al. Evaluation of the new body fluid mode on the Sysmex XE-5000 for counting leukocytes and erythrocytes in cerebrospinal fluid and other body fluids. Clin Chem Lab Med 2010;48(5):665–75.

16. Kresie L, Benavides D, Bollinger P, et al. Performance evaluation of the application of body fluids on the Sysmex XE-2100 series automated hematology analyzer. Lab Hematol 2005;11:24–30.

17. Lehto T, Leskinen P, Hedberg P, et al. Evaluation of the Sysmex XT-4000i for the automated body fluid analysis. Int J Lab Hematol 2014;36:114–23.

18. Lippi G, Cattabiani C, Benegiamo A, et al. Evaluation of the fully automated hematological analyzer Sysmex XE-5000 for flow cytometric analysis of peritoneal fluid. J Lab Autom 2013;18:240–4.

19. Mahieu S, Vertessen F, Van Der Planken M. Evaluation of ADVIA 120 CSF assay (Bayer) vs. chamber counting of cerebrospinal fluid specimens. Clin Lab Haematol 2004;26:195–9.

20. Paris A, Nhan T, Cornet E, et al. Performance evaluation of the body fluid mode on the platform Sysmex XE-5000 series automated hematology analyzer. Int J Lab Hematol 2010;32:539–47.

21. Perne A, Hainfellner J, Womastek I, et al. Performance evaluation of the Sysmex XE-5000 hematology analyzer for white blood cell analysis in cerebrospinal fluid. Arch Pathol Lab Med 2012;136:194–8.

22. Sandhaus L, Ciarlini P, Kidric D, et al. Automated cerebrospinal fluid cell counts using the Sysmex XE-5000. Am J Clin Pathol 2010;134:734–8.

23. Tejerina P, Serrando M, Ramirez J. Automated cerebrospinal fluid cell counts in the Sysmex XN-Series. Int J Lab Hematol 2014;36(Suppl 1):1–136.

24. Ziebig R, Lun A, Sinha P. Leukocyte counts in cerebrospinal fluid with the automated hematology analyzer CellDyn 3500 and the urine flow cytometer UF-100. Clin Chem 2000;46:242–7.

25. Zimmermann M, Ruprecht K, Kainzinger F, et al. Automated vs. manual cerebrospinal fluid cell counts: a work cost analysis comparing the Sysmex XE-5000 and the Fuchs-Rosenthal manual counting chamber. Int J Lab Hematol 2011;33:629–37.

26. Butch AW, Wises PK, Wah DT, et al. A multicenter evaluation of the Iris iQ200 automated urine microscopy analyzer body fluids module and comparison with hemacytometer cell counts. Am J Clin Pathol 2008;129:445–50.

27. Walker T, Nelson L, Dunphy B, et al. Comparative evaluation of the Iris iQ200 body fluid module with manual hemacytometer count. Am J Clin Pathol 2009;131:333–8.

28. Clinical and Laboratory Standards Institute. Defining, establishing, and verifying reference intervals in the clinical laboratory. Approved guideline. 3rd edition. Wayne (PA): Clinical and Laboratory Standards Institute; 2008. CLSI document CD28–A3.

29. Bourner G, De La Salle B, George T, et al. ICSH guidelines for the verification and performance of automated cell counters for body fluids. Int J Lab Hematol 2014. [Epub ahead of print].

30. College of American Pathologists. Hemocytometer fluid count (HFC) and automated body fluid (ABF2) surveys. Participant Summaries; 2007-2009.
31. Chinchilli VM, Gruemer HD. The correlation coefficient in the interpretation of laboratory data. Clin Chim Acta 1994;229:1–3.
32. Omuse G, Makau P. Interference of cerebrospinal fluid white blood cell counts performed on the Sysmex XT-4000i by yeast and bacteria [letter to the editor]. Int J Lab Hematol 2013;35:e5–7.
33. Galagan KA, Blomberg D, Cornbleet PJ, et al. Color atlas of body fluids: an illustrated field guide based on proficiency testing. Northfield (IL): College of American Pathologists; 2006.
34. Stokes BO. Principles of cytocentrifugation. Lab Med 2004;35(7):434–7.
35. Kjeldsberg C, Knight J. Body fluids: laboratory examination of cerebrospinal, seminal, serous, and synovial fluids. 3rd edition. Chicago: ASCP Press; 1993.
36. Zimmermann M, Otto O, Gonzalex J, et al. Cellular origin and diagnostic significance of high-fluorescent cells in cerebrospinal fluid detected by the XE-5000 hematology analyzer. Int J Lab Hematol 2013;35:580–8.
37. Labaere D, Boeckx N, Geerts I, et al. Validation and implementation of the Sysmex XN 2000 body fluid module for white blood cell differential count in serous fluids. Int J Lab Hematol 2014;36(Suppl 1):1–136.
38. Labaere D, Boeckx N, Geerts I, et al. Detection of malignant cells in serous body fluids by counting high-fluorescent cells on the Sysmex XN2000. Int J Lab Hematol 2014;36(Suppl 1):1–136.
39. Jerz J, Donohue R, Mody R, et al. Detection of malignancy in body fluids: a comparison of the hematology and cytology laboratories. Arch Pathol Lab Med 2014; 138(5):651–7.
40. Bonadio WA, Smith DS, Goddard S, et al. Distinguishing cerebrospinal fluid abnormalities in children with bacterial meningitis and traumatic lumbar puncture. J Infect Dis 1990;162:251–4.
41. Novak RW. Lack of validity of standard corrections for white blood cell counts of blood-contaminated cerebrospinal fluid in infants. Am J Clin Pathol 1984;82:95–7.
42. Burger B, Zimmermann M, Mann G, et al. Diagnostic cerebrospinal fluid examination in children with acute lymphoblastic leukemia: significance of low leukocyte counts with blasts or traumatic lumbar puncture. J Clin Oncol 2003;21(2):184–8.
43. Gajjar A, Harrison P, Sandlund J, et al. Traumatic lumbar puncture at diagnosis adversely affects outcome in childhood acute lymphoblastic leukemia. Blood 2000;96(10):3381–4.
44. te Loo DM, Kamps W, van der Does-van den Berg A, et al. Prognostic significance of blasts in the cerebrospinal fluid without pleiocytosis or a traumatic lumbar puncture in children with acute lymphoblastic leukemia: experience of the Dutch Childhood Oncology Group. J Clin Oncol 2006;24(15):2332–6.
45. Byington CL, Kendrick J, Sheng X. Normative cerebrospinal fluid profiles in febrile infants. J Pediatr 2011;158(1):130–4.
46. Piraino B, Ballie GR, Bermardini J, et al. Peritoneal dialysis-related infection recommendations; 2005 update. Perit Dial Int 2005;2005:107–31.
47. Runyon B. Management of adult patients with ascites due to cirrhosis: an update. Hepatology 2009;49:2087–107.
48. Sugiuchi H, Ando Y, Manabe M, et al. Measurement of total and differential white blood cell counts in synovial fluid by means of an automated hematology analyzer. J Lab Clin Med 2005;146:36–42.

Digital Image Analysis of Blood Cells

Lydie Da Costa, MD, PhD[a,b,c,d,*]

KEYWORDS

- ANC • Automated blood cells analyzers • Differentials • Digital image • CellaVision

KEY POINTS

- The performance of modern hematology analyzers is suboptimal in identifying specific blast cells, whereas manual review is still required in the presence of immature granulocyte flags or abnormal white blood cell distribution.
- The Beckman Coulter HematoFlow analyzer is a promising new technique but cytology remains the gold standard because to date it is the only modality to reach a definitive diagnosis in many cases.
- Automated microscopy count shows good correlation with the reference manual microscopy count and may replace the regular microscope in high-volume hematology laboratories and in adult samples.

INTRODUCTION

The complete blood cell (CBC) count is one of the most commonly ordered laboratory tests. Blood cell differential counts, and morphologic analysis of white blood cells (WBC), red blood cells (RBCs), and platelets, are an important diagnostic value in malignant and benign hemopathies. The acute myeloid leukemia (AML) classification is still based on cytology and cytology is an important diagnostic criterion in the myelodysplastic syndromes and classification of their different subtypes. Most of the RBC and platelet disorders have unique features for either red cell or platelet morphology, which can then guide the selection of additional tests. Thus, it is imperative to guarantee high levels of consistency and quality and maintenance of expertise in hematology laboratories. The interpretation of manual blood cell differential count, WBC, RBC, and platelet cytology is one of the most important and difficult tasks in a hematology laboratory; unfortunately, it is also less recognized and valued than flow cytometry or molecular biology.

Conflicts of interest: The author has nothing to disclose.
[a] AP-HP, Robert Debré, 48 Boulevard Sérurier, Paris F-75019, France; [b] Sorbonne Paris Cité, Paris 7, Paris F-75010, France; [c] Inserm U1149, Bichat-Claude Bernard, CRI, Paris F-75018, France; [d] Laboratoire d'excellence des globules rouges, GR-Ex, Paris France
* Robert Debré, 48 Boulevard Sérurier, Paris 75019, France.
E-mail address: lydie.dacosta@rdb.aphp.fr

In performing automated blood cell differential counting, hematology analyzers can flag abnormalities in RBCs and reticulocytes, WBCs, and platelets, which trigger examination of a peripheral blood smear. Until the last century, all the blood smears that required an examination were analyzed manually by light microscopy. Manual light microscopic examination is still the gold standard and, according to the Clinical and Laboratory Standards Institute guidelines in the United States, requires the manual differential count of 200 cells performed by 2 experienced laboratory staff members (technologists, scientists, biologists). However, manual blood smear examination is time consuming, labor intensive, and as stated requires highly experienced, well-trained laboratory staff. Furthermore, it remains subjective and it is difficult to apply proper quality control. There is substantial variability between staff members and even in the microscopic examination of the same smear by the same person at different times; manual cell counting remains subject to significant statistical variance because of the low number of cells counted.[1–4] In addition, constant budget pressures have resulted in staff reductions for many hematology laboratories, with more work being done by fewer laboratory staff members. The development of analytical platforms capable of analyzing thousands of samples per day has prompted research and development for the automation of the manual morphologic analysis of blood cells.

HISTORY OF DIGITAL IMAGING INSTRUMENTS FOR PERIPHERAL BLOOD

The first automated morphologic analysis system was the Cydac Scanning Microscope System (Cydac, Uppsala, Sweden) in 1966.[5] Further developments lead to the LARC (leukocyte automatic recognition computer) (Corning Medical, Raleigh, NC), the Hematrak (Geometric Data, Wayne, PA), the Coulter Diff3 and Diff4 (Coulter S-Plus WBC histogram, Coulter Electronics, Hialeah, FL), and the ADC 500 (Abbott Laboratories, Abbott Park, IL).[6] However, these systems were too slow; with limited automation and, most importantly, did not prove their superiority, or at least their equivalence, compared with the reference method, the manual microscopy examination. In the early 2000s, CellaVision (CellaVision AB, Lund, Sweden) produced a new generation of automated morphologic analysis system for peripheral blood smears and fluids, initially called Diffmaster Octavia (2001), DM8, DM96 (2004) (**Fig. 1**), and recently the CellaVision DM1200.

DIGITAL IMAGE MICROSCOPY WITH THE CELLAVISION INSTRUMENT

Barcode-labeled, May Grünwald Giemsa (MGG)/Wright Giemsa/Wright stained glass slides are placed into a magazine. The DM96 instrument can be loaded with up to 8 magazines, each containing up to 12 slides, and operates with a

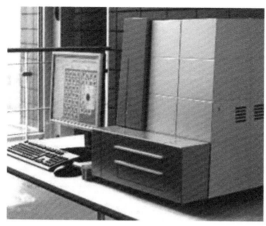

Fig. 1. DM96: an automated instrument for the differential counting of WBCs, and red cell and platelet morphology analysis. (*From* Cornet E, Perol JP, Troussard X. Performance evaluation and relevance of the CellaVision DM96 system in routine analysis and in patients with malignant hematological diseases. Int J Lab Hematol 2008;30(6):536–42; with permission.)

continuous feed (in case of emergency, magazines can be loaded instantaneously). This analyzer scans slides at low power, identifying WBCs, and then takes digital images at high magnification. The images are analyzed by an artificial neural network based on size, shape, color, and content of cells. The cells are then pre-classified according to WBC class and morphology particularities. They are shown on a computer screen for validation or reclassification if the cells have been misclassified. Better classification agreements are obtained with automated slide maker/stainers compared with manually produced smears, particularly for the smudge cell category ($P = .002$).[7,8] **Table 1** recapitulates the different features of the Cella-Vision DM8, DM96, and DM1200 (Sysmex, Kobe, Japan). DM8 and DM96 have the same technology but the DM96 is completely automated in contrast with the DM8 (see **Table 1**).

Blood Cell Analysis and Counting

Red blood cell analysis

The system allows the review of RBC features and platelet count and morphology.[7,9–14] For this type of evaluation, the DM96 provides an image, which corresponds with 8 areas of the smear viewed at 100× objective. The DM96 classifies only 6 RBC features (polychromasia, hypochromia, microcytosis, macrocytosis, anisocytosis, and poikilocytosis) with a scale from 0 to 3. We and others pointed out that macrocytosis was often wrongly reported when red cells overlapped in the digital field.[7–10] However, in our study, abnormal RBC morphology has been noted by the user in all 110 RBC pathologic blood smears, even when the anomalies were present at low frequencies.[7] The DM was unable to analyze only 3 RBC pathologic blood smears, 1 with a parasitemia of 0.1% and 2 cases with rare targets cells reported on microscopic analysis. To correct the previous disappointing version of the CellaVision system for RBC morphology analysis, the new upgraded RBC software analysis offers an extended analysis of the most common red cell abnormalities and seems promising. It can recognize most of the RBC shape anomalies with red light on the anomaly and a function when the user clicks on the anomaly, which dashes the normal RBC and highlights the abnormal RBC. It is convenient to

Table 1
Features of the CellaVision DM automated digital image instruments: DM8, DM96, and DM1200

	DM8	DM96	DM1200
Number of slides per hour	20	30	20
Loading of the slides	Manual	Automated	Automated
Barcode-labeled reading	No	Yes	Yes
Oil distribution	Manual	Automated	Automated
Number of slides per magazine	8	12	12
Continuous feeding	No	Yes Only 1 magazine by 1 possible	Only 1 magazine by 1 possible
Software	CellaVision DM software	CellaVision DM software, optional CellaVision Remote Review software, and optional Competency software package	CellaVision DM software, optional CellaVision Remote Review software, and optional Competency software package

diagnose the RBC anomalies and to appreciate the number of abnormal RBCs in a reduced time evaluation.

Platelet analysis

The instrument is able to provide a platelet count if this feature is selected. In the DM96, the user is asked to count the number of platelet cells per field (or subimage). A calculated estimate of the platelet concentration is then made based on the counts per field and a platelet estimate factor. Platelet count from the DM96 system gave a correlation coefficient (r^2) of 0.94 compared with manual platelet count and an r^2 of 0.92 compared with the automated hematology instrument. The automated morphologic analysis system may replace the time-consuming micromethod platelet count in the near future with the possibility to store the data for patients, but further studies are needed to confirm this possibility.[12] Most of the abnormal platelet morphology (eg, macroplatelets and giant platelets, gray platelets) has been accurately identified by the DM technology.[7,12] However, in our study on the DM8, almost all platelet aggregates, along with fibrin, were not classified by the DM as thrombocytic agglutinates except if they were present in great numbers in the smear or if the user recognized them on the RBC digitalized field.[7] In a recent survey about the DM96,[15] the difficulties in accurately appreciating the platelets and the RBC morphology were the most frequently cited limitations, noted in 60.7% and 53.6% respectively. Further upgraded CellaVision systems may have improved on this limitation but no study has been yet published.

Automated white blood cell differential counts and digital images of white blood cells

The CellaVision instruments are able to provide an automated microscopy WBC differential count and WBC morphology analysis. The CellaVision instruments are used in the workflow of hematology laboratories after automated hematology analyzers, which provide an automated WBC differential count, absolute neutrophil count

(ANC), scattergrams, and flags. The analysis of all these parameters may lead to the making of a blood smear, most often automatically, followed by either a fast scan of the smear or a manual/automated microscopy count and morphology analysis. The involvement of the CellaVision instruments in the workflow of a hematology laboratory is summarized next.

Automated white blood cell differential count Modern hematology analyzers combine various techniques such as absorption, spectrometry, impedance, conductivity measurement, and recently flow cytometry, for CBC counting and WBC differential counting.[16–29] The recent automated hematology analyzers are in good correlation with each other. Three recent publications have compared the performance of various instruments, namely CELL-DYN Abbott Sapphire (Abbott Diagnostics, Santa Clara, CA), Beckman Coulter UniCel DxH800 and LH780 (Beckman Coulter, Brea, CA),[30] Siemens Advia 120[24] or Advia 2120[16] (Siemens Healthcare Diagnostics, Eschborn, Germany), XE-2100[24] or XN2000[16] (Sysmex, Kobe, Japan), and UniCel DxH800 (Beckman Coulter, Brea, CA).[24] In the study by Meintker and colleagues,[24] both CELL-DYN Abbott Sapphire and Beckman Coulter UniCel DxH800 were compared with the Siemens Advia 120 and with the Sysmex XE-2100. The WBC, platelet, and RBC counts showed good correlations among the different analyzers ($r^2 > 0.99$).[24] In the automated WBC differential counts, neutrophils and eosinophils showed good correlations, whereas monocytes correlated poorly between the 4 instruments (**Fig. 2**). Basophil counts were unreliable with all analyzers. Higher percentages of lymphocytes and lower percentages of monocytes are obtained by microscopic examination compared with the analyzers' average. This discrepancy is related to an erroneous classification of immature, small monocytes or artifact of the smear with the monocytes located on the border of the blood smear.[24,30] None of the analyzers showed perfect flagging of atypical cells. Technologists and biologists often need to rely on immature granulocyte flags in order to detect blast cells and cannot rely on the blast flags alone in addition to the scrupulous analysis of the complete hemograms and scattergrams. The manual or automated microscopic analysis of blood smears validates the presence of blast cells and estimates their numbers. However, in all hematology analyzers, the manual and automated WBC counts and differentials in severely leukopenic samples are challenging. A new method called HematoFlow combines an automated blood cell analyzer (DxH800, Beckman Coulter) and flow cytometer (5-color cytometer, FC500, Beckman Coulter) using 6 flow cytometry CD36, CD2, CD294, CD19, CD16, and CD45 antibodies[29] and analysis software (Beckman Coulter) with an autogating program. Leukocytes are identified in 17 categories (B lymphocytes, CD16-negative T lymphocytes, CD16-positive T lymphocytes, T and natural killer lymphocytes, total lymphocytes, CD16-negative monocytes, CD16-positive monocytes, total monocytes, immature granulocytes, total eosinophils, mature neutrophils, total neutrophils, B blasts, T blasts, monoblasts, myeloblasts, total basophils). One study analyzed the correlation between HematoFlow and the Sysmex XE-2100, showing a good coefficient correlation for the neutrophil count ($r^2 = 0.9$), which was even better than the one obtained with the DxH800 ($r^2 = 0.87$).[22] The HematoFlow analysis of leukopenic samples was faster than the automated and manual methods with a total time of 90 minutes for the 20 leukopenic samples (0.04×10^9/L to 0.99×10^9/L) using HematoFlow compared with 115 minutes using the regular automated hematology analyzer and performing a manual microscopy count. However, the automated microscopy differential counts were not compared with the ones obtained by the HematoFlow technique. This technique may be useful in leukopenic samples from patients diagnosed with leukemia in

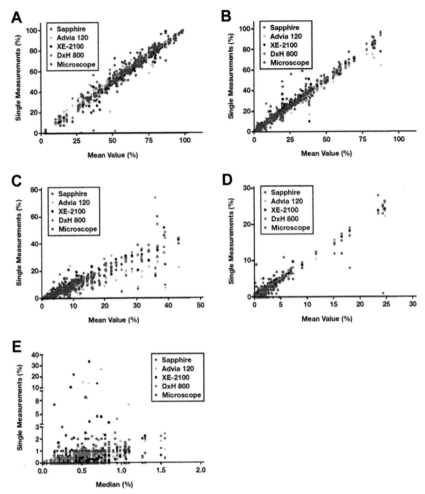

Fig. 2. Interinstrument evaluation of parameter: regression of individual measurements to the mean/median of all analyzers. (*A*) Neutrophils, (*B*) lymphocytes, (*C*) monocytes, (*D*) eosinophils, (*E*) basophils. (*From* Meintker L, Ringwald J, Rauh M, et al. Comparison of automated differential blood cell counts from Abbott Sapphire, Siemens Advia 120, Beckman Coulter DxH 800, and Sysmex XE-2100 in normal and pathologic samples. Am J Clin Pathol 2013;139(5):641–50; with permission.)

regular follow-up to save time relative to the time-consuming and often unreliable manual microscopy count. A manual or automated microscopy analysis should still validate the flow analysis and the measurement of minimal residual disease with the blast number evaluation, to determine the presence or absence of blasts in the follow-up of particular patients.[21,22,31]

Absolute neutrophil count The ANC is calculated based on the following calculation: (sum of the percentage of segmented neutrophils and band cells) × (WBC/100). The automated blood cell analyzers are able to accurately count the absolute number of neutrophils with a strong correlation with the manual differential count in the normal interval.[26,32] Neutropenia is associated with an increased risk of severe infection, which is responsible for the high risk of mortality if untreated.[33] The accuracy of the blood cell automated analyzers to count very low numbers of neutrophils is diminished but the manual count is likely inaccurate at very low neutrophil counts as well. The reference method for the low neutrophil count is the counting of 400 leukocytes by microscopic examination in 2 blood smears (Wayne, PA, Clinical and Laboratory Standards Institute, 2007), which is frequently impossible in samples with very low leukocyte counts. A study[34] recently compared the accuracy of ANC in 106 samples from patients with ANC less than 0.2×10^9/L between different automated blood cells instruments, including two 5-part differential hematology analyzers (Sysmex XE-2100, Sysmex, Kobe, Japan) and Advia 2120i (Siemens Healthcare Diagnostics, Deerfield, IL), two 3-part differential analyzers (Sysmex K4500 and Advia 60), the automated system for examination of microscopic slides (CellaVision DM96, CellaVision, Lund, Sweden), and a flow cytometric (FCM) neutrophil count using monoclonal antibodies.[34] Both 5-part differential hematology analyzers (Sysmex XE-2100 and the Advia 2120i) were able to estimate with satisfactory accuracy the ANCs of samples containing fewer than 0.1×10^9/L. There was a strong correlation for the ANC between each 5-part differential hematology analyzers, and the FCM with $r^2 = 0.978$ and $r^2 = 0.968$ respectively. The correlation between CellaVision DM96 neutrophil count and the FCM even at very low cell counts was comparable with the one obtained with the automated blood cell analyzers with $r^2 = 0.958$.

Should the automated ANC be validated systematically when it is less than a defined cutoff[17] (first ANC $<1 \times 10^9$/L or WBC count $<4 \times 10^9$/L) with a microscopic examination? This strategy is recommended if there are flags from the instrument, such as immature granulocytes, blasts, and abnormal scattergram in the Sysmex XE-2100, which indicate a failure to classify leukocytes.[35,36] Another important question regarding the ANC is whether the ANC can be used as a stand-alone test. It is used in hematology/oncology practice during chemotherapy in order to confirm that the ANC is sufficient to proceed to the treatment. It is faster than the manual differential cell count or using an automated image recognition system such as CellaVision, which needs a blood smear, coloration, and microscopic examination. We recently showed using a Sysmex XN (Sysmex, Kobe, Japan) (article in preparation) a strong correlation between the manual differential cell count and the ANC without any change in the correlation depending on the age of the patients, which is crucial in our regular pediatrics practice. The ANC may be an interesting tool for oncology/hematology practice in order to reduce the delay between the sample collection and the blood test result for the clinician, who could reduce the delay before the beginning of the chemotherapy. The turnaround time for all differentials was reduced by 75% ($P = .042$) using the ANC as a stand-alone test.[37] The investigators concluded that ANC can be used as a separate, stand-alone test in hematology/oncology because "the test result's relevance is more important than the volume of information provided and that determines clinicians' use."

Digital Image Instrument Advantages

Accuracy
Various studies have compared WBC differentials obtained on automated microscopy systems with those obtained on either automated hematology analyzers or with manual microscopic counting.[4,7–9,11,38] An important parameter is the accuracy of the DM system in identifying and classifying digitized cells. Accuracy is defined by the total number of cells classified correctly, divided by the total number of cells classified. The accuracy depends on the preclassification agreement (percentage of WBCs classified by the DM in a category and validated by the user as belonging to

this category) and the postclassification agreement (percentage of WBCs classified by the DM in disagreement with the final result validated by the user). Additional factors such as influence of the blood smearing technique, age, particular diseases, and the time of analysis have also been investigated.

In all the studies, WBC differential produced by the automated digital cell morphology system showed acceptable accuracy and reliability (**Tables 2** and **3**) with up to 98% accuracy.[7–9,11] Only a few cells analyzed in the DM96 or in DM8 were either not identified (2.6% and 2% unidentified cells according to Cornet and colleagues[11] and Billard and colleagues,[7] respectively) or misclassified (14%, 10.8%, 8% misclassified by the DM96 according to Kratz and colleagues[8] and Briggs and colleagues,[9] and by the DM8 according to Billard and colleagues,[7] respectively) at the preclassification stage. After reclassification of the cells, good correlation between the automated digital image counting on the DM96 and manual microscopy counting for the most common hematological parameters has been reported (see **Tables 2** and **3**). Depending on the WBC category, with direct microscopy being used as the reference method and excluding all clinically insignificant discrepant results caused by nomenclature differences, Kratz and colleagues[8] established a sensitivity varying from 95% (immature granulocyte category) to 100% (blasts or unusual RBCs or the nucleated RBC category) and a specificity from 88% (immature

Table 2
Accuracy of the CellaVision DM96

Cell Class	Kratz et al,[8] 2005 N = 120 Blood Smears; 9194 Cells	Cornet et al,[11] 2008 N = 440 Blood Smears; 62,904 Cells	Briggs et al,[9] 2009 N = 132 Blood Smears
	% Preclassification/% Postclassification/Correlation (r^2)		
Neutrophils (segmented and band neutrophils)	NA/NA/0.96	95.6/98/NA	99.5/NA/0.98
Segmented neutrophils	92.5/82.8/0.88	NA	NA
Band neutrophils	57.1/54.2/0.68	NA	NA
Lymphocytes	96.4/95.3/0.94	99/99/NA	94.9/NA/0.96
Monocytes	81.4/74.8/0.66	92/98/NA	87.6/NA/0.8
Eosinophils	63.2/93.6/0.73	96/98/NA	79.9/NA/0.67
Basophils	80.0/85.1/NA	80/83/NA	54.1/NA/0.05
Blasts	65.1/84.8/NA	NA/NA/0.9	76.6/NA/0.99
Immature myeloid cells	53.2/63.8/NA	58/86/NA	NA/NA/0.95
Metamyelocyte	—	—	32.6/NA/0.93
Myelocyte	—	—	37.7/NA/0.37
Promyelocyte	—	—	77.6/NA/0.42
Nucleated RBC	86.7/79.9/NA	56/82/NA	89.6/NA/0.97

% Preclassification is the percentage of the cells in the various WBC subtypes as preclassified with the DM96, in which the technologist agreed with the instrument's preclassification (ie, percentage of original suggestions that were correct).

% Postclassification is the percentage of the cells in the various WBC subtypes released by the technologist that were preclassified correctly by the DM96 (ie, percentage of final results preclassified correctly by the CellaVision) according to Kratz and colleagues.[8]

r^2 is the correlation of direct microscopic WBC differential results with the final reclassified results from the CellaVision DM96.

Abbreviation: NA, data not available.
Data from Refs.[8,9,11]

Table 3
Sensitivity and specificity of the DM96

Cell Identified on a Slide	Sensitivity (%)	Specificity (%)	False-positive (%)	False-negative (%)	Positive Predictive Value (%)	Negative Predictive Value (%)
Promyelocyte/myelocyte and/or metamyelocyte						
Kratz et al,[8] 2005 (n = 9194 cells)	95	88	12	5	NA	NA
Promyelocyte	87.76	99.86	NA	NA	13.07	100
Myelocyte	66.78	99.81	NA	NA	59.21	99.86
Metamyelocyte Rollins-Laval et al,[38] 2012 (n = 211,218 cells in an adult cancer center)	48.67	99.83	NA	NA	70.52	99.58
Blasts						
Kratz et al,[8] 2005	100	94	6	0	NA	NA
Rollins-Laval et al,[38] 2012	64.7	99.8	NA	NA	57.72	99.89
Nucleated RBC						
Kratz et al,[8] 2005	100	97	3	0	NA	NA
Rollins-Laval et al,[38] 2012	98.38	99.63	NA	NA	77.57	99.98

Data from Kratz A, Bengtsson HI, Casey JE, et al. Performance evaluation of the CellaVision DM96 system: WBC differentials by automated digital image analysis supported by an artificial neural network. Am J Clin Pathol 2005;124(5):770–81; and Rollins-Raval MA, Raval JS, Contis L. Experience with CellaVision DM96 for peripheral blood differentials in a large multi-center academic hospital system. J Pathol Inform 2012;3:29.

granulocyte category) to 97% (unusual RBCs or the nucleated RBC category). In the adult samples, the DM96 preclassified the blast category correctly in 65.1% (84.8% in the final result released by the technologist)[8] to 76.6%. The technologist to DM96 or DM8 blast correlation showed an r^2 of 0.57[11] to 0.63[9] in adult samples and 0.66 in pediatric acute lymphoblastic leukemia (ALL) samples respectively (**Fig. 3**A).[7] The r^2 increased to 0.9,[11] 0.96,[7] and 0.99[9] after DM blast reclassification. However, the number of blasts identified by the DM in adults and infants was often underestimated (see **Fig. 3**A)[7,9–11] with lymphoid blast cells, often being inappropriately categorized as lymphocytes. In our experience of studying the CellaVision performance compared with the manual microscopy method in 521 pediatric samples, the preclassification agreement in ALL samples was 74% because of the high proportion of cells misclassified: 39% of lymphoid blast cells were identified as lymphocytes and 10% as variant lymphocytes (see **Fig. 3**B). In AML pediatric samples, the number of blasts was underestimated as well, but the correlation between the DM96 and the manual method was higher than for ALL samples ($r^2 = 0.88$ vs $r^2 = 0.66$) in the preclassification agreement. Even after reclassification by the user, the number of blasts provided by the DM increased but was still less than the number provided by the manual microscopic counting method. Classification of normal WBCs as blast cells decreases specificity. However, the sensitivity in pediatric samples was high because 94% of the samples with a low number of blasts (<3%) were correctly analyzed.[7] A recent study analyzed 72 blood cell slides in pediatrics. The global accuracy was higher than in our study (95.4% vs 87%). However, the investigators did not compare the DM96 results with the reference manual method but with the final results obtained after reclassification of the cells.[38] New standardized studies with the upgraded version of CellaVision

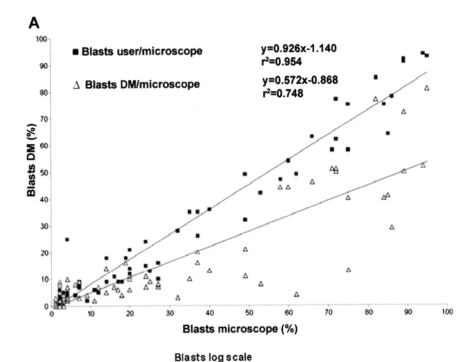

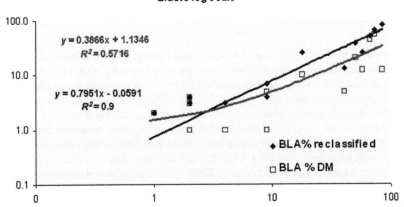

Fig. 3. (*A*) Blast correlation between the manual microscopy count and the CellaVision system in pediatric samples (top panel) and in adult samples (bottom panel). (*B*) Example of misclassification by the DM between lymphocytes and blast categories in B-cell ALL in pediatric samples. The presented cells have been classified as lymphocytes despite being recognizable as blasts (×100 magnification). (*From* [*A*] Billard M, Lainey E, Armoogum P, et al. Evaluation of the CellaVision DM automated microscope in pediatrics. Int J Lab Hematol 2010;32(5):530–8; with permission and Cornet E, Perol JP, Troussard X. Performance evaluation and relevance of the CellaVision DM96 system in routine analysis and in patients with malignant hematological diseases. Int J Lab Hematol 2008;30(6):536–42, with permission; and [*B*] Billard M, Lainey E, Armoogum P, et al. Evaluation of the CellaVision DM automated microscope in pediatrics. Int J Lab Hematol 2010;32(5):530–8; with permission.)

B

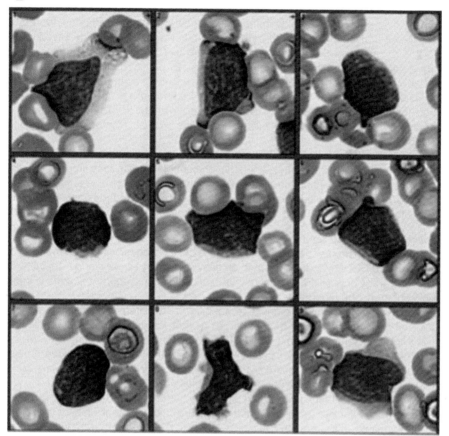

Fig. 3. (*continued*)

are needed in pediatrics, and should also take into account that automated WBC differentials are not as accurate as the manual microscopy method.

Time saving

One of the major advantages of the CellaVision method compared with the manual microscopy method is the shorter time required to deliver a WBC differential to the physician.[7–9,11,38] Total analysis time, which includes both time for the CellaVision instrument to perform the preclassification and for the laboratory technician to perform the reclassification of cells, depends on the sample (age and the disorder of the patient as well as the number of WBCs) and the user (training level of the user on the DM and the degree of experience in manual differential counting).[7–9,11,38] In pediatrics, the average time necessary for a user to reclassify WBCs and perform the morphologic analysis of the CBCs (WBCs, RBCs, and platelets) on 138 healthy samples has been described for the CellaVision instrument as 3 min/smear in samples from infants 0 to 1 month old and as 2 min/smear in samples from older patients. The average time to read a blood film with the DM96 has been found to be 2.7 min/slide compared with 5.8 min/slide with the manual microscope according to Briggs and colleagues,[9] whereas the time of analysis was longer with the

DM96 (6.4 min/slide) compared with manual microscope analysis (5.1 min/slide) according to Kratz and colleagues.[8] However, Kratz and colleagues[8] performed timing studies on smears requiring only manual differential counting, which may not reproduce the normal workflow of a laboratory. When they analyzed the time saved in the 50% of the samples flagged by the automated cell analyzer that required a full manual differential and the 50% that required just a scan of the smear but not a fully manual count, the results were more favorable for the automated digital imaging approach, especially for the less experienced technologists (no differences were found for the most experimented technologists).[8] Variability of results caused by different levels of experience of the technologists was also noted by Briggs and colleagues.[9]

In addition to the regular WBC differentials there are other cell counting procedures that may benefit from digital image analysis; for example, to diagnose storage cell diseases, microscopic examination of 100 lymphocytes is required. The automated microscope analysis reduced the time of analysis of 100 lymphocytes by at least 10 minutes per slide compared with traditional manual counting.[7]

Quality of testing and teaching

The CellaVision instrument allows storage of the digital images, with a storage capacity of 4000 (20 GB) individual slides and an easy secondary storage and retrieval with external storage media. This function has important implications for patient care, training of staff, and laboratory quality.

Digital technology allows retrieval of specific WBC differential analyses and of abnormal cellular morphology of specific cell types such as WBC, RBC, and platelet for individual patients over time. This retrieval is exceptionally challenging with the manual microscopy approach. Digital imaging allows analysis of the malignant blast cell clone for an individual and provides the opportunity of following its evolution over time, both as percentage of blast cells and as specific blast morphology.

Automated digital image technology is a powerful tool for the training of new staff members (technologists, residents, biologists). Specific cells that present particular challenges in their interpretation can be presented to the laboratory staff both for initial training and for verification of continued competence. Remedial actions can be targeted to specific criteria for cellular identification that need to be reinforced in individual staff members.

The CellaVision instrument provides a specific software package (CellaVision Competency Software) that can be used for external quality assessment of clinical laboratories but is also used for continuing professional development and education, with the objective of improving individual performance of WBC differential and interpretation.[15,39]

Ergonomics

Surveys of staff working with automated digital image instruments have shown overall better ergonomic features compared with manual microscopy, with less fatigue for back and eye (96.5% of agreement in a recently published survey).[15] Less dizziness and physical fatigue using digital images were also highlighted as major benefits.[15]

Digital image limitations

Limitations of digital image analysis have been reported.[7–9,11] Among them, the CellaVision instrument failed if the quality of blood smears was poor (suboptimal staining or slide making). Eleven slides out of 120 (10 of 11 manually spread) were unreadable in the CellaVision DM96 instrument in Kratz and colleagues'[8] study. In addition, the instrument may select the wrong areas on the slide for review, which may be too dense

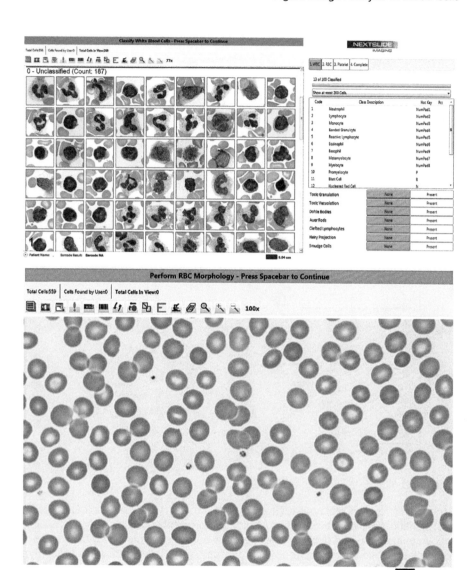

Fig. 4. A new automated digital imaging system, the NextSlide Digital Review Network (NextSlide). (Top panel) Example of unidentified WBC review on the screen in the NextSlide Digital Review Network system on the left. Morphology codes for WBC can be entered or edited on the right. (Bottom panel) A screen shot for RBC and platelet morphology evaluation from the NextSlide Digital Review Network system (×100 magnification). (*A*) Correlation between the NextSlide Digital Review Network system and the manual differential count for the WBC categories, precursors, blasts, and atypical lymphocytes. (*B*) Correlation between the NextSlide Digital Review Network system and the CellaVision DM96 differential count for the WBC categories, precursors, blasts, and atypical lymphocytes. (*From* Yu H, Ok CY, Hesse A, et al. Evaluation of an automated digital imaging system, NextSlide Digital Review Network, for examination of peripheral blood smears. Arch Pathol Lab Med 2012;136(6):660–7; with permission.)

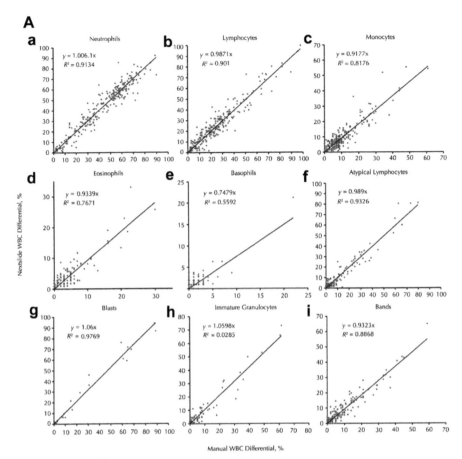

Fig. 4. (*continued*)

or too sparse for a correct analysis (for picture examples see Billard and colleagues[7]). Blast identification, in particular of lymphoblasts from acute leukemia samples, is often inaccurate in automated digital image analyzers both in adults and infants because of the misclassification of the blasts as lymphocytes.[7,11] The misclassification of lymphoblasts by the DM technology is often underestimated.[7,9–11,40] In some myelodysplastic syndrome samples, the time to reclassify cells is sometimes so long that it is easier to survey the entire smear in manual mode; the same applies for ALL samples. Another limitation concerns platelet aggregates, which are presently not identified using the CellaVision instrument unless they were present in great numbers in the smear. These limitations may be overcome in the future with the improvement of the technology but, in particular in pediatrics, which associates a higher prevalence of ALL compared with the adult population and a higher risk of platelet aggregates on the smear, the use of a digital image system may be limited.

OTHER AUTOMATED DIGITAL IMAGING SYSTEMS: NEXTSLIDE AND EASYCELL ASSISTANT

A new automated digital imaging system, NextSlide Digital Review Network (NextSlide Imaging, Cleveland, OH, and University of Massachusetts Memorial Medical Center [Worcester]) recently came on the market. It consists of a high-resolution scanner

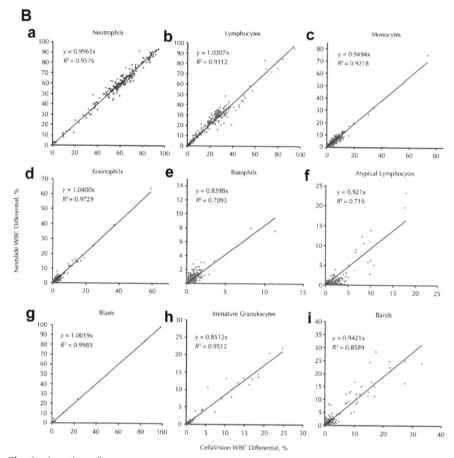

B

a Neutrophils
y = 0.9961x
R² = 0.9576

b Lymphocytes
y = 1.0307x
R² = 0.9312

c Monocytes
y = 0.9494x
R² = 0.9218

d Eosinophils
y = 1.0400x
R² = 0.9729

e Basophils
y = 0.8398x
R² = 0.7093

f Atypical Lymphocytes
y = 0.921x
R² = 0.719

g Blasts
y = 1.0019x
R² = 0.9989

h Immature Granulocytes
y = 0.8512x
R² = 0.9512

i Bands
y = 0.9421x
R² = 0.8589

Nextslide WBC Differential, %

CellaVision WBC Differential, %

Fig. 4. (continued)

and a hosted software application suite running in a data center accessed through the Internet. Slides are loaded on a tray for scanning. Each tray holds 5 slides. The throughput of the instrument is 26 slides/h and a single slide may be loaded for urgent cases. It has been evaluated in adult and neonatal samples, with an accuracy for each WBC category from 94.6% to 99.7% and an excellent correlation for blasts with manual WBC differential counts of up to $r^2 = 0.98$ and, with the DM96, WBC differential counts of up to $r^2 = 0.999$ (**Fig. 4**).[28]

The EasyCell assistant (Medica Corporation, Bedford, MA) is a fully automated imaging system that can locate 100 to 200 white cells on a peripheral smear and preclassify them in defined classes before the final operator review. It also provides smear images for platelet/RBC morphology. Up to 30 slides can be loaded into a carousel, with the capability of loading STAT slides as well. Each slide can be scanned for WBCs in 4.5 minutes, although collection of WBC together with platelet and RBC images takes 5.5 minutes. Up to 10,000 smears can be stored electronically.

SUMMARY

Major progress has been made in the automation of hematology laboratories prompted by both commercial competition among instrument vendors and continuous pressure to reduce costs. The development of analytical platforms capable of analyzing thousands of samples per day has prompted research and development for the automation of the manual morphologic analysis of blood cells. Automated digital imaging systems provide high-quality images faster and with better ergonomic features compared with manual microscopy analysis. In the future, remote automated digital system review will be extended to a larger number of laboratories, including public institutions. However, digital image systems have some limitations of which users need to be aware. Although digital methods may eventually replace conventional microscopy, it is essential that laboratories maintain the competence and capability of performing manual microscopic analysis, especially in order to confirm the presence of blasts.

ACKNOWLEDGMENTS

The author thanks Jean-Pierre Pérol (Sysmex Europe) for his support in the DM study, and Dr Anne Beauchamp-Nicoud and Dr Odile Fenneteau for their read-through of the article and for constructive suggestions.

REFERENCES

1. Koepke JA, Dotson MA, Shifman MA. A critical evaluation of the manual/visual differential leukocyte counting method. Blood Cells 1985;11(2):173–86.
2. Rumke CL. The imprecision of the ratio of two percentages observed in differential white blood cell counts: a warning. Blood Cells 1985;11(1):137–40.
3. Rumke CL. Imprecision of ratio-derived differential leukocyte counts. Blood Cells 1985;11(2):311–4, 5.
4. Smits SM, Leyte A. Clinical performance evaluation of the CellaVision Image Capture System in the white blood cell differential on peripheral blood smears. J Clin Pathol 2014;67(2):168–72.
5. Prewitt JM, Mendelsohn ML. The analysis of cell images. Ann N Y Acad Sci 1966; 128(3):1035–53.
6. Tatsumi N, Pierre RV. Automated image processing. Past, present, and future of blood cell morphology identification. Clin Lab Med 2002;22(1):299–315, viii.
7. Billard M, Lainey E, Armoogum P, et al. Evaluation of the CellaVision DM automated microscope in pediatrics. Int J Lab Hematol 2010;32(5):530–8.
8. Kratz A, Bengtsson HI, Casey JE, et al. Performance evaluation of the CellaVision DM96 system: WBC differentials by automated digital image analysis supported by an artificial neural network. Am J Clin Pathol 2005;124(5):770–81.
9. Briggs C, Longair I, Slavik M, et al. Can automated blood film analysis replace the manual differential? An evaluation of the CellaVision DM96 automated image analysis system. Int J Lab Hematol 2009;31(1):48–60.
10. Ceelie H, Dinkelaar RB, van Gelder W. Examination of peripheral blood films using automated microscopy; evaluation of Diffmaster Octavia and CellaVision DM96. J Clin Pathol 2007;60(1):72–9.
11. Cornet E, Perol JP, Troussard X. Performance evaluation and relevance of the CellaVision DM96 system in routine analysis and in patients with malignant hematological diseases. Int J Lab Hematol 2008;30(6):536–42.
12. Gao Y, Mansoor A, Wood B, et al. Platelet count estimation using the CellaVision DM96 system. J Pathol Inform 2013;4:16.
13. Surcouf C, Delaune D, Samson T, et al. Automated cell recognition in hematology: CellaVision DM96 TM system. Ann Biol Clin (Paris) 2009;67(4):419–24.

14. Maenou I, Tabe Y, Bengtsson HI, et al. Performance evaluation of the automated morphological analysis of erythrocytes by CellaVision DM96. Clin Lab 2013; 59(11–12):1413–7.

15. VanVranken SJ, Patterson ES, Rudmann SV, et al. A survey study of benefits and limitations of using CellaVision DM96 for peripheral blood differentials. Clin Lab Sci 2014;27(1):32–9.

16. Depoorter M, Goletti S, Latinne D, et al. Optimal flagging combinations for best performance of five blood cell analyzers. Int J Lab Hematol 2014;36(3): 279–88.

17. Barnes PW, McFadden SL, Machin SJ, et al. The international consensus group for hematology review: suggested criteria for action following automated CBC and WBC differential analysis. Lab Hematol 2005;11(2):83–90.

18. Bourner G, Dhaliwal J, Sumner J. Performance evaluation of the latest fully auto-mated hematology analyzers in a large, commercial laboratory setting: a 4-way, side-by-side study. Lab Hematol 2005;11(4):285–97.

19. Cherian S, Levin G, Lo WY, et al. Evaluation of an 8-color flow cytometric refer-ence method for white blood cell differential enumeration. Cytometry B Clin Cytom 2010;78(5):319–28.

20. Genevieve F, Godon A, Marteau-Tessier A, et al. Automated hematology analy-sers and spurious counts Part 2. Leukocyte count and differential. Ann Biol Clin (Paris) 2012;70(2):141–54.

21. Kim AH, Lee W, Kim M, et al. White blood cell differential counts in severely leuko-penic samples: a comparative analysis of different solutions available in modern laboratory hematology. Blood Res 2014;49(2):120–6.

22. Kim JE, Kim BR, Woo KS, et al. Evaluation of the leukocyte differential on a new automated flow cytometry hematology analyzer. Int J Lab Hematol 2012;34(5): 547–50.

23. Longair I, Briggs C, Machin SJ. Performance evaluation of the Celltac F haema-tology analyser. Int J Lab Hematol 2011;33(4):357–68.

24. Meintker L, Ringwald J, Rauh M, et al. Comparison of automated differential blood cell counts from Abbott Sapphire, Siemens Advia 120, Beckman Coulter DxH 800, and Sysmex XE-2100 in normal and pathologic samples. Am J Clin Pathol 2013;139(5):641–50.

25. Park BG, Park CJ, Kim S, et al. Comparison of the Cytodiff flow cytometric leuco-cyte differential count system with the Sysmex XE-2100 and Beckman Coulter UniCel DxH 800. Int J Lab Hematol 2012;34:584–93.

26. Stamminger G, Auch D, Diem H, et al. Performance of the XE-2100 leucocyte dif-ferential. Clin Lab Haematol 2002;24(5):271–80.

27. Takubo T, Tatsumi N, Satoh N, et al. Evaluation of hematological values obtained with reference automated hematology analyzers of six manufacturers. Southeast Asian J Trop Med Public Health 2002;33(Suppl 2):62–7.

28. Yu H, Ok CY, Hesse A, et al. Evaluation of an automated digital imaging system, NextSlide Digital Review Network, for examination of peripheral blood smears. Arch Pathol Lab Med 2012;136(6):660–7.

29. Faucher JL, Lacronique-Gazaille C, Frebet E, et al. "6 markers/5 colors" extended white blood cell differential by flow cytometry. Cytometry A 2007; 71(11):934–44.

30. Tan BT, Nava AJ, George TI. Evaluation of the Beckman Coulter UniCel DxH 800, Beckman Coulter LH 780, and Abbott Diagnostics Cell-Dyn Sapphire hematology analyzers on adult specimens in a tertiary care hospital. Am J Clin Pathol 2011; 135(6):939–51.

31. Jo Y, Kim SH, Koh K, et al. Reliable, accurate determination of the leukocyte differential of leukopenic samples by using Hematoflow method. Korean J Lab Med 2011;31(3):131–7.

32. Harris N, Jou JM, Devoto G, et al. Performance evaluation of the ADVIA 2120 hematology analyzer: an international multicenter clinical trial. Lab Hematol 2005; 11(1):62–70.

33. Lin MY, Weinstein RA, Hota B. Delay of active antimicrobial therapy and mortality among patients with bacteremia: impact of severe neutropenia. Antimicrob Agents Chemother 2008;52(9):3188–94.

34. Amundsen EK, Urdal P, Hagve TA, et al. Absolute neutrophil counts from automated hematology instruments are accurate and precise even at very low levels. Am J Clin Pathol 2012;137(6):862–9.

35. Friis-Hansen L, Saelsen L, Abildstrom SZ, et al. An algorithm for applying flagged Sysmex XE-2100 absolute neutrophil counts in clinical practice. Eur J Haematol 2008;81(2):140–53.

36. Sireci AN, Herlitz L, Lee K, et al. Validation and implementation of an algorithm for reporting the automated absolute neutrophil count from selected flagged specimens. Am J Clin Pathol 2010;134(5):720–5.

37. Jatoi A, Jaromin R, Jennings L, et al. Using the absolute neutrophil count as a stand-alone test in a hematology/oncology clinic: an abbreviated test can be preferable. Clin Lab Manage Rev 1998;12(4):256–60.

38. Rollins-Raval MA, Raval JS, Contis L. Experience with CellaVision DM96 for peripheral blood differentials in a large multi-center academic hospital system. J Pathol Inform 2012;3:29.

39. Horiuchi Y, Tabe Y, Idei M, et al. The use of CellaVision competency software for external quality assessment and continuing professional development. J Clin Pathol 2011;64(7):610–7.

40. Roumier T, Valent A, Perfettini JL, et al. A cellular machine generating apoptosis-prone aneuploid cells. Cell Death Differ 2005;12(1):91–3.

Platelets

The Few, the Young, and the Active

Carol D'Souza, FIBMS[a], Carol Briggs, FIBMS[b], Samuel J. Machin, FRCP[c],*

KEYWORDS

- Automated platelet counting • Reticulated platelets • MPV

KEY POINTS

- Many cell counters use novel approaches, ranging from the use of fluorescent dyes to monoclonal antibodies, to improve the accuracy and precision of the platelet count in patients with severe thrombocytopenia.
- The determination of the percentage of immature platelets (immature platelet fraction) can be helpful in the determination of the underlying cause of a low platelet count.
- Several companies are developing new cell counters based on digital image analysis; these instruments may allow better platelet analysis, especially in cases with platelet clumping.

INTRODUCTION

Circulating platelets are produced from megakaryocytes primarily in the bone marrow. Megakaryocytes, like all other blood cells, develop from a master stem cell.[1] All hematopoietic progenitors express cell surface markers CD34 and CD41; commitment to the megakaryocyte lineage is indicated by the expression of CD61 (integrin β3 and GP111a) and elevated CD41 (integrin α11b, GP11b) levels.[1]

There is evidence that megakaryocytes are also found in mammalian lungs and that the lungs are sites for thrombopoiesis.[2]

Unlike other maturing blood cells, megakaryocytes develop by a mechanism of internal cell growth, known as *endomitosis*. During this process, the megakaryocyte begins the mitotic cycle but without dissolution of the nuclear membrane and without cytokinesis resulting in doubling of the cell DNA content. Most megakaryocytes undergo at least 3 endomitotic cycles to attain a DNA content of 16N.[1] During the final stages of development, the megakaryocyte cytoplasm undergoes reorganization

Financial Disclosure and Conflicts of Interest Obligations: S.J. Machin and C. Briggs have received an unrestricted educational grant from Sysmex in recent years.
[a] Biomedical Sciences, Faculty of Science & Technology, University of Westminster, 115 New Cavendish Street, London W1W 6UW, UK; [b] Department of Haematology, University College Hospital London, 60 Whitfield Street, London W1T 4EU, UK; [c] Haemostasis Research Unit, Department of Haematology, University College London, 1st Floor, 51 Chenies Mews, London WC1E 6HX, UK
* Corresponding author.
E-mail address: samuel.machin@ucl.ac.uk

Clin Lab Med 35 (2015) 123–131
http://dx.doi.org/10.1016/j.cll.2014.11.002
labmed.theclinics.com

Abbreviations	
CBC	Complete blood count
CNS	Central nervous system
EDTA	Ethylenediaminetetraacetic acid
GP	Glycoprotein
ICSH	International Council for Standardization in Haematology
IPF	Immature platelet fraction
ISLH	International Society for Laboratory Hematology
L-PLT	Large platelet
MPC	Mean platelet component
MPV	Mean platelet volume
NRBC	Nucleated red blood cell
PCDW	Platelet component distribution width
PCT	Plateletcrit
PDW	Platelet distribution width
PLT	Platelet count
PLT-F	Fluorescent platelet count
PLT-I	Impedance platelet count
PLT-O	Optical platelet count
PMP	Platelet microparticles
POC	Point of care
RBC	Red blood cells
rPLT	Reticulated platelets
WBC	White blood cells

into beaded cytoplasmic extensions called proplatelets, which then develop into platelets. Young immature platelets like reticulocytes contain intracellular inclusions, such as RNA, that is gradually lost as they circulate.[1] Green and colleagues[3] (2014) have stated that "it is widely believed that younger, newly made platelets have greater functional capacity than those that have been in circulation for at least 1 day." Mature platelets, although small in size, normally between 2 and 20 μm, when compared with red blood cells or white blood cells (WBC), play an important role in both the body's inflammatory response and with the rapid response in primary hemostasis.

Recent research has demonstrated that both megakaryocytes and platelets release microparticles (PMP).[4] PMP are heterogeneous in size ranging from 0.1 to 1.0 μm and share the common glycoprotein receptors chiefly GP11b-111a (integrin α11bβ3) and GP 1b/1X. PMP are thought to be rich in membrane receptors for coagulation factors and play an important role in blood coagulation and inflammation. Elevated levels of PMP have been detected in patients with disseminated intravascular coagulation, coronary heart disease, transient ischemic attacks, cancer, and diabetes mellitus.[5] Several flow cytometry methods for the measurement of PMP have been published; but although there are a large number of publications, the lack of standardization makes comparison between methods difficult. There is now an appreciation that cells other than platelets, such as endothelial cells and leukocytes, shed microparticles and not all methods may distinguish the cell of origin.[5]

HISTORY OF PLATELET COUNTING TECHNIQUES

Platelet size initially eluded them to being included in the early automated technology. However, this has now been overcome by setting thresholds for different cells; there is now a reference method for platelet counting recommended by both the International Council for Standardization in Haematology (ICSH) and the International Society for Laboratory Hematology.[6]

Historically, through the 1970s, manual platelet counts were common practice. The method using a Neubauer hemocytometer and red cell lysing fluid are well documented.[7] For any platelet count (PLT), it is important to have fresh blood samples taken in suitable anticoagulant. Ethylenediaminetetraacetic acid (EDTA) is the anticoagulant of choice for blood cell counts. The ICSH's guidelines recommend dipotassium EDTA,[6] although, in some patients this has been known to cause in vitro platelet clumping resulting in erroneously low PLTs.[7] Manual platelet counting using phase contrast microscopy, the gold standard in platelet counting[7] until the mid-1970s, has now widely been replaced with multiparameter analytical instruments. Multiparameter analyzers using photoelectric and impedance technologies had been around since the mid 1950s. However, although they were able to produce seven parameters, comprising the complete blood count (CBC), they did not include a PLT. The drivers for including PLTs with the automated analytical systems came following the increased frequency of low PLTs induced by chemotherapeutic agents and the increase in demand for platelet concentrates following bone marrow and stem cell transplantation.

In the 1970s, Technicon produced the Hemolog 8, a continuous flow analyzer that used a separate channel for platelet counting. This analyzer used a photoelectric method for platelet counting following red cell lysis using urea. However, as with previous Technicon instrumentation, calibration was unstable; therefore, the technology was not widely adapted.

In the 1980s, the Clay Adams Ultra-Flo 100 platelet counter was the first dedicated analyzer to use hydrodynamic focusing.[8] A steady flow of diluent is drawn through an aperture, and the cell suspension is injected into the center of the moving fluid in a fine stream. This approach reduces the chances of 2 cells passing through the aperture at the same time, and there was clear discrimination between the red cells and platelets. Coulter's electrical aperture impedance technology came with the introduction of the Coulter model S-Plus series in the 1980s.[9] This series produced accurate and reliable PLTs; this parameter was added to the automated CBC profile, making this a more economical option than the dedicated platelet-only counter. Platelets on this analytical system were counted between 2 fixed thresholds, 2 and 20 fL, correlating to the platelet size.

The Coulter S-plus series discriminated platelets and red blood cells based on signal size. Following on from this, the Coulter S-plus 11 series added the mean platelet volume (MPV) and the platelet distribution width (PDW) by taking the average of the signal heights and the spread of the platelet signals. This Coulter principle was later incorporated into several other instruments and further developed by different manufacturers, Toa (now Sysmex), ABX (now Horiba), and Sequoia-Turner (now Abbott), and still applies today with some modifications in threshold settings. However, one manufacturer, Bayer Corporation, formally Technicon and now Siemens, incorporated a system of optical detection based on light scatter for the cell counting and CBC. Cells pass through a stream onto which a laser light is focused. As each cell passes through the sensing zone of the flow cell, it scatters the focused light. Scattered light is detected by a photodetector and converted into an electrical impulse. The number of impulses generated is directly proportional to the number of cells passing through the sensing zone in a given time.

Table 1 demonstrates that, although all main line analyzers offer PLT and related platelet indices, they have relied on various modifications of the impedance technology without further advances in technology. A small minority, however, have taken bold steps to introduce novel technologies with new parameters linked to clinical advances. In the multiparameter analyzers of the twenty-first century, a combination of

Table 1
Current automated analyzers available for PLT and related platelet parameters in diagnostic hematology (2014)

Manufacturer	Analyzer	Platelet Counting Principle	Related Platelet Parameters
Abbott	CELL-DYN Series	Impedance with floating thresholds, optical and immunologic	MPV, IPF
Beckman Coulter	DxH	Impedance fixed thresholds, with extended histogram analysis	MPV, PCT, PDW
Beckman Coulter	LH series	Impedance	MPV, PCT, PDW
Horiba (ABX Diagnostics)	ABX Pentra	Impedance with floating thresholds	MPV
Mindray	BC-6800	Focus flow DC and optical	MPV, PDW, PCT, P-LCR, IPF
Nihon Kohden	Celltac F (MEK-8222)	Impedance mobile thresholds	PCT, MPV, PDW
Siemens (Bayer Corporation)	Advia	Optical	L-PLT, MPV, PDW, PCT, MPC, PCDW
Sysmex Corporation	XN series	Impedance with floating thresholds, optical and fluorescence	PLT-I, PLT-F, IPF
Sysmex Corporation	XE series	Impedance with floating thresholds and optical	PLT-I, PLT-O, IPF

Abbreviations: IPF, immature platelet fraction; L-PLT, large platelet; MPC, mean platelet component; PCDW, platelet component distribution width; PCT, plateletcrit; PLT-F, fluorescent platelet count; PLT-I, impedance platelet count; PLT-O, optical platelet count.

counting principles and staining technologies is incorporated into the automated system; each analyzer is now driven by information technology and complex rules and algorithms that assist with providing the most accurate PLT and related platelet indices.

NOVEL TECHNOLOGIES
The Few

Achieving accurate PLTs at the low level, that is, less than 20 to 30 × 10^9/L, is essential in preventing spontaneous bleeding and in reducing the need for platelet transfusions.

Regular daily prophylactic platelet transfusion is the standard of care for patients with severe thrombocytopenia. The usual threshold is set for counts of 5 to 20 × 10^9/L in patients who have no clinical signs of bleeding and are apyrexial nonseptic, and on whom no invasive procedure is planned for the next 24 to 36 hours. The therapeutic strategy has recently potentially changed with patients undergoing autologous hemopoietic stem cell transplantation not receiving regular prophylactic platelet transfusions and only being transfused when bleeding has occurred (a so-called therapeutic strategy). This strategy, however, depends on the clinical staff being well educated and experienced in this new approach and being able to detect and react in a timely way to the first signs of central nervous system (CNS) bleeding.[10]

As a PLT decreases to less than 80 × 10^9/L, there is a progressive increase in the skin bleeding time. Generally speaking, most types of major surgery can be undertaken when the PLT is more than 50 × 10^9/L. However, for CNS neurosurgical procedures and ophthalmic surgery, a count more than 80 × 10^9/L is optimally required with appropriate platelet transfusion support. For multiple trauma patients with massive blood loss (defined as the loss of one blood volume within the last 24-hour period), one should anticipate when the PLT will decrease to less than 50×10^9/L and target achieving a count more than 100×10^9/L with regular platelet transfusions.

Automated analyzer manufacturers have introduced various mechanisms that have reduced inaccuracies in the PLT, where there are large platelets or interferences from small red cells, red cell fragments, or white cell debris. Sysmex with the new XN series modular system has introduced a dedicated fluorescent channel for platelets, Platelet-F.[11,12] In cases whereby the PLT is flagged by the impedance method or a reflex rule set up by the laboratory has been triggered, the XN will automatically analyze the sample in a new fluorescent channel, which extends the counting time 5-fold, increasing both the accuracy and precision. The Platelet-F channel will stain and count platelets using a platelet-specific, patented fluorescent dye called Fluoro-cell PLT. This reagent contains oxazine and stains the rough-surface endoplasmic reticulum and mitochondria. This staining has demonstrated good correlation with CD41/CD61–stained platelets and minimizes interferences from microcytic red cells, red cell fragments, and white cell debris.[12] The immature platelet fraction (IPF) is now calculated in this channel compared with the previous Sysmex XE series whereby this was performed as part of the reticulocyte analyses and used a combination of polymethine and oxazine dyes (**Fig. 1**).

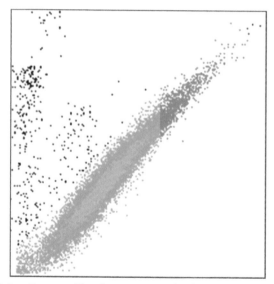

Fig. 1. XN Platelet-F scattergram. Blue dots represent platelets; green dots represent IPF. x-axis, side florescence; y-axis, forward scatter. (*Courtesy of* Sysmex, Kobe, Japan; with permission.)

The Siemens Advia systems use laser light scattered at 2 different angles: a low-angle light scatter at 2° to 3° and a high-angle light scatter at 5° to 15°. The information produced from this technology is then converted to volume, which equates to the size of the platelet and refractive index equating to platelet density. The system is then able to count and differentiate normal from abnormal platelets, red cell fragments, and debris using a volume set between 1 and 60 fL and refractive index set at 1.35 to 1.40. Large platelets (L-PLTs) are identified and displayed on the printout as *L-PLT* (**Fig. 2**).

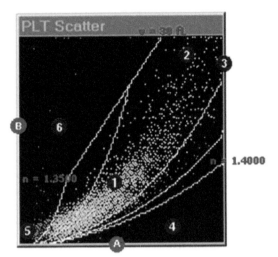

Fig. 2. Siemen's Advia scattergram. (1) Platelets, (2) large platelets, (3) red blood cells (RBC), (4) RBC fragments, (5) debris, and (6) RBC ghosts. The PLT scatter cytogram is the graphical representation of 2 light-scatter measurements: the high-angle, high-gain light scatter is plotted on the x-axis (*A*), and the low-angle, high-gain light scatter is plotted on the y-axis (*B*). (*Courtesy of* Siemens, Washington, DC; with permission.)

Throughout their development, Beckman Coulter, using impedance technology, has relied on fixed thresholds for both red cells and platelets. With the DxH 800 automated analyzer, Beckman Coulter has incorporated and introduced data fusion technology, merging of multiple cellular measurements, flexible algorithms, and statistical processes to enhance the impedance count. Particles between 2 and 25 fL are counted as platelets. The pulses are obtained from all 3 red cell and platelet apertures to obtain 256 channel size distribution histograms for each aperture. The histograms are fused, and high and low points are identified in the distribution. A log normal curve is fitted to these points. The curves have a range of 0 to 70 fL and the PLT, MPV, and PDW are derived from this curve. The DxH 800 analyzer also incorporates information from the WBC histograms and the nucleated red blood cell analysis to support PLT correction caused by interfering substances, such as giant platelets or platelet clumps and white cell debris.[13]

The Abbott CELL-DYN (CD) (4000 and Sapphire) has incorporated into their automated analyzer the immunoPLT method, which the user is able to select during analysis if the PLT is low. Here platelets are labeled using CD61 antibodies contained within a lyophilized pellet inside special evacuated tubes (Beckton Dickenson, San Jose, CA). Following incubation, the PLT is performed within a fixed volume and includes platelet and red cell coincidence. This method has been shown to provide accurate PLT, due to targeting the platelet specific membrane marker, especially in thrombocytopenic patients.[14]

The Young

Immature platelets, also known as reticulated platelets (rPLTs), contain RNA and can, therefore, be detected by a variety of RNA staining dyes. Sysmex was the first diagnostic analyzer manufacturer to introduce the IPF. In the XE series, this was identified by flow cytometry and the use of nucleic acid dyes, in the form of a combination of polymethine and oxazine in the reticulocyte/optical platelet channel. Stained cells then pass through a laser beam, and forward scattered light and fluorescence intensity are measured. Both mature and immature rPLTs are identified by the intensity of forward scatter (cell volume) and fluorescence (RNA content). The resulting scattergram is divided into the platelet area and the red cell/reticulocyte area; the IPF is then measured in the high-fluorescing, large-platelet section of the scattergram.

On the XN modular series, the IPF is measured in a dedicated platelet channel still using optical fluorescence and using a specific platelet RNA dye, oxazine. The IPF is expressed as a percentage of the total optical PLT to represent the rate of platelet production.[12]

The other manufacturer to provide an IPF parameter is Abbott with the CD-Sapphire referred to here as *rPLTs*. The rPLT is measured as part of the reticulocyte estimation after staining with a proprietary fluorescent CD4K30 dye,[15] which stains the RNA in both red cells and platelets. Cells pass through a laser beam at different angles of light scatter and green fluorescence. A variable gate is applied to separate the red cell and platelet populations. Within the platelet gate, mature PLT and rPLT are discriminated by the scatter and the green fluorescent light. The rPLT is expressed as a percentage of the total PLT.[14]

Clinical utility of the IPF has been established in the laboratory diagnosis and monitoring of thrombocytopenia caused by increased platelet destruction and autoimmune thrombocytopenic purpura. The IPF is increased in diseases in which there is increased platelet destruction or consumption and decreased in bone marrow failure. Individual instruments may have slightly different reference ranges, and these should be established by the manufacturer and validated by the laboratory.

The Active

Platelet activation is a complex process that involves many receptors and signaling pathways and is thought to be linked to the specific changes in the surface glycoproteins. Most analytical techniques to detect platelet activation currently rely on flow cytometry, however, within the Siemens Advia analyzer; as well measuring the PLT and related platelet parameters the analytical system also evaluates some activation-related parameters, the mean platelet component (MPC).[16] The MPC is designed to reveal degranulation. In addition, the Advia also provides platelet component distribution width, a parameter related to the alteration in platelet shape through activation and expression of P-selectin. However, the age of the sample is critical as changes occur over storage time.

MEAN PLATELET VOLUME

All current automated hematology analyzers produce the MPV parameter. The normal range varies between 7–12 fL, although this parameter has not been standardised. Recently released platelets are larger and haemostatically more active. Platelet activation leads to changes in platelet shape and an increase in platelet swelling (sphering) resulting in an increased MPV. With impedance analyzers the MPV and PDW are derived from the platelet distribution curve and therefore should be interpreted carefully as they will be influenced by the anticoagulant used, platelet swelling and possible time delay in sample analysis.

Normally there is an inverse relationship between the MPV and the PLT, the lower the PLT the higher the MPV. There is evidence that the MPV is an important risk factor for arterial thrombosis, acute myocardial infarction, diabetes and venous thromboembolism.[17] The MPV has also been evaluated as a diagnostic tool in different thrombocytopenic conditions.[18]

FUTURE DEVELOPING TECHNOLOGY

Although currently in development for point of care (POC), image analysis could become the standard practice within diagnostic automated laboratories during the twenty-first century. Moving away from impedance or flow technology, these technologies incorporate image analysis. The main challenge for image analysis technology is in obtaining a single layer of cells to enable the cells to be captured for identification. A fixed volume of blood is used; thousands of images are captured; and using complex algorithms, the cells are differentiated and cell counts are calculated to produce a CBC.

The Bloodhound integrated hematology system from Constitution Medical, now Roche, produces a CBC from 1 μL of blood spread on a slide in adjacent rows to form a monolayer blood smear; this enables each cell to be identified and analyzed for classification. The slide is stained with a proprietary Romanowsky stain to allow for multispectral image analysis, using 4 wavelengths of light to illuminate the slide. Computer-driven morphologic descriptors of cell size, color, optical density, and instrument statistical classifiers are used to locate, group, and count all the cells present. It has the ability to produce 26 parameters within the CBC, including the MPV, calculated from the mean of each platelet volume in the high-power image scanning. Bloodhound technology uniquely combines a slide maker, stainer, digital image–based cell locator, and cell counter within a 42 × 56-in instrument.[19]

Other developing technologies obtain a monolayer of cells for identification by:

1. Using a bead column with standard height, Abbott POC
2. Using viscoelastic focusing, PixCell Medical Technologies

In the Abbott technology, a fluorescent dye is incorporated into the microfluidic column; using multiple wavelengths of light, different cells and cellular content can be identified. Platelets will be identified by a different fluorescent signal to those used for plasma, red or white cells, so small and large platelets will be separated from other cells. In the same way, platelet clumping is detected because of a different signal output.[20]

PixCell Medical HemoScreen technology uses viscoelastic focusing to align the cells in a single layer within the microfluidic column. A proprietary stain is used for white cell differentiation. Thousands of cells are captured, and image-processing algorithms are used to differentiate the cells and calculate the cell numbers. Platelet clumps are differentiated from other cells on the image capture, and there is the possibility to count the number of platelets within the clump. Platelet parameters and rPLTs are not currently included in the developmental data on any of these developing technologies.[20]

SUMMARY

The PLT has been incorporated in to the routine CBC for more than 50 years. Technology is rapidly evolving so that the accuracy and precision of the PLT, particularly in severe thrombocytopenic patients, has improved greatly. This improvement allows a more established set of rules for giving prophylactic and therapeutic platelet transfusions. Additional useful platelet parameters have become available, including MPV and rPLTs, which aid in the diagnostic and management decisions. In the future, POC platelet analysis should become available at the bedside and in the clinic for more rapid diagnostic and management decisions.

REFERENCES

1. Michelson A. Platelets. Chapter 2. In: Italiano J Jr, Hartwig J, editors. Megakaryocyte development and platelet formation. 3rd edition. London: Elsevier; 2013. p. 27.
2. Weyrich AS, Zimmerman GA. Platelets in lung biology. Annu Rev Physiol 2013;75: 569–91.
3. Green LA, Chen S, Seery C, et al. Beyond the platelet count: immature platelet fraction and thromboelastometry correlate with bleeding in patients with immune thrombocytopenia. Br J Haematol 2014;166:592–600.
4. Michelson A. Platelets. Chapter 22. In: Nieuwlan R, van der Pol E, Gardiner C, et al, editors. Platelet derived microparticles. 3rd edition. London: Elsevier; 2013. p. 453–5.
5. Kottke-Marchant K, Bruce D. Laboratory hematology practice. Chapter 5. In: Briggs C, Machin SJ, editors. Automated platelet analysis. Hoboken, NJ: Wiley Blackwell; 2013. p. 56.
6. Briggs C, Harrison P, Machin SJ. Continuing developments with the automated platelet count. Int J Lab Hematol 2007;29:77–91.
7. Brecher G, Schneiderman M, Cronkite EP. The reproducibility of the platelet count. Am J Clin Pathol 1953;23:15–21.
8. Guthrie DL, Lam KT, Priest CJ. The ultra-flo 100 platelet counter: a new approach to platelet counting. Clin Lab Haematol 1980;2(3):231–42.
9. Brecher G, Schneiderman M, Williams GZ. Evaluation of red blood cell counter. Am J Clin Pathol 1956;26:1439–49.
10. Wandt H, Schaefer-Eckart K, Wendelin K, et al. Therapeutic platelet transfusion versus routine prophylactic transfusion in patients with haematological malignancies: an open-label, multicentre, randomised study. Lancet 2012;380:1309–16.
11. Sysmex Corporation. XN series, PLT – F channel performance specifications. Japan: Sysmex Corporation; 2012.
12. Briggs C, Longair I, Kumar P, et al. Performance evaluation of the Sysmex haematology XN modular system. J Clin Pathol 2012;65:1024–30. http://dx.doi.org/10.1136/jclinpath-2012-200930.
13. Beckman Coulter Inc. Advancements in technology: derivation of platelet parameters. Unicel DxH 800 coulter cellular analysis system. Brea, CA: Beckman Coulter Inc.; 2010.
14. Michelson A. Platelets. Chapter 27. In: Harrison P, Briggs C, editors. Platelet counting. 3rd edition. London: Elsevier; 2013. p. 554–7.
15. Meintker L, Haimerl M, Ringwald J, et al. Measurement of immature platelets with Abbott CD- sapphire and Sysmex XE-5000 in haematology and oncology patients. Clin Chem Lab Med 2013;51(11):2125–31.
16. Giacomini A, Legovini P, Antico F, et al. Assessment of in vitro platelet activation by Advia 120 platelet parameters. Lab Hematol 2003;9(3):132–7.
17. Machin SJ, Briggs C. Mean platelet volume: a quick, easy determinant of thrombotic risk. J Thromb Haemost 2010;8(1):146–7.
18. Bowles KM, Cooke LJ, Richards EM, et al. Platelet size has diagnostic predictive value in patients with thrombocytopenia. Clin Lab Haematol 2005;27(6):370–3.
19. Available at: http://www.roche-rdh.com/. Accessed October 13, 2014.
20. D'Souza C. Invited Presentation Abstracts. International Journal of Laboratory Hematology 2014;36:1–29. http://dx.doi.org/10.1111/ijlh.12265.

Clinical Utility of Reticulocyte Parameters

Elisa Piva, MD[a],*, Carlo Brugnara, MD[b], Federica Spolaore, MD[a], Mario Plebani, MD[a]

KEYWORDS

- Reticulocyte • Immature reticulocyte fraction • Reticulocyte maturation
- Reticulocyte hemoglobin content • Reticulocyte volume
- Reticulocyte hemoglobin concentration

KEY POINTS

- Automated reticulocyte counts provide an acceptable precision and bias while parameters and indices improve the evaluation of erythropoiesis. Nevertheless, standardization and harmonization should be encouraged.
- Immature reticulocyte fraction (IRF) indicates the younger fraction of reticulocytes, reflecting erythropoietic activity. Recovery of bone marrow following bone marrow transplantation, erythropoiesis-stimulating agent therapy, or chemotherapy is reflected by increased IRF within a few days.
- Reticulocyte haemoglobin content is a real-time indicator of bone marrow iron status, and reflects the balance between iron and erythropoiesis. It is not however the appropriate measure in assessing iron adequacy in the presence of genetic microcytosis.
- Reticulocyte cell volume has a clinical utility similar to that of reticulocyte hemoglobin content, in evaluation and monitoring of anemia.

HISTORY OF RETICULOCYTES OVER THE LAST 150 YEARS

The Mid 1800s: Discovery of "Granulated" Erythrocytes

The first description of reticulocytes was made in 1865 by Wilhelm Heinrich Erb (1840–1921), a German neurologist who was a leading physician and eminent figure of his time. Thanks to his scientific interest in toxicology and histology early on in his career, he observed the effects of acetic and picric acid on the development of erythrocytes, thus discovering a population of "granulated" erythrocytes.[1] The "granular" cells were described as larger than normal erythrocytes. He studied granulated erythrocytes of calves, cats, normal adult animals, and human fetuses. He described observations on granulated erythrocytes after hemorrhage and in patients with

The authors have nothing to disclose.

[a] Department of Laboratory Medicine, University-Hospital of Padova, Via Nicolò Giustiniani 2, 35128 Padova, Italy; [b] Department of Laboratory Medicine, Boston Children's Hospital, Harvard Medical School, 300 Longwood Avenue, BA 760, Boston, MA 02115, USA
* Corresponding author.
E-mail address: elisa.piva@sanita.padova.it

Clin Lab Med 35 (2015) 133–163
http://dx.doi.org/10.1016/j.cll.2014.10.004
0272-2712/15/$ – see front matter © 2015 Elsevier Inc. All rights reserved.

Abbreviations	
ACD	Anemia of chronic disease
ANC	Absolute neutrophil count
BCB	Brilliant cresyl blue
CBC	Complete blood count
CD71	Transferrin receptor
CERA	Continuous erythropoietin receptor activator
CHCMr	Reticulocyte hemoglobin concentration
CHCr	Mean cellular hemoglobin concentration of reticulocytes
CHr	Reticulocyte hemoglobin content
CKD	Chronic kidney disease
CV	Coefficient of variation
CVg	Between-subject biological variation
CVw	Within-subject biological variation
EQA	External quality assessment
ESA	Erythropoiesis-stimulating agent
FDA	Food and Drug Administration
FID	Functional iron deficiency
FS	Forward scatter
GdSE	Hematology Study Group of Italian Society Of Laboratory Medicine
Hb	Hemoglobin
HFR	High-fluorescence reticulocyte
HS	Hereditary spherocytosis
HSCT	Hematopoietic stem cell transplantation
Hypo-He	Hypochromic erythrocytes
ID	Iron deficiency
IPF	Immature platelet fraction (reticulated platelets)
IRF	Immature reticulocyte fraction
IRF-D	IRF doubling time
LFR	Low-fluorescence reticulocyte
MCHr	Mean cellular Hb content of reticulocytes
MCVr	Reticulocyte mean cellular volume
MFR	Medium-fluorescence reticulocyte
MRV	Mean reticulocyte volume
MVC	Volume of mature red cells
NCCLS-ICSH	Clinical and Laboratory Standards Institute and International Council for Standardization in Hematology
NMB	New methylene blue
Ret-He	Reticulocyte hemoglobin equivalent
RET-Y	Reticulocyte hemoglobin parameter
RHCc	Reticulocyte hemoglobin cellular content
RHE	Reticulocyte hemoglobin expression
RPI	Reticulocyte production index
RSf	Red blood cell size factor
SIMeL	Italian Society Of Laboratory Medicine
sTfR	Soluble transferrin receptor

certain chronic diseases, especially after iron therapy. Erb, however, erroneously regarded these cells as transitional forms between white and red corpuscles.

The Late 1800s: Discussions About the Meaning of the Granular Basophilic Filamentous Substance

An eminent investigator in this field was the German researcher and Nobel Prize winner Paul Ehrlich (1854–1915). Ehrlich was a visionary in hematology. He was the first to discover polymorphonuclear leukocytes, making it possible to classify them as eosinophils, basophils, and neutrophils. He also described the properties of the granular basophilic filamentous substance of reticulocytes, which led to his growing interest in the microchemical study of blood cells by means of a basic dye procedures; he used methylene blue as a staining technique for the erythrocytes in films made from the blood of patients with pernicious anemia. Ehrlich described the stained material as fine, dense, and elegant networks. He considered the baso-philic substance as a feature of senescent erythrocytes rather than of young ones.[2] Ehrlich's observations were soon confirmed by many other investigations carried out in Germany, Italy, France, and North America. The reticular substance was first regarded as a degenerative material, a "coagulation necrosis" or a substance pro-duced by the action of certain deleterious agents on corpuscles.

The Early 1900s: Reticulocytes Are Young Red Cells

It was Theobald Smith (1859–1934) who contradicted Erlich's postulate and brilliantly asserted that reticulocytes represented young red cells. Smith was an American bacteriologist who, studying blood diseases in animals, particularly the mechanism by which parasites are transmitted, observed variations in the number of these cells in relation to pathologic conditions such as anemia. The foregoing studies regarding the granular erythrocyte led to some confusion in nomenclature.[3]

Whereas the German, Italian, and French investigators designated these cells as erythrocytes with "substantia granulo-filamentosa," the Americans used such terms as "reticulated red cell" or "vital-staining erythrocyte." In 1922, Edward Bell Krumb-haar (1883–1966), the eminent leader of several American medical societies, first coined the term "reticulocyte" when he stated that: "Erythrocytes revealing a more or less extensive reticulum (granular filamentous substance) by the methods of vital staining may be conveniently designated 'reticulocytes'."[4] In another article, he stated: "Variations in the reticulocyte percentage in disease naturally depend on the intensity of the demand and the capacity of the bone marrow to respond," postulating principles that seem to clarify the clinical meaning of reticulocytes in various diseases. Until this time, research on reticulocytes had focused mainly on their morphology, the technical methods of staining, and the properties of granular substance. The evidence of different quantities of granular filamentous substance signified a hallmark of reticu-locyte maturation and the presence of various subpopulations among circulating reticulocytes.

The Mid 1900s: Studies on Biochemical Characteristics and Reticulocyte Maturation

A large body of literature concerning reticulocytes accumulated in this time.[5] Lud-wig Heilmeyer (1899–1969), a German internist, proposed the still well-known clas-sification of reticulocytes maturity in 1932 (**Fig. 1**).[6] Clark Wright Heath (1900–1986), a researcher at Harvard University in the 1940s, focused his research on the life of reticulocytes and the duration of their presence in the body's circulatory system. In 1944, Pierre Dustin (1914–1993), a Belgian pathologist, showed that granular "retic-ulated" substance is RNA.[7] A few years later, in 1947, Giovanni Astaldi (1914–2002), an Italian hematologist, classified reticulocytes into 3 stages of maturity, as in the current maturation classification used in flow cytometry. Since the 1950s many investigators have focused their research on erythropoiesis and reticulocytes.[8] In 1918 Irving M. London, Professor of Medicine Emeritus at Harvard and MIT, in collaboration with David Shemin and David Rittenberg, demonstrated that reticulo-cytes synthesize hemoglobin (Hb) and absorb iron.[9] Over the years acridine orange, a fluorescent dye, replaced the supravital stain, improving the sensitivity of

Reticulocyte maturation stages according to Heilmeyer classification

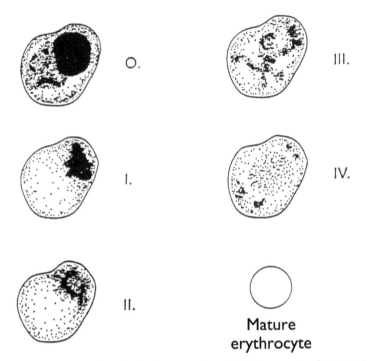

Fig. 1. Maturation stages of reticulocytes according to Heilmeyer classification: Group 0: nucleated erythrocyte (orthochromatic normoblast), stained strongly for reticulin and the nucleus. This cell type is not included in the reticulocyte count. Group I: non-nucleated red cells, appearing with a dense clumped reticulum; they comprise 0.1% of the population of reticulocytes in normal individuals. Group II: extended network of loose reticulum; they comprise 0.7% of the reticulocyte population in normal individuals. Group III: scattered granules with residual reticulum network; they comprise 32% of the reticulocyte population in normal individuals. Group IV: scattered granules; they comprise 61% of the reticulocytes in normal individuals. (*Adapted from* Pradella M, Rizzotti P. La Medicina di Laboratorio, volume IX n 2: I reticolociti. Padova, Italy: Piccin Nuova Libraria SpA; 2000. p. 30; with permission.)

microscopic counts.[10] Today, understanding the maturation process in reticulocytes and the mechanisms for erythroid development at the molecular level represent a fascinating field for research.

DEFINITION OF RETICULOCYTES
Origin of the Term and Definition

The reticulocyte derives its name from the reticulum of RNA and protein precipitated by the fixation and staining that appears microscopically after treatment with supravital dyes.[11,12] The reticulum network or granules represent precipitated rough endoplasmic reticulum with associated polyribosomes. Based on the morphologic characteristics, the original definition of human reticulocytes was that of mature red cells that form a reticulum network or granules on exposure to supravital stains, such as new methylene blue (NMB) or brilliant cresyl blue (BCB).[6,13] Based on the physiologic characteristics, Bessis[14] proposed the term "proerythrocyte." In 1976 Gilmer and Koepke defined the basic criteria for morphologic identification of reticulocytes.[15] Although this definition has been revised several times, in 1997 it was chosen to be the universal standard by the Clinical and Laboratory Standards Institute and the International Council for Standardization in Hematology (NCCLS-ICSH).[16]

Morphology

With a Romanowsky-type stain, such as May-Grünwald Giemsa or Wright stain, the RNA disappears during alcohol fixation and reticulocytes appear slightly larger than mature erythrocytes, with a uniform blue-gray color (polychromasia). On exposure to NMB, a heterocyclic aromatic chemical compound, or BCB, a basic dye of the oxazin class, the RNA precipitates and becomes visible, showing the characteristic scattered granules under the microscope.

Morphologic Standardization of Reticulocytes

The NCCLS-ICSH definition states that reticulocytes must have at least 2 blue-staining granules, visible without fine microscope adjustment and located away from the cell margin to avoid confusion with Heinz bodies.[16] The benefit of this official definition is the standardization of the reticulocyte morphology, but it does not take into account the wide use of fluorescent dyes presently used in measuring reticulocyte mRNA.

Properties

Reticulocytes, in comparison with mature erythrocytes, show:[17]

- Greater volume: approximately +24%
- Slightly higher Hb content: approximately +3%
- Lower Hb concentration: approximately −16.7%
- Constant volume ratio between reticulocytes and erythrocytes: approximately 1.24

RETICULOCYTE MATURATION

When the late-stage erythroblast loses its nucleus, the cell becomes a reticulocyte that usually remains in the bone marrow for 3 days and is subsequently released into the circulation, where its maturation is completed in 1 day.[18,19] Maturation is a continuum, presenting morphologic, biochemical, and functional changes that lead to membrane remodeling, volume changes, and elimination of internal or membrane-bound organelles and ribosomes.[20] In **Fig. 2**, a scanning electron micrograph of reticulocytes shows the irregular forms that these cell membranes can assume. Lobular-shaped reticulocytes are larger and less dense and deformable, with more adhesiveness in comparison with mature erythrocytes.[21,22] Immature, early reticulocytes are biochemically more active than mature ones, and some activities such as hexokinase, pyruvate kinase, glucose-6-phosphate dehydrogenase, and oxygen transport, are increased.[23] In the bone marrow, cellular functions such as Hb production and absorption of iron are maintained.[24] The membrane receptors for transferrin (CD71) decrease from the youngest to less mature reticulocytes, as evaluated by flow cytometry with CD71 intensity expression. Nucleic acid stains, such as the DRAQ5 fluorochrome, also decrease during reticulocyte maturation, reflecting the loss of RNA.[25]

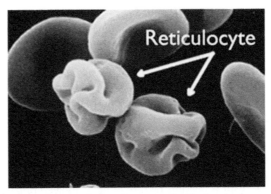

Fig. 2. Scanning electron micrograph showing normal reticulocyte shapes; the lobular membrane of the reticulocyte is shown by the arrows. (*Courtesy of* Professor Amos Cohen, Tel-Aviv University Sackler School of Medicine, Tel-Aviv, Israel.)

Because Hb synthesis occurs only in the younger reticulocytes found in the bone marrow, circulating reticulocytes are unable to synthesize Hb and cannot further increase their Hb content, which is usually greater than that of erythrocytes, whereas the Hb concentration is lower.[17,18,26]

Maturation of reticulocytes is a complex mechanism that involves enucleation, caused by chromatin condensation, vesicular trafficking, and selective autophagy.[27] The maturation is complete when the basophilic filamentous substance that characterizes the reticulocyte disappears.[28] Subcellular structures such as the mitochondria, ribosomes, and endosomal vesicles are eliminated by physiologic events such as macroautophagy and mitoptosis, a mitochondrial death program.[29,30]

Plasma membrane remodeling is achieved through an exosomal pathway. Early reticulocyte maturation is characterized by the selective elimination of unwanted plasma membrane proteins (CD71, CD98, and β1 integrin) through the endosome-exosome pathway. By contrast, late maturation is characterized by the generation of large glycophorin A–decorated vesicles of autophagic origin.[31,32]

Recent advances in the study of reticulocyte maturation suggest that the small amount of RNA that remains in reticulocytes might still be essential for reticulocyte maturation to form normal biconcave erythrocytes.[33] The transition from the discoid shape of reticulocytes to biconcave erythrocyte is a key step in the maturation process. During the maturational remodeling of the membrane cytoskeleton, by vesiculation and endocytosis, reticulocytes lose about 24% of their volume and surface area, and increase their stability and deformability.[34] Recently the dynamic process of reticulocyte maturation has been studied in cord blood, assessing the phenotypic changes in reticulocytes that correlate with the morphologic, biochemical, and functional development of human reticulocytes. The study highlights the change from a "wrinkled globular" shape in the youngest $CD71_{high}$ and $CD71_{medium}$ to the proto-biconcave and biconcave shapes found in the CD71-negative reticulocytes.[35] Several investigators have asserted that, as biconcave-like geometries confer a greater deformability, the loss of the globular shape first detected in the $CD71_{low}$ reticulocytes contributes to their decreased stiffness. These results are in agreement with previous findings of Chasis and Schrier,[22] who demonstrated the increases of deformability and mechanical stability in later stages of reticulocyte development, speculating on the fact that biomechanical changes are due to membrane skeleton remodeling, especially the assembly of spectrin and the 4.1R complex.

The maturation process is thus associated with the briefly described molecular changes, but attempts have also been made to classify the maturity of reticulocytes at a morphologic level, based on the quantity of the reticulum and distribution of "granular filamentous substance" in their cytoplasm.[36]

The first attempt was made by Heilmeyer and Westharer,[37] who divided the cells into 4 groups (the fourth being the most mature), designated by Roman numerals and characterized by a progressive reduction in the compactness of the reticulum. Therefore, reticulocyte maturation according to the Heilmeyer classification assesses the relative proportion of mRNA (see **Fig. 1**).

According to Lowenstein,[38] in steady-state erythropoiesis the circulating reticulocytes are more than 60% in Group IV, 30% in Group III, and less than 1% in Groups I or II.

Stress Erythropoiesis

When erythropoiesis is acutely increased above baseline (stress erythropoiesis), the immature, larger, more stained form of reticulocytes (stress reticulocytes) are released into the peripheral blood where they appear as polychromatophilic elements among erythrocytes. All polychromatophils are reticulocytes; however, not all reticulocytes are polychromatophils on a Wright-stained blood smear. Under stress, reticulocyte production can be increased 15- to 20-fold above the steady-state values of 2×10^6 reticulocytes per second, accomplished by increased production and shortening of marrow maturation time, with the reticulocyte final maturation occurring in the circulation, thus increasing reticulocyte circulation time.[39,40] Stress reticulocytosis is seen in bone marrow regeneration following autoimmune hemolysis, chemotherapy-induced anemia, administration of therapy in nutritional anemia, and use of erythropoiesis-stimulating agents (ESAs).[26,41,42]

BIOLOGICAL AND PREANALYTICAL VARIATION OF RETICULOCYTE MEASUREMENTS

Biological and preanalytical variations can potentially affect test performance and clinical interpretation of laboratory results.[43,44] In 1998 Sandberg and colleagues[45] assessed the within-subject (CVw) and between-subject (CVg) reticulocyte biological variation in 13 healthy subjects for 7 weeks, using 2 different instruments (Sysmex R-1000 and Bayer H*3). The value of CVw was 11% on both instruments, whereas the CVg value was different for the 2 instruments (33% for the Sysmex R-1000% and 26% for Bayer H*3). For both methods, the 3 fractions of maturation, low-fluorescence (LFR), middle-fluorescence (MFR), and high-fluorescence (HFR), presented biological variation similar to those of the reticulocyte count, whereas the variability of reticulocyte Hb content (CHr), reticulocyte mean cellular volume (MCVr), and reticulocyte Hb concentration (CHCMr) was smaller, comparable with those of the corresponding erythrocyte parameters and in agreement with normal erythropoiesis. The index of individuality obtained for both methods was less than 0.5 for the reticulocyte parameters, whereas for MCVr it was 0.6. According to Costongs and colleagues,[46] this biological variation is similar to that of leukocytes, with the within-subject variation being inversely related to cellular life span. Biological variability of reticulocytes was also assessed over a period of 7 consecutive days in 20 healthy subjects. CVw and CVg were 5.8% and 32.4%, respectively, as the average of results from 5 different instruments.[47] Within-day variation in reticulocyte percentage was also described, although these data were not confirmed by other studies.[48,49] Several reports have described gender-related and age-related differences in reticulocyte counting.[50–53] In their experience the authors have not seen significant gender differences in reticulocyte counts (data not shown). Menarche and menopause do not cause variations in reticulocyte counts.[54] During pregnancy, reticulocytes decrease slightly from the 24th to 28th week and then increase again.[55]

Preanalytical variation represents the major source of inaccurate laboratory results. Variations caused by the application of tourniquets during the blood collection process did not generate any meaningful differences in the reticulocyte count.[56] Reticulocyte counts are significantly decreased after 24 hours of storage at room temperature because of in vitro maturation of the reticulocytes. At constant temperatures of 4°C the counts remain unchanged, with certain limitations for parameters derived or calculated from cellular volumes. In a study of sample stability, a small but statistically insignificant drop in CHr values over 24 hours was demonstrated.[57–59] Storage-induced variation of reticulocyte parameters is greater with Siemens ADVIA systems than with Sysmex analyzers.[60]

In a study by Kouri and colleagues,[61] several preanalytical uncertainty components were estimated, combined with data on analytical variation and biological variation taken from the literature. Measurement uncertainties obtained for reticulocytes (41%) were larger than those obtained for platelet and leukocyte counts (24% and 31%, respectively). Uncertainty for reticulocytes was greater in preanalytical, sample-related components, particularly because of transportation and storage. The sample-related uncertainty was 13% while the analytical component of measurement uncertainty was 12%. The high sample-related uncertainty, which exceeded that of the analytical component, requires that reticulocytes be analyzed without delay.

MICROSCOPIC RETICULOCYTE COUNTING

Until the 1990s, the standard method of counting reticulocytes was based on the visual detection of granules and RNA ribosomal networks, stained by supravital dyes. There are several sources of imprecision in the manual counting of reticulocytes, including different procedures, staining variation, distributional variability for quality of blood film, intraobserver and interobserver variations, and inadequate number of cells counted. The NMB method and procedure described in the NCCLS-ICSH H44-A2 guidelines still remains the recommended method for agreement/correlation assessments when evaluating the performances of automated techniques. Standardized NMB staining procedures have been suggested to improve the accuracy and reliability of reticulocyte manual counting.[62]

AUTOMATED RETICULOCYTE ANALYSIS

Automated reticulocyte counts are widely used in the clinical laboratory, owing to the greater precision, accuracy, and reproducibility than those obtained using microscopy. In 1988 the TOA Medical Electronics Co. Ltd, later known as Sysmex, introduced the Sysmex R-1000, the first automated and dedicated reticulocyte analyzer. The reticulocyte RNA content was detected by fluorochrome Auramina O, while the cell size was determined by forward light scattering using an argon ion laser as the light source.[63] In the mid 1990s, Sysmex fully integrated reticulocyte counting into the automated complete blood count (CBC) in high-throughput hematology analyzers. The Abbott CELL-DYN 4000 was the first hematology analyzer launched with fully automated reticulocyte measurement performed during routine cell blood count and differential.[64] The most important benefit of automated methods is the greater precision of the counts. By analyzing a much greater number of reticulocytes (more than 10,000), the statistical error is minimized. Visual microscopy is still recommended as the comparability method for reticulocytes, despite studies showing that the coefficient of variation (CV) ranges from 20% to 40%. When the reticulocyte percentages are between 0.6% and 2.7%, many studies have yielded a CV of less than 10% for automated counting, with a higher CV for counts lower than 0.2%.[65] Fully automated methods have eliminated interobserver variability and subjectivity and have substantially reduced turnaround time. Variability resulting from staining, dilution, and incubation are also strictly controlled in automatic analyzers, but problems still exist. Automated methods use a wide variety of reagents for reticulocyte RNA, and these show different sensitivity on the binding to RNA and other cellular components. The most commonly used automated reticulocyte analyzers and the parameters they provide are listed in **Table 1**. Initial comparative evaluations showed significant differences between methods, which were, however, considered equivalent for daily routine reticulocyte enumeration.[66] Methods using the fluorescent dye thiazole orange provide different reticulocyte counts than those using the supravital dye methylene blue.[67] Buttarello and colleagues[68] evaluated the performance of 5 automated reticulocyte analyzers and compared results with the microscopic reference method. Agreement was satisfactory for all automated methods considered, even though there was a tendency to overestimate low reticulocyte counts. Another parallel evaluation of 5 fully automated analyzers, according to the NCCLS-ICSH H44-A document, was carried out by the Hematology Study Group (GdSE) of the Italian Society of Laboratory Medicine (SIMeL). The comparison of reticulocyte enumeration for ADVIA 120 (Siemens Healthcare Diagnostics, Deerfield, IL, USA), CELL-DYN 4000 (Abbott Diagnostics, Santa Clara, CA, USA), LH 750 (Beckman Coulter, Brea, CA, USA), Pentra 120 (Horiba Medical, Montpellier, France), and XE 2100 (Sysmex Corp, Kobe, Japan) confirmed a close correlation with the microscopic method (r^2 from 0.89 to 0.96).[69,70]

Reference reticulocyte values obtained using fluorescence are reported to be higher than those obtained using automated methods with supravital dyes.[71] Method-specific reference intervals are not interchangeable and thus do not allow for easy monitoring of patients across different laboratories. The distribution in the general population of reticulocyte counts, reported as either a percentage or as a number per volume of blood (10^9/L), is skewed; thus, the reference range should be calculated as the central 95% of results.[72] The comparison of reference ranges in adults reported by different investigators is shown in **Table 2**.[17,73–79]

The main sources of inaccurately high reticulocyte counts are cellular interferences (such as a high number of lymphocytes, cellular fragments, giant platelets, platelet/red cell coincidence, orthochromatic erythroblasts present, platelet clumps), erythrocyte inclusions (such as Howell-Jolly bodies, Heinz bodies, Pappenheimer bodies, parasites such as malaria and babesia, basophilic stippling bodies, Hb H inclusion bodies), autofluorescence due to drugs, as anthracyclines, or porphyria, presence of paraproteins, cold agglutinins, and hemolysis.[80]

RETICULOCYTE MATURITY AND INDICES

Automated reticulocyte counts not only provide enhanced precision and accuracy but also perform reliable measurements of mRNA content and cellular indices such as volume, Hb concentration, and content. These novel parameters have prompted interest and studies regarding their clinical usefulness, the utility of reporting such counts, and their interpretation.

Immature Reticulocyte Fraction

Assessment of reticulocyte maturity is based on the intensity of either fluorescence or light scattering/absorbance, which depends on RNA content. Different populations

Table 1
State of art of the reticulocyte parameters provided for most hematology analyzers. Principles of methodology and techniques

Corporation and Instrument	Method and Dye	Parameters Provided by Reticulocyte Measurements	Notes
Abbott Diagnostics			
CELL-DYN **SAPPHIRE**	Fluorescence detection Multiangle laser light-scattering detection	IRF (immature reticulocyte fraction) MCVr (mean cellular volume of reticulocytes), MCHr (mean cellular Hb content of reticulocytes), CHCr (cell hemoglobin concentration of reticulocytes)	Fully automated
	Dye: Cyanine dye (Sybr II)		
Beckman Coulter Inc			
UNICEL **DxH 800**	Flow cytometric digital analysis using different angles of light-scattering detection, impedance, radiofrequency	IRF, MRV[a] (mean reticulocyte volume), HLR[b] (high light scatter reticulocytes), RDWR-CV[b] (reticulocyte distribution width, coefficient of variation), RDWR-SD[b] (reticulocyte distribution width, standard deviation), RSF[b] (red cell size factor, square root of MCV×MVR)	Fully automated
COULTER LH **700 SERIES**	Light scattering, impedance, and conductivity (VCS technology)	IRF, MRV[a], HLR, RDWR-CV, RDWR-SD, RSF	Fully automated
COULTER **LH 500**	Light scattering, impedance, and conductivity (VCS technology)	IRF, MRV[a]	Fully automated
COULTER **HmX**	Light scattering, impedance, and conductivity (VCS technology)	IRF, MRV[a]	Manual operation required
	Dye: New methylene blue		
Horiba Medical			
PENTRA **NEXUS DX** **ABX PENTRA** **XLR**	DHSS technology: focused flow cytometry and sequential measurements of impedance, absorbance, and fluorescence	IRF, MRV[a], CRC% (corrected reticulocyte count) RETH% (high-fluorescence reticulocytes) RETM% (medium-fluorescence reticulocytes), RETL% (low-fluorescence reticulocytes), IMR% (immature reticulocytes), MFI% (mean fluorescence index) RHCc[a] (reticulocyte hemoglobin cellular content)	Fully automated

(continued on next page)

Table 1
State of art of the reticulocyte parameters provided for most hematology analyzers. Principles of methodology and techniques (*continued*)

Corporation and Instrument	Method and Dye	Parameters Provided by Reticulocyte Measurements	Notes
ABX PENTRA DX 120	Fluorescence detection	IRF, MRV RETH%[b], RETM%[b], RETL%[b], IMR%[b], MFI%[b], CRC%[b]	Fully automated
	Dye: Thiazole orange		
Mindray			
BC 6800	Fluorescence and light scattering (with sphering cells)	IRF, H-RET% (high-adsorbance reticulocytes) M-RET% (medium-adsorbance reticulocytes), L-RET% (low-adsorbance reticulocytes), MVR[b] (mean volume of reticulocytes), RHE[b] (reticulocyte hemoglobin content)	Fully automated
	Dye: Asymmetric cyanine		
Siemens Health Care Diagnostics			
ADVIA 2120	Absorbance and optical light scatter detection	MCVr[a], CHr, CHCMr[a], RDWr, HDWr, CHDWr, H-RET%, M-RET%, L-RET%, IRF[b]	Fully automated
ADVIA 120	Absorbance and optical light scatter detection	MCVr[a], CHr, CHCMr[a], RDWr, HDWr, CHDWr, H-RET%, M-RET%, L-RET%, in development IRF	Fully automated The production was discontinued
	Dye: Oxazine 750		
Sysmex			
XN -SERIES	Fluorescence and light scattering	IRF, Ret-He[a] (reticulocyte hemoglobin equivalent) DELTA-He (delta hemoglobin equivalent) RPI (reticulocyte production index)	Fully automated
XE 5000 XT 4000i	Fluorescence and light scattering	IRF, Ret-He[a], RPI	Fully automated
XT 2000i XE 2100	Fluorescence and light scattering	IRF, Ret-He[a], RPI	Fully automated The production was discontinued for XE 2100
	Dye: Polymethine		

[a] Direct measurement.
[b] Research-use-only parameter.

are discriminated by a software-based algorithm that usually clusters reticulocytes into 3 areas according to stain intensity. High-fluorescence light scatter/absorbance reticulocytes correspond to young or immature reticulocytes, whereas maturing reticulocytes have medium-fluorescence light scatter/absorbance, and older reticulocytes have low-fluorescence light scatter/absorbance. These 3 classes are called HFR, MFR, and HFR, respectively, but their acronyms vary among analyzers, as reported in **Table 1**.

Table 2
Reference ranges for absolute reticulocyte count and reticulocyte parameters in adults, as reported by different investigators

Authors,[Ref.] Year	Reticulocytes and Parameters	Company/Instrument				
		CELL-DYN 4000	GEN*S	PENTRA 120	H*3	SE 9500
d'Onofrio et al,[17] 1995 (N = 64)	MCVr (fL) CHr (pg)				103.2–126.3 25.9–30.6	
Van den Bossche et al,[73] 2002 (F: N = 175; M: N = 142)	Reticulocytes (10⁹/L) IRF	F 21–98 M 30–110 0.14–0.35	F 24–73 M 30–90	F 22–95 M 31–130	F 19–64 M 2–69	F 16–66 M 16–70
			LH 750		ADVIA 120	XE 2100
GdS-Simel-Emat, 2003 (N = 127)[a]	Reticulocytes (10⁹/L) IRF MCVr (fL) CHr (pg)	29–146 0.16–0.42	18–117 0.19–0.43 91–111	30–148 0.07–0.19 98–120	30–111 0.04–0.23 100–114 28.0–35.1	18–104 0.01–0.13
Noronha and Grotto,[74] 2005 (N = 50)	Reticulocytes (10⁹/L) IRF					20.5–122.8 0.01–0.18
Bovy et al,[75] 2005 (N = 57)	Reticulocytes (10⁹/L) MCVr (fL) CHr (pg)				38.3–65.1 103.3–109.9 32.2–32.8	
Canals et al,[119] 2005 (N = 196)	Ret-He (pg)					30.2–36.7
Banfi et al,[76] 2006 (N = 73)	MRV (fL) IRF		93–117.8 0.19–0.42			
Garzia et al,[121] 2007 (N = 55)	CHr (pg) Ret-He (pg)				29.2–33.6	30.5–35.5
Piva et al,[70] 2007 (N = 126); data not published[a]	Reticulocytes (10⁹/L) MCVr (fL) CHr (pg) Ret-He (pg)				22–85 98–115 30.2–35.9	27–90 30.7–37.0
		CELL-DYN Sapphire				
Hoffmann et al,[77] 2012 (N = 182)	Reticulocytes (10⁹/L) MCVr (fL) MCHr (pg) MCHCr (g/dL) MCHCr (mmol/L)	24–106 92–116 26.0–35.1 27.3–32.5 16.9–20.1				
Costa et al,[78] 2012 (N = 151)	MCVr (fL) MCHr (pg) MCHCr (mmol/L)	86.2–102.4 26.2–31.9 17.4–19.8				
						XE 5000
Nunes et al,[79] 2014 (N = 120)	Reticulocytes (10⁹/L) IRF Ret-He (pg)					28–68 0.03–0.14 32.2–39.2

Abbreviations: F, female; M, male; MCHCr, mean cellular Hb concentration of reticulocytes. For other abbreviations in column 2, see Table 1 column 3.

  [a] Healthy adults for reference population were selected according to H44A2 criteria. Reference ranges (95% interval, nonparametric method) are calculated from the selected reference population in a parallel evaluation of the listed instruments. GdS-Simel-Emat is the Hematology Study Group of Italian Society of Laboratory Medicine.

  Data from Refs.[17,70,73–79,119,121]

Originally called the reticulocyte maturity index, the immature reticulocyte fraction (IRF) is the internationally accepted term to quantify the younger fraction of reticulocytes.[81–83] Because automated methods use different dyes with varying sensitivities to reticulocyte RNA stain, in an attempt to harmonize the results obtained by the different automated methods, it has been proposed that instruments that identify 3 populations of differing maturity should define the IRF as the sum of the populations of high and medium stain intensity (ie, the immature reticulocytes). The expression should be as a fraction (0.00–1.00). The consensus meeting, organized by the International Society of Laboratory Hematology, assessed the clinical usefulness of the IRF parameter, and its effectiveness when IRF is evaluated in correlation with the absolute reticulocyte count. The workshop recommended that manufacturers indicate information such as imprecision and the expected reference range of each maturity class in addition to potential interferences with IRF measurements. The manufacturers should also provide adequate quality control material and intermethod comparison over the complete IRF reference range.[84] These recommendations and goals have not been fulfilled.[85] Few studies have compared the performance of automated methods in estimating the immature reticulocyte fraction. Results highlight substantial differences in the reference intervals that should be strictly method dependent.[86] Even though standardization and diagnostic efficiency still require substantial improvement, a level of intermethod agreement seems to have been achieved for some instruments.[87,88] In a recent study, the values of IRF determined in elite athletes with 2 different technologies have shown good correlation.[89] The IRF is included in many existing reticulocyte external quality assessment (EQA) schemes; however, fixed blood represents a more stable material than fresh blood, and may mask imprecision among instruments when measuring reticulocyte IRF.[70,90] Reporting of IRF for clinical use has been approved by the Food and Drug Administration (FDA) on some analyzers.

Clinical Utility of the Immature Reticulocyte Fraction

The IRF has been proposed as an early marker of engraftment in bone marrow or hematopoietic stem cell transplantation and bone marrow regeneration following chemotherapy.[82] Several studies have demonstrated that increases in IRF are an indicator of engraftment that precedes other parameters, such as absolute neutrophil counts (ANC), reticulated platelets (immature platelet fraction [IPF]), or reticulocyte counts.[91–94] In patients undergoing autologous stem cell transplantation (HSCT) for a variety of underlying diseases and with different conditioning regimens, IRF doubling time (IRF-D), defined as the first of 2 consecutive days during which the IRF value doubles from nadir, can predict myeloid engraftment several days before ANC exceeds 0.100×10^9/L.[95–97] In a large group of patients undergoing allogeneic HSCT from related or nonrelated donors, IRF greater than 10% occurred 1 to 4 days sooner than an ANC greater than 0.100×10^9/L in most instances.[98] Therefore, most investigators consider an IRF value greater than 10% to indicate early marrow recovery.

In successfully autologous and allogeneic HSCT, monitoring of the IRF in the posttransplant period shows that this parameter increases before ANC counts do, and remains at higher levels than in IPF.[99,100] IPF exhibited variations caused by platelet transfusion, and concomitant complication such as sepsis.[101] IRF may be not only the first sign of hematologic recovery but also a very strong indicator of postchemotherapy aplasia in children with cancer, serving as an additional parameter of impaired bone marrow function.[102]

IRF has been proposed as an early marker of CD34$^+$ mobilization for peripheral stem cell harvesting to optimize the timing for stem cell collection following growth factor mobilization or cytotoxic drug therapy.[103]

IRF increases in response to treatment with ESAs before there is an increase of reticulocyte number in renal failure, AIDS, and myelodysplastic syndromes. Thus, changes in IRF during ESA therapy indicate erythropoietic stimulation.[104]

Many investigators have reported data concerning the clinical utility of IRF in the diagnosis and monitoring of anemias.[105,106] A study by Mullier and colleagues[107] showed that IRF, in combination with reticulocyte count, may be useful in hereditary spherocytosis (HS) diagnosis, as HS is characterized by a high reticulocyte count without an equally elevated IRF. A reticulocytes/IRF ratio higher than 7.7 is used as a precondition for the screening of all HS cases using a diagnostic algorithm that includes microcytic erythrocytes and hypochromic erythrocytes (Hypo-He) measured by the Sysmex XE 5000 analyzer. Persjin and colleagues[108] subsequently optimized the HS algorithm and applied it as a screening tool.

IRF in conjunction with the reticulocyte number provides essentially the same information as the reticulocyte production index (RPI), making its manual calculation unnecessary. To clarify the concept, the RPI was proposed to correct the reticulocyte percentage for peripheral blood maturation time based on the hematocrit value. The correction was an empirical method to evaluate the "correct" reticulocyte percentage when intense erythroid stimulation, or shift in circulating reticulocyte maturity (due to a premature release from the marrow) occur. The result of early release is an increase in reticulocyte count, without any increase in erythropoietic activity. These reticulocytes spend more time in the circulation before maturation occurs. Early release shortens the fraction of time that reticulocytes mature in the marrow and proportionally prolongs their maturation time in circulation. The RPI was proposed for evaluating erythropoiesis and classifying anemias. An RPI greater than 3 was associated with hemolytic anemia (ie, HS), recent hemorrhage, and response to therapy. A RPI of less than 2 was associated with hypoproliferative disorders (ie, aplastic anemia) and ineffective erythropoiesis, as seen in megaloblastic anemias.

Because the IRF increases earlier than the reticulocyte number, it is useful in monitoring the efficacy of therapy in nutritional anemias such as megaloblastic or iron deficiency (ID) anemias.

As a feature of ineffective erythropoiesis, IRF is increased while reticulocyte count is reduced or normal, as demonstrated in some cases of myelodysplastic syndrome or in dyserythropoietic anemia.[65]

The clinical utility of IRF has been reported in a variety of conditions, such as: the monitoring of anemia treatment and neonatal transfusion needs; the prognosis in prematurity and in AIDS anemias; renal transplant engraftment from erythropoietin production; the detection of occult or compensated hemorrhages or hemolysis, and aplastic crisis in hemolytic anemias; and the diagnosis and monitoring of aplastic anemias.[62] The IRF is a promising parameter that needs consolidation into clinical practice.

Reticulocyte Indices

Mean cell Hb, mean cell volume, and mean cell Hb concentration can now be determined in conjunction with the automated counting of reticulocytes by several hematologic analyzers.

Reticulocyte Mean Cell Hemoglobin Content

Reticulocyte mean cell Hb, a measurement of the Hb content of reticulocytes expressed in pg/cell, was first measured by Bayer H3 instruments and abbreviated as CHr.[109,110] CHr is the product of the cellular volume and the cellular Hb concentration. The volume and Hb concentration of individual reticulocytes are independently determined from measurement of light scatter at 2 different angles (high angle, 5°–15° and low angle, 2°–3°), after isovolumetric sphering of stained reticulocytes. The isovolumetric sphering has great importance in the application of the Mie theory. According to this theory, the light-scattering detection at high angle reflects the refractive index of the cells that, in reticulocytes and erythrocytes, can be related to Hb concentration, while light scattering detected at low angle is proportional to cell volume.[111] A similar methodology is used in the ADVIA 120 and ADVIA 2120 analyzers (Siemens Healthcare Diagnostics). Reticulocyte mean cell Hb has become available in other fully automated hematology analyzers that provide reticulocyte count and maturity, as reported in **Table 1**. The methodology develop by Sysmex for the XE and later for the XN series of automated hematology analyzers provides the reticulocyte Hb equivalent or Ret-He parameter, formerly defined as reticulocyte hemoglobin parameter (RET-Y). This parameter is measured using a photodiode through the light-scattering signals detected at the forward scatter (FS). RET-Y has been assessed as the mean channel number of the FS light signal histogram within the reticulocyte population. However, the FS signal depends on many cell characteristics, such as size and volume if the cell is spherical, shape and orientation, refractive index or density, internal structure and cell complexity, and staining.[112–116]

The first study on RET-Y raw data showed a better comparison with CHr ($r = 0.94$) than with MCVr ($r = 0.88$) and, during intravenous iron therapy for ID anemia, a significant shift according to CHr change. For the RET-Y the study demonstrated a high degree of efficiency in differentiating moderate or severe ID anemia from the healthy state.[117]

Subsequently, the RET-Y behavior was examined in large groups of anemic patients, in which RET-Y was expressed as Ret-He. The RET-Y demonstrated an excellent curvilinear relationship with CHr, and the arbitrary units of RET-Y were mathematically transformed into pg/cell as the Ret-He. As a result, a natural log transformation of RET-Y (ie, Ret-He) has become an alternative measure of reticulocyte Hb content.[118] For clinical application within the United States, the CHr was approved by the FDA in August 1997 (K#971998), while the Ret-He was cleared in May 2005 (K#050589).

Many studies have found a good agreement of Ret-He with CHr in patients with both ID and chronic renal failure, and have shown similar clinical value for these 2 parameters.

Because the methodologies used to determine CHr and Ret-He are fundamentally different, it is not a surprise that some studies have shown poor correlation or lack of interchangeability between these two values.[119–124]

The mean cellular Hb content of reticulocytes (MCHr) and the mean cellular Hb concentration of reticulocytes (CHCr) have become available in the CELL-DYN Sapphire analyzer from Abbott. These indices are calculated from light-scattering signals by applying the Mie theory and using a 3-dimensional laser. The study performance has shown that the CELL-DYN Sapphire parameters measured generally correlated well with those of the ADVIA 120, but the MCHr has shown significant systematic differences.[77,125]

The reticulocyte hemoglobin expression (RHE) is available in the BC 6800 Mindray analyzer for research use only (Mindray BioMedical Electronics Co., Shenzhen, China), while reticulocyte Hb cellular RHCc is provided in the new generation of Pentra blood cell analytical systems (Horiba Medical). RHE and RHCc need to be evaluated and comparison studies performed to verify whether the new indices are comparable with those obtained by other instruments.

Beckman Coulter provides a new parameter, the red blood cell size factor (RSf), that seems to be in agreement with CHr. The RSf parameter, expressed as femtoliters, joins together the mean volume of mature red cells (MCV) and the mean volume of reticulocytes (MRV), according to the following mathematical formula: $RSf = \sqrt{(MCV \times MVR)}$.[126]

Clinical Utility of Reticulocyte Hemoglobin Content

Iron deficiency

ID is the most common nutritional deficiency worldwide.[127] For all ages, the consequences of ID are relevant; in children, intellectual disability and cognitive delays have been described. As iron has great importance for the maintenance of cellular metabolism in tissues such as the heart, liver, kidneys, muscles, and brain, ID is emerging as a comorbidity finding in many diseases such as chronic heart failure and chronic renal insufficiency.[128,129] Traditionally the diagnosis of ID is based on the determination of biochemical parameters, such as ferritin and transferrin saturation, but their usefulness is limited to uncomplicated ID, usually caused by poor nutrition or chronic occult blood loss. Many factors, including inflammation, infections, and malignancies, all of which may elevate the serum ferritin, complicate the interpretation of the classic laboratory biomarkers of iron status. New markers, such as the serum transferrin receptor or hepcidin, have some limitations as far as their usefulness in particular clinical settings is concerned, such as in renal patients receiving ESA therapy.[130–132]

Because the life span of the reticulocytes is 4 days, the measurement of reticulocyte Hb content can directly reflect the functional availability of iron in that time frame.[133–135] The clinical utility of the CHr in the diagnosis of ID was evaluated in 2002 by Mast and colleagues[136] in patients without anemia or iron therapy, and the reference standard for ID was based on the lack of stainable iron in the bone marrow aspirates. The diagnostic power was limited in patients presenting with macrocytosis or red cell diseases. However, the prediction of the absence of bone marrow iron stores was demonstrated by a CHr less than 28 pg, which showed a better negative predictive value for iron depletion than MCVr, serum ferritin less than 50 mg/L, or transferrin saturation less than 13%. Studies concerning ID in pediatric patients have demonstrated that the measurement of reticulocyte Hb content is helpful in identifying ID before the development of anemia.[137,138] In the ambulatory primary care setting, a CHr threshold of less than 27.5 pg seems to be a valuable screening tool for ID in healthy 9- to 12-month-old infants.[139] As CHr is reduced in microcytic anemia because of hemoglobinopathies such as α- and β-thalassemias without ID, an accurate clinical history should be obtained to rule out hemoglobinopathies. An algorithm that includes CHr has been proposed to discriminate subjects with thalassemic traits and early ID. The algorithm is based on Hb/CHr and the micro/hypo ratio, which is used to identify subjects with thalassemic traits.[140] In another algorithm, the addition of CHr to screen for ID seems to increase the diagnostic accuracy, enabling early detection and treatment of iron deficiency without the need for additional costly iron studies.[141]

In a recent Scandinavian study, CHr was confirmed as a useful tool for evaluating iron status in young infants, and also as a sensitive and specific marker for predicting later anemia. Accordingly, early reticulocyte Hb measurements may prevent cognitive impairment in children.[142] The clinical usefulness of CHr in diagnosing ID in pregnant women at term has been demonstrated by Ervasti and colleagues,[143] who suggested criteria for the practical use of CHr and the quantification of hypochromic erythrocytes.

Iron depletion is an important issue for the management of blood donors, and thus requires a rapid identification of donors at risk of or developing ID. A reticulocyte Hb content less than 28 pg seems to be an early and reliable tool for early detection of iron depletion and impaired hemoglobinization that may occur in frequent blood donors.[144,145] However, subsequent work determined that the sensitivity and specificity of CHr were not high enough to be used in blood donors at risk for ID.[146]

More recently, Karlsson[147] showed that the specificity of CHr was less than that of MCHr, ferritin, soluble transferrin receptor (sTfR), or the Ferritin index in screening elderly chronically anemic patients for ID anemia. The reference standard for diagnosis of ID anemia used in this study was the absence of bone marrow iron. However, this group consisted of both pure ID anemia and ID anemia complicated by anemia of chronic disease (ACD). A second study performed in 2013 by Joosten and colleagues[148] confirmed the previous one.

Functional iron deficiency and iron-sequestration syndromes

Functional ID (FID) occurs when iron stores are transiently unable to meet the demands of an increased erythropoiesis, such as that occurring during ESA treatment. Because responsiveness to ESAs is markedly affected by the baseline iron stores,[149] FID is one of the most important factors limiting ESA responsiveness, especially in patients with borderline to low iron stores. A decrease in reticulocyte Hb content, measured as CHr in an H*3 Bayer/Siemens blood analyzer, was observed by Brugnara and colleagues[150] in healthy volunteers after treatment with recombinant human erythropoietin, suggesting that this could be an early marker of FID.

Iron-sequestration syndromes occur in chronic diseases when iron is not available for erythropoiesis, because of inappropriately high serum hepcidin values, which determines iron sequestration in the reticuloendothelial system macrophages.[151–154] One of the major determinants of ACD is iron sequestration.

In patients with chronic kidney disease (CKD) and anemia who are undergoing ESA treatment, repletion of iron stores should be ensured before and during therapy. Iron levels must be adequate to optimize Hb production in a balance with erythropoiesis stimulation.[155] The Kidney Disease Outcomes Quality Initiative of the National Kidney Foundation has provided evidence-based clinical practice guidelines in which CHr is considered an appropriate test to assess adequacy of iron for erythropoiesis.[156] In the British guidelines for laboratory diagnosis of FID, CHr is one of the recommended tests, with a proposed cutoff CHr value of less than 29 pg.[157] Three studies, however, have suggested using a different cutoff value of 32 pg to identify FID, because some patients presenting with CHr greater than 29 pg have responded to intravenous iron therapy.[158–160] A study by Buttarello and colleagues[161] has proposed cutoff values of 31.2 pg for CHr and 30.6 pg for Ret-He in patients undergoing long-term hemodialysis. Low Ret-He or low CHr values are predictive of response to intravenous iron. A comparison of iron therapy management based on serum transferrin saturation and ferritin versus iron therapy based on CHr demonstrated a substantial reduction in the use of intravenous iron when CHr was used.[159] Responders to intravenous iron therapy have been better identified in another study using both the percentage of Hypo-He greater than 6% and CHr of 29 pg or less.[162] Ret-He can be used to monitor the efficacy of the treatment using continuous erythropoietin receptor activator (CERA) in dialysis-dependent (HD) patients with end-stage renal disease. In a randomized study in HD patients receiving CERA monthly, Ret-He decreased and reached its lowest value after 7 days, indicating iron requirements. In the setting of CERA-induced erythropoiesis, Ret-He is an indicator of accelerated iron utilization in comparison with hepcidin, ferritin, and transferrin saturation.[163] The Agency for Healthcare Research and Quality, as part of the management strategies for iron deficiency in stage 3 to 5 CKD patients (both nondialysis and dialysis) has recently generated a comprehensive review on the use of newer versus classic laboratory bio-markers of iron status.[164] Under this rigorous scrutiny, considerable variability in study methods was identified, resulting in substantial limitations of the available data, with high risk of bias, and low utility in informing clinical practice. Despite these limitations, the document states that in HD CKD patients, CHr and percentage of Hypo-He may have better predictive ability for a response to intravenous iron treatment than trans-ferrin saturation less than 20% or ferritin less than 100 ng/mL. Furthermore, the document highlights results from the randomized controlled trials cited earlier, which demonstrated that better iron management guided by CHr leads to a reduction in the number of iron status tests and intravenous iron treatments. The clinical applica-tion of these results suggest that CHr may reduce potential harm from intravenous iron treatment by lowering the frequency of iron testing, although there is still insufficient evidence for the potential harm associated with testing or test-associated treatment.[164]

Several studies have assessed the value of reticulocyte Hb in conjunction with other parameters to diagnose ID states. The so-called Thomas plot combines retic-ulocyte Hb content with the sTfR/ferritin ratio to distinguish ID and FID from iron-sequestration syndromes, such as ACD.[118,165] A subsequent variation of this plot uses CHr in combination with hepcidin-25.[166] Unfortunately, owing to a lack of uni-form recognized reference materials for both sTfR and hepcidin, the use of this plot is extremely limited. Other studies have assessed the usefulness of both hepcidin and reticulocyte Hb in ACD. In patients with active rheumatoid arthritis, clinical utility to detect ID for Ret-He was demonstrated when hepcidin levels fell between 2.4 and 7.6 nmol/L. An algorithm based on the test characteristics and values was proposed by the investigators to identify anemic patients who may benefit from iron treat-ment.[167] Ret-He was evaluated in patients with ACD or other iron-restricted states. Ret-He at the cutoff of 25 pg was able to distinguish ID and iron-sufficient subjects.[122]

Serum hepcidin was shown not to be clinically useful or superior to more standard iron status tests for managing iron therapy in HD patients with ESA treatment; reticulocyte Hb content and percentage of hypochromic red blood cells were shown to be more use-ful, either alone or in combination with transferrin saturation and ferritin levels.[168,169]

The clinical utility of reticulocyte Hb content has been well established as a reliable marker of FID in hemodialysis patients, exhibiting high specificity and sensitivity in the management of intravenous iron therapy. Although ESA treatment has been approved for anemia in several settings outside CKD, appropriate studies still need to be per-formed to assess the suitability of CHr and/or percentage of Hypo-He concerning the detection of FID in other disease-related anemias, and in the reduction of ESA doses and duration of treatment.[170–174]

Clinical utility of reticulocyte hemoglobin in monitoring the efficacy of treatment in iron deficiency anemia and iron deficiency detection during recovery from megaloblastic anemia

Reticulocyte Hb improves the monitoring of erythropoietic response to intravenous iron administration in ID anemia. As shown in **Fig. 3**, in a patient with ID anemia CHr is a very early marker of the efficacy of intravenous iron administration. Response can be demonstrated on the second day of treatment because of the increase of CHr and reticulocyte volume, which precede changes in reticulocyte number. CHr and MCVr continue to increase in the following days, reaching the normal values on the fifth day, when for the first time the reticulocyte number also increases. The response to oral iron treatment occurs with a longer time

DAY

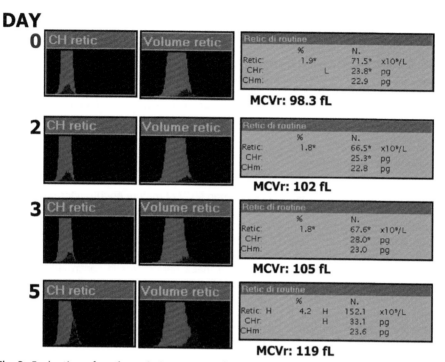

Fig. 3. Evaluation of erythropoiesis response: changes of the reticulocyte indices following intravenous iron administration. Histograms of red blood cells (*red area*) and reticulocytes (*blue area*) hemoglobin content and volume. Panels on the right show reticulocyte percentage and number (10^9/L), hemoglobin erythrocyte content (CHm) and reticulocyte hemoglobin content (CHr) values (pg), and the reticulocyte volume value (MCVr) (fL). Values at day 0: CHm 22.9 pg, CHr 23.8 pg, MCVr 98.3 fL, reticulocytes 1.9%, and reticulocytes 71.5 × 10^9/L. Values at day 2: CHm 22.8 pg, CHr 25.3 pg, MCVr 102 fL, reticulocytes 1.8%, and reticulocytes 66.5 × 10^9/L. Values at day 3: CHm 23.0 pg, CHr 28.0 pg, MCVr 105 fL, reticulocytes 1.8%, and reticulocytes 67.6 × 10^9/L. Values at day 5: CHm 23.6 pg, CHr 33.1 pg, MCVr 119 fL, reticulocytes 4.2%, and reticulocytes 152.1 × 10^9/L. The hemoglobin content and volume of reticulocytes increased significantly after intravenous iron therapy, reaching the normal values on day 3. Reticulocyte indices allow for real-time evaluation of iron-deficient erythropoiesis and for monitoring response to iron replacement therapy. *, sample related flag, due to anemia. (*Courtesy of* Mauro Buttarello, MD, Dipartimento dei servizi di diagnosi e cura, Laboratorio Analisi, Adria, Rovigo, Italy.)

lag, and CHr increases after 2 weeks. Nevertheless, abnormally low CHr makes it possible to identify patients who are not responding well to oral iron. Baseline values for CHr and high-fluorescence reticulocytes and their variation after 2 and 4 weeks of intravenous iron therapy allow correct identification of ID and response to intravenous iron therapy (96% sensitivity and 100% specificity for the latter).[175] During hematologic recovery following vitamin B_{12} administration, a low CHr of less than 26 pg on the third day indicated ID and the concomitant need for treatment with iron and vitamin B_{12}.[176]

Limitations in Clinical Utility of the Reticulocyte Hemoglobin Content

The reticulocyte Hb content presents some diagnostic limitations: it is decreased in thalassemia syndromes, whereby the reduction in CHr seems to be correlated with the degree of impairment in β-chain synthesis, and in other microcytic anemias resulting from congenital Hb diseases.[177] It can also be elevated in ID patients with confounding megaloblastic anemia because of the high mean reticulocyte volume associated with megaloblastosis.[178] It is increased by drugs inducing transient or permanent macrocytosis, such as chronic hydroxyurea treatment in patients with sickle cell disease.[179]

Therefore, it is important that CHr values be interpreted in the context of the patient's overall erythrocyte physiology, including knowledge of recent blood transfusions, iron therapy, vitamin B_{12} or folate deficiency, chemotherapy, and the results of Hb analysis.[137]

Reticulocyte Mean Volume

All automated reticulocyte counting assays can determine MCVr based on light scattering. On average, MCVr is 24% higher than MCV of mature erythrocytes, showing a Gaussian distribution, without differences between sexes. As shown in **Table 2**, in the adult population MCVr presents differences among various instruments. Reference intervals should therefore be determined according to the use of specific methods or analyzers, and these should not be interchangeable in the monitoring of patients.[180] If the clinical usefulness of these parameters is confirmed by future studies, quality control procedures and appropriate reference materials to calibrate the method will be needed.[90] The MCVr multiplied by the number of reticulocytes gives the "hematocrit" values of the reticulocytes.[181] Some analyzers provide the measure of MCVr dispersion, such as the distribution width of reticulocytes, that is, the CV of volumes, which under normal conditions is very close to that of mature erythrocytes.

Clinical Utility of Reticulocyte Cell Volume

Few studies are available on the clinical utility of reticulocyte cell volume. Reticulocyte cell volume is decreased in ID anemia and thalassemia syndromes, but reticulocyte count is usually lower in ID anemia, whereas IRF may be higher in thalassemia. Reticulocyte volume increases in ID anemia during iron treatment and decreases with the development of ID erythropoiesis, such as reticulocyte Hb content.[109,178] In macrocytic anemia, the reticulocyte volume is larger than that of normal reticulocytes, demonstrating megaloblastic erythropoiesis. Treatment with vitamin B_{12} or folate induces a rapid normalization of the volume of reticulocyte, reflecting the efficacy of replacement therapy. In response to B_{12} treatment, the reticulocyte volume is smaller than in predominant erythrocytes. An inversion of the MCVr/MCV ratio has been reported. Owing to their different life spans, the circulating reticulocytes produced after 17 days of treatment had an MCVr of 108.8 fL, whereas the MCV was still 109.8 fL.[17]

MCVr has been measured in sickle cell anemia: induction of fetal Hb synthesis by hydroxyurea therapy was associated with increased hydration of sickle reticulocytes, assessed as MCVr.[175,182,183]

RETICULOCYTE REPORTING

It should be standard for all clinical laboratories to report reticulocytes as absolute counts, because this parameter gives more accurate information on erythropoiesis than the simple reticulocyte percentage.[184] Automated absolute reticulocyte counts have resulted in phasing out the old-fashioned "hematocrit correction" of reticulocyte percentage. As previously stated, the obsolete RPI, which corrected the reticulocyte count both for hematocrit and maturation time, can be replaced with IRF, as it offers the same clinical significance.

What Information Should Be Reported to Clinicians and How?

Information overload is a major concern in reporting new hematologic parameters, given the large number of parameters already reported in the routine CBC. Laboratories should report the reticulocyte count as the absolute number of reticulocytes, accompanied by properly determined and method-specific reference ranges. The percentage value may be optional, but is still important in monitoring the bone marrow response when plasma volume is fluctuating, as happens in blood boosting in athletes or in kidney diseases. The clinical utility of reticulocyte cellular parameters such as IRF and reticulocyte Hb content has been proved, whereas MCVr may be optional, even though it could in some instances provide useful information. Physicians seem to be more interested in the reticulocyte percentage and absolute number, as shown by a study aimed at ascertaining which components of reticulocyte count reports are perceived as useful in clinical practice.[184] A subset analysis by specialty indicated that a small number of pediatric hematologist-oncologists, hematologist-oncologists, and nephrologists also wanted the IRF to be included in reports.[185] It may be useful for laboratories to consider providing an interpretation of the reticulocyte analysis. As an example, if the absolute reticulocyte count and IRF are simultaneously increased, an interpretative comment could be added to emphasize the increase for erythropoietic activity. The comment could help physicians to assess cases of suspected hemolytic anemia or in monitoring the treatment of anemia.

SUMMARY

Automated flow-cytometric analysis has led to a significant advance in reticulocyte counting, providing the reticulocyte immature reticulocyte fraction (IRF), the reticulocyte volume and the hemoglobin content and concentration. IRF assesses reticulocyte maturation by the intensity of the staining that reflects the mRNA content. IRF has been proposed as an early marker of engraftment in bone marrow or hematopoietic stem cell transplantation and bone marrow regeneration following chemotherapy. Reticulocyte hemoglobin content is useful in assessing the functional iron available for erythropoiesis during the previous 3–4 days, while reticulocyte volume is a useful indicator when monitoring the therapeutic response of anemias.

REFERENCES

1. Erb W. Zur Entwicklungsgeschichte der roten Blutkörperchen. Virch Arch Pathol Anat Physiol 1865;34:138–93.
2. Ehrlich P. Uber einige Beobachtungen am anämischen Blut. Berl Klein Wschr 1881;18:43.
3. Smith T. On changes in the red blood corpuscles in pernicious anemia of Texas cattle fever. Trans Assoc Am Physicians 1891;6:263–77.
4. Krumbhaar EB, Chanutin A. Studies on experimental plethora in dogs and rabbits. Exp Biol Med 1922;19:188–90.
5. Heilmeyer L. Blutfarbostoffwechselstudien. Probleme, Methoden, und Kritik der Whippleschen Theorie. Dtsch Arch Klein Med 1931;171:123–53.
6. Heath CW, Daland GA. Staining of reticulocytes by brilliant cresyl blue. Arch Intern Med 1931;48:133–45.
7. Dustin P. Contribution à l'étude histophysiologique et histochimique des globules rouges des vertébrés. Arch Biol 1944;55:285–92.
8. Astaldi G, Tolentino P. Studies in vitro on maturation of erythroblasts in normal and pathological conditions. J Clin Pathol 1949;2:217–22.

9. London IM, Shemin D, Rittenberg D. Synthesis of heme in vitro by the immature non-nucleated mammalian erythrocytes. J Biol Chem 1950;183:749–55.
10. Vander JB, Harris CA, Ellis SR. Reticulocyte counts by means of fluorescence microscopy. J Lab Clin Med 1963;62:132–40.
11. Seip M. Reticulocyte studies. Acta Med Scand 1953;282(Suppl):9–164.
12. Houwen B. Reticulocyte maturation. Blood Cells 1992;18:167–86.
13. Brecher G. New methylene blue as a reticulocyte stain. Am J Clin Pathol 1949; 19:895.
14. Bessis M. Cellules du sang normal et pathologique. Paris: Masson et Cie; 1972. p. 166–278.
15. Gilmer PR Jr, Koepke JA. The reticulocyte: an approach to definition. Am J Clin Pathol 1976;66:262–7.
16. Koepke JA, Broden PN, Corash L, et al. NCCLS document H44-A-Methods for Reticulocyte Counting (Flow Cytometry, and Supravital Dyes); Approved Guideline 1997;17(15).
17. d'Onofrio G, Chirillo R, Zini G, et al. Simultaneous measurement of reticulocyte and red blood cell indices in healthy subjects and patients with microcytic and macrocytic anemia. Blood 1995;85:818–23.
18. Skadberg O, Brun A, Sandberg S. Human reticulocytes isolated from peripheral blood: maturation time and hemoglobin synthesis. Lab Hematol 2003;9: 198–206.
19. Koury MJ, Koury ST, Kopsombut P, et al. In vitro maturation of nascent reticulocytes to erythrocytes. Blood 2005;105:2168–74.
20. Bertles J, Beck W. Biochemical aspects of reticulocyte maturation. J Biol Chem 1962;237:3770–7.
21. Mel HC, Prenant M, Mohandas N. Reticulocyte motility and form: studies on maturation and classification. Blood 1977;49:1001–9.
22. Chasis JA, Schrier SL. Membrane deformability and the capacity for shape change in the erythrocyte. Blood 1989;74:2562–8.
23. Lakomek M, Schröter W, De Maeyer G, et al. On the diagnosis of erythrocyte enzyme defects in the presence of high reticulocyte counts. Br J Haematol 1989;72:445–51.
24. London IM, Shemin D, Rittenberg D. Heme synthesis and red blood cell dynamics in normal humans and in subjects with polycythemia vera, sickle-cell anemia, and pernicious anemia. J Biol Chem 1949;179:463–84.
25. Wangen JR, Eidenschink Brodersen L, Stolk TT, et al. Assessment of normal erythropoiesis by flow cytometry: important considerations for specimen preparation. Int J Lab Hematol 2014;36:184–96.
26. Brugnara C, Kruskall MS, Johnstone RM. Membrane properties of erythrocytes in subjects undergoing multiple blood donations with or without recombinant erythropoietin. Br J Haematol 1993;84:118–30.
27. Sandoval H, Thiagarajan P, Dasgupta SK, et al. Essential role for Nix in autophagic maturation of erythroid cells. Nature 2008;454:232–5.
28. Chen M, Sandoval H, Wang J. Selective mitochondrial autophagy during erythroid maturation. Autophagy 2008;4:926–8.
29. Shimizu S, Honda S, Arakawa S, et al. Alternative macroautophagy and mitophagy. Int J Biochem Cell Biol 2014;50:64–6.
30. Geminard C, de Gassart A, Vidal M. Reticulocyte maturation: mitoptosis and exosome release. Biocell 2002;26:205–15.
31. Ney PA. Normal and disordered reticulocyte maturation. Curr Opin Hematol 2011;18:152–7.

32. Griffiths RE, Kupzig S, Cogan N, et al. Maturing reticulocytes internalize plasma membrane in glycophorin A-containing vesicles that fuse with autophagosomes before exocytosis. Blood 2012;119:6296–306.
33. Lee E, Choi HS, Hwang JH, et al. The RNA in reticulocytes is not just debris: it is necessary for the final stages of erythrocyte formation. Blood Cells Mol Dis 2014;53:1–10.
34. Liu J, Guo X, Mohandas N, et al. Membrane remodeling during reticulocyte maturation. Blood 2010;115:2021–7.
35. Malleret B, Xu F, Mohandas N, et al. Significant biochemical, biophysical and metabolic diversity in circulating human cord blood reticulocytes. PLoS One 2013;8(10):e76062.
36. Kono M, Kondo T, Takagi Y, et al. Morphological definition of CD71 positive reticulocytes by various staining techniques and electron microscopy compared to reticulocytes detected by an automated hematology analyzer. Clin Chim Acta 2009;404:105–10.
37. Heimeyer L, Westharer R. Reifungssstadien an uberlebenden reticulocyte in vitro und ihre bedentung fur die schatzung der taglichen hamoglobin produktion in vivo. Ztsch Klein Med 1932;121:361–9.
38. Lowenstein LM. The mammalian reticulocyte. Int Rev Cytol 1959;8:135–74.
39. Manwani D, Bieker JJ. The erythroblastic island. Curr Top Dev Biol 2008;82:23–53.
40. Chasis JA, Mohandas N. Erythroblastic islands: niches for erythropoiesis. Blood 2008;112:470–8.
41. Baldini M, Panaciulli I. The maturation rate of reticulocytes. Blood 1960;15:614–29.
42. Kuse R. The appearance of reticulocytes with medium or high RNA content is a sensitive indicator of beginning granulocyte recovery after aplasiogenic cytostatic drug therapy in patients with AML. Ann Hematol 1993;66:213–4.
43. Ricos C, Alvarez V, Cava F, et al. Current databases on biological variation: pros, cons and progress. Scand J Clin Lab Invest 1999;59:491–500.
44. Fraser CG. Biological variation: from principles to practice. Washington, DC: AACC Press; 2001. p. 151.
45. Sandberg S, Rustad P, Johannesen B, et al. Within-subject biological variation of reticulocytes and reticulocyte-derived parameters. Eur J Haematol 1998;61:42–8.
46. Costongs GM, Janson PC, Bas BM, et al. Short-term and long-term intra-individual variations and critical differences of haematological laboratory parameters. J Clin Chem Clin Biochem 1985;23:69–76.
47. Buttarello M. Variabilità dei parametri ematologici. Riv Med Lab 2003;4:88–91.
48. Tsuda I, Tatsumi N. Reticulocytes in human preserved blood as control material for automated reticulocyte counters. Am J Clin Pathol 1990;94:109–10.
49. Jones AR, Twedt D, Swaim W, et al. Diurnal change of blood count analytes in normal subjects. Am J Clin Pathol 1996;106:723–7.
50. Tarallo P, Humbert JC, Mahassen P, et al. Reticulocytes: biological variations and reference limits. Eur J Haematol 1994;53:11–5.
51. Carter JM, McSweeney PA, Wakem PJ, et al. Counting reticulocytes by flow cytometry: use of thiazole orange. Clin Lab Haematol 1989;11:267–71.
52. Tarallo P, Humbert JC, Fournier B, et al. Reticulocytes: reference limits. Clin Lab Haematol 1996;18(S1):13–4.
53. Otterman ML, Nijboer JM, van der Horst IC, et al. Reticulocyte counts and their relation to hemoglobin levels in trauma patients. J Trauma 2009;67:121–4.

54. Paterakis GS, Voskaridou E, Loutradi A, et al. Reticulocyte counting in thalassemic and other conditions with the R-1000 Sysmex analyzer. Ann Hematol 1991;63:218–22.
55. Howells MR, Jones SE, Napier JA, et al. Erythropoiesis in pregnancy. Br J Haematol 1986;64:595–9.
56. Lippi G, Salvagno GL, Solero GP, et al. The influence of the tourniquet time on hematological testing for antidoping purposes. Int J Sports Med 2006;27:359–62.
57. Cavill I, Kraaijenhagen R, Pradella R, et al. In vitro stability of the reticulocyte count. Clin Lab Haematol 1996;18:9–11.
58. Lippi G, Salvagno GL, Solero GP, et al. Stability of blood cell counts, hematologic parameters and reticulocytes indexes on the Advia A120 hematologic analyzer. J Lab Clin Med 2005;146:333–40.
59. Lombardi G, Lanteri P, Colombini A, et al. Stability of haematological parameters and its relevance on the athlete's biological passport model. Sports Med 2011; 41:1033–42.
60. Imeri F, Herklotz R, Risch L, et al. Stability of hematological analytes depends on the hematology analyser used: a stability study with Bayer Advia 120, Beckman Coulter LH 750 and Sysmex XE 2100. Clin Chim Acta 2008;397:68–71.
61. Kouri T, Siloaho M, Pohjavaara S, et al. Pre-analytical factors and measurement uncertainty. Scand J Clin Lab Invest 2005;65:463–75.
62. Arkin CF, Davis BH, Bessman BH, et al. NCCLS. Methods for Reticulocyte Counting (Automated Blood Cell Counters, Flow Cytometry, and Supravital Dyes); Approved Guideline. 2nd Edition. NCCLS Document H44-A 2. Wayne (PA): NCCLS; 2004.
63. Tichelli A, Gratwohl A, Driessen A, et al. Evaluation of the Sysmex R-1000. An automated reticulocyte analyzer. Am J Clin Pathol 1990;93:70–8.
64. d'Onofrio G, Kim YR, Schulze S, et al. Evaluation of the Abbott Cell Dyn 4000 automated fluorescent reticulocyte measurements: comparison with manual, FACScan and Sysmex R1000 methods. Clin Lab Haematol 1997;19(4):253–60.
65. D'Onofrio G, Zini G, Rowan RM. Reticulocyte counting: methods and clinical applications. In: Rowan RM, van Assendelft OW, Preston FE, editors. Advanced Laboratory Methods in Haematology. London: Arnold Publisher; 2002. p. 78–126.
66. Van Petegem M, Cartuyvels R, de Schouwer P, et al. Comparative evaluation of three flow cytometers for reticulocyte enumeration. Clin Lab Haematol 1993;15: 103–11.
67. Siekmeier R, Bierlich A, Jaross W. Determination of reticulocytes: three methods compared. Clin Chem Lab Med 2000;38:245–9.
68. Buttarello M, Bulian P, Farina G, et al. Flow cytometric reticulocyte counting. Parallel evaluation of five fully automated analyzers: an NCCLS-ICSH approach. Am J Clin Pathol 2001;115:100–11.
69. Buttarello M, Cappelletti P, Biasioli B, et al. Risultati della sperimentazione multistrumentale in ematologia automatizzata: lo stato dell'arte. Riv Med Lab 2004; 5(Suppl 3):136–41.
70. Piva E, Brugnara C, Chiandetti L, et al. Automated reticulocyte counting: state of the art and clinical applications in the evaluation of erythropoiesis. Clin Chem Lab Med 2010;48:1369–80.
71. Davis BH, Bigelow NC, Koepke JA, et al. Flow cytometric analysis: multiinstitutional interlaboratory correlation study. Am J Clin Pathol 1994;102:468–77.
72. Horowitz G, Altaie S, Boyd CJ, et al. Defining, establishing, and verifying reference intervals in the clinical laboratory. Wayne (PA): CSLI; 2008. CLSI/NCCLS C28-A3 document.

73. Van den Bossche J, Devreese K, Malfait R, et al. Reference intervals for a complete blood count determined on different automated haematology analysers: Abx Pentra 120 Retic, Coulter Gen-S, Sysmex SE9500, Abbott Cell Dyn 4000 and Bayer Advia 120. Clin Chem Lab Med 2002;40:69–73.
74. Noronha JF, Grotto HZ. Measurement of reticulocyte and red blood indices in patients with iron thalassemia minor. Clin Chem Lab Med 2005;43:195–7.
75. Bovy C, Gothot A, Krzesinki JM, et al. Mature erythrocytes indices: new markers of iron availability. Haematologica 2005;90:549–51.
76. Banfi G, Mauri C, Morelli B, et al. Reticulocyte count, mean reticulocyte volume, immature reticulocyte fraction, and mean sphered cell volume in elite athletes: reference values and comparison with the general population. Clin Chem Lab Med 2006;44:616–22.
77. Hoffmann JJ, van den Broek NM, Curvers J. Reference intervals of extended erythrocyte and reticulocyte parameters. Clin Chem Lab Med 2012;50:941–8.
78. Costa O, Van Moer G, Jochmans K, et al. Reference values for new red blood cell and platelet parameters on the Abbott Diagnostics Cell-Dyn Sapphire. Clin Chem Lab Med 2012;50:967–9.
79. Nunes LA, Grotto HZ, Brenzikofer R, et al. Hematological and biochemical markers of iron status in a male, young, physically active population. Biomed Res Int 2014;2014:349182.
80. Zandecki M, Genevieve F, Gerard J, et al. Spurious counts and spurious results on haematology analysers: a review. Part II: white blood cells, red blood cells, haemoglobin, red cell indices and reticulocytes. Int J Lab Hematol 2007;29: 21–41.
81. Davis BH, Ornvold K, Bigelow NC. Flow cytometric reticulocyte maturity index: a useful laboratory parameter of erythropoietic activity in anemia. Cytometry 1995; 22:35–9.
82. Davis BH. Immature reticulocyte fraction (IFR): by any name, a useful clinical parameter of erythropoietic activity. Lab Hematol 1996;2:2–8.
83. Davis BH, Bigelow NC. Automated reticulocyte analysis. Clinical practice and associated new parameters. Hematol Oncol Clin North Am 1994;8:617–30.
84. Davis BH. Report on the ISLH-sponsored Immature Reticulocyte fraction (IRF) Workshop. Lab Hematol 1997;3:261–3.
85. Davis BH, DiCorato M, Bigelow NC, et al. Proposal for the standardization of flow cytometric reticulocyte maturity index measurements. Cytometry 1993;14: 318–26.
86. Buttarello M, Bulian P, Farina G, et al. Five fully automated methods for performing immature reticulocyte fraction: comparison in diagnosis of bone marrow aplasia. Am J Clin Pathol 2002;117:871–9.
87. Davis BH, Bigelow NC, van Hove L. Immature reticulocyte fraction and reticulocyte counts, comparison of Cell-Dyn 4000, Sysmex R-3000, thiazole flow cytometry, and manual counts. Lab Hematol 1996;2:144–8.
88. Briggs C, Grant D, Machin JS. Comparison of the automated reticulocyte counts and immature reticulocyte fraction measurements obtained with the ABX Pentra 120 Retic blood analyzer and the Sysmex XE-2100 automated haematology analyzer. Lab Hematol 2001;7:75–80.
89. Banfi G, Corsi M, Melegati G. The values of immature reticulocytes fraction in élite athletes measured by means of two different methodologies are concordant. J Sports Med Phys Fitness 2006;46:163–4.
90. Briggs C. Quality counts: new parameters in blood cell counting. Int J Lab Hematol 2009;31:277–97.

91. d'Onofrio G, Tichelli A, Foures C, et al. Indicators of haematopoietic recovery after bone marrow transplantation: the role of reticulocyte measurements. Clin Lab Haematol 1996;18:45–53.

92. Testa U, Rutella S, Martucci R, et al. Autologous stem cell transplantation: evaluation of erythropoietic reconstitution by highly fluorescent reticulocyte counts, erythropoietin, soluble transferrin receptors, ferritin, TIBC and iron dosages. Br J Haematol 1997;96:762–75.

93. Torres Gomez A, Sánchez J, Lakomsky D, et al. Assessment of hematologic progenitor engraftment by complete reticulocyte maturation parameters after autologous and allogeneic hematopoietic stem cell transplantation. Haematologica 2001;86:24–9.

94. Noronha JF, De Souza CA, Vigorito AC, et al. Immature reticulocytes as an early predictor of engraftment in autologous and allogeneic bone marrow transplantation. Clin Lab Haematol 2003;25:47–54.

95. Das R, Rawal A, Garewal G, et al. Automated reticulocyte response is a good predictor of bone-marrow recovery in pediatric malignancies. Pediatr Hematol Oncol 2006;23:299–305.

96. Takami A, Shibayama M, Orito M, et al. Immature platelet fraction for prediction of platelet engraftment after allogeneic stem cell transplantation. Bone Marrow Transplant 2007;39:501–7.

97. Grazziutti ML, Dong L, Miceli MH, et al. Recovery from neutropenia can be predicted by the immature reticulocyte fraction several days before neutrophil recovery in autologous stem cell transplant recipients. Bone Marrow Transplant 2006;37:403–9.

98. Molina JR, Sanchez-Garcia J, Torres A, et al. Reticulocyte maturation parameters are reliable early predictors of hematopoietic engraftment after allogeneic stem cell transplantation. Biol Blood Marrow Transplant 2007;13:172–82.

99. Yamaoka G, Kubota Y, Nomura T, et al. The immature platelet fraction is a useful marker for predicting the timing of platelet recovery in patients with cancer after chemotherapy and hematopoietic stem cell transplantation. Int J Lab Hematol 2010;32:208–16.

100. Gonçalo AP, Barbosa IL, Campilho F, et al. Predictive value of immature reticulocyte and platelet fractions in hematopoietic recovery of allograft patients. Transplant Proc 2011;43:241–3.

101. Morkis IV, Farias MG, Rigoni LD, et al. Assessment of immature platelet fraction and immature reticulocyte fraction as predictors of engraftment after hematopoietic stem cell transplantation. Int J Lab Hematol 2014. [Epub ahead of print].

102. Luczyński W, Ratomski K, Wysocka J, et al. Immature reticulocyte fraction (IRF): an universal marker of hemopoiesis in children with cancer? Adv Med Sci 2006; 51:188–90.

103. Remacha AF, Martino R, Sureda A, et al. Changes in the reticulocyte fraction during peripheral stem cell harvesting: role in monitoring stem cell collection. Bone Marrow Transplant 1996;17:163–8.

104. Dunlop LC, Cohen J, Harvey M, et al. The immature reticulocyte fraction: a negative predictor of the harvesting of CD34 cells for autologous peripheral blood stem cell transplantation. Clin Lab Haematol 2006;28:245–7.

105. Torres Gomez A, Casano J, Sanchez J, et al. Utility of reticulocyte maturation parameters in the differential diagnosis of macrocytic anemias. Clin Lab Haematol 2003;25:283–8.

106. Lesesve JF, Daliphard S, Callat MP, et al. Increase of immature reticulocyte fraction in myelodysplastic syndromes [letter]. Clin Lab Haematol 2004;26:301–2.

107. Mullier F, Lainey E, Fenneteau O, et al. Additional erythrocytic and reticulocytic parameters helpful for diagnosis of hereditary spherocytosis: results of a multi-centre study. Ann Hematol 2011;90:759–68.
108. Persijn L, Bonroy C, Mondelaers V, et al. Screening for hereditary spherocytosis in routine practice: evaluation of a diagnostic algorithm with focus on non-splenectomised patients. Ann Hematol 2012;91:301–2.
109. Brugnara C, Laufer MR, Friedman AJ, et al. Reticulocyte hemoglobin content (CHr): early indicator of iron deficiency and response to therapy. Blood 1994; 83:3100–1.
110. Brugnara C, Hipp MJ, Irving PJ, et al. Automated reticulocyte counting and measurement of reticulocyte cellular indices. Evaluation of the Miles H*3 blood analyzer. Am J Clin Pathol 1994;102:623–32.
111. Mohandas N, Kim YR, Tycko DH, et al. Accurate and independent measurement of volume and hemoglobin concentration of individual red cells by laser light scattering. Blood 1986;68:506–13.
112. Mullaney PF, Dean PN. Cell sizing: a small-angle light scattering method for sizing particles of low relative refractive index. Appl Opt 1969;8:2361–2.
113. Latimer P, Brunsting A, Pyle BE, et al. Effects of asphericity on single particle scattering. Appl Opt 1978;17:3152–8.
114. Sharpless TK, Bartholdi M, Melamed MR. Size and refractive index dependence of simple forward-angle scattering measurements in a flow system using sharply focused illumination. J Histochem Cytochem 1977;25:845–56.
115. Salzmann GC, Crowell JM, Martin JC, et al. Cell classification by laser light scattering: identification and separation of unstained leukocytes. Acta Cytol 1975; 19:374–7.
116. Kamentsky LA. Cytology automation. Adv Biol Med Phys 1973;14:93–161.
117. Buttarello M, Temporin V, Ceravolo R, et al. The new reticulocyte parameter (RET-Y) of the Sysmex XE 2100: its use in the diagnosis and monitoring of post-treatment sideropenic anemia. Am J Clin Pathol 2004;121:489–95.
118. Thomas L, Franck S, Messinger M, et al. Reticulocyte hemoglobin measurement—comparison of two methods in the diagnosis of iron-restricted erythropoiesis. Clin Chem Lab Med 2005;43:1193–202.
119. Canals C, Remacha AF, Sarda MP, et al. Clinical utility of the new Sysmex XE2100 parameter—reticulocyte hemoglobin equivalent—in the diagnosis of anemia. Haematologica 2005;90:1133–4.
120. Brugnara C, Schiller B, Moran J. Reticulocyte hemoglobin equivalent (Ret He) and assessment of iron-deficient states. Clin Lab Haematol 2006;28:303–8.
121. Garzia M, Di Mario A, Ferraro E, et al. Reticulocyte hemoglobin equivalent: an indicator of reduced iron availability in chronic kidney diseases during erythropoietin therapy. Lab Hematol 2007;13:6–11.
122. Maconi M, Cavalca L, Danise P, et al. Erythrocyte and reticulocyte indices in iron deficiency in chronic kidney disease: comparison of two methods. Scand J Clin Lab Invest 2009;69:365–70.
123. Maconi M, Danise P, Cavalca L, et al. Flow cytometric reticulocyte counting: a comparison between two methods. J Clin Lab Anal 2010;24:252–5.
124. Miwa N, Akiba T, Kimata N, et al. Usefulness of measuring reticulocyte hemoglobin equivalent in the management of haemodialysis patients with iron deficiency. Int J Lab Hematol 2010;32:248–55.
125. Ermens AA, Hoffmann JJ, Krockenberger M, et al. New erythrocyte and reticulocyte parameters on CELL-DYN Sapphire: analytical and preanalytical aspects. Int J Lab Hematol 2012;34:274–82.

126. Urrechaga E. Clinical utility of the new Beckman-Coulter parameter red blood cell size factor in the study of erythropoiesis. Int J Lab Hematol 2009;31:623–9.
127. McLean E, Cogswell M, Egli I, et al. Worldwide prevalence of anaemia, WHO vitamin and mineral nutrition information system, 1993-2005. Public Health Nutr 2009;12:444–5.
128. Klip IT, Comin-Colet J, Voors AA, et al. Iron deficiency in chronic heart failure: an international pooled analysis. Am Heart J 2013;165:575–82.
129. Cohen-Solal A, Leclercq C, Deray G, et al. Iron deficiency: an emerging therapeutic target in heart failure. Heart 2014;100:1414–20.
130. Jacobs A, Worwood M. Clinical and biochemical implications. Ferritin in serum. N Engl J Med 1975;292:951–6.
131. Goodnough LT, Skikne B, Brugnara C. Erythropoietin, iron, and erythropoiesis. Blood 2000;96:823–33.
132. Rushton DH, Barth JH. What is the evidence for gender differences in ferritin and haemoglobin? Crit Rev Oncol Hematol 2010;73:1–9.
133. Brugnara C. A hematologic "gold standard" for iron-deficient states? Clin Chem 2002;48:981–2.
134. Brugnara C. Iron deficiency and erythropoiesis: new diagnostic approaches. Clin Chem 2003;49:1573–8.
135. Brugnara C, Adamson J, Auerbach M, et al. Iron deficiency: what are the future trends in diagnostics and therapeutics? Clin Chem 2013;59:740–5.
136. Mast AE, Blinder MA, Lu Q, et al. Clinical utility of the reticulocyte hemoglobin content in the diagnosis of iron deficiency. Blood 2002;99:1489–91.
137. Brugnara C, Zurakowski D, Di Canzio J, et al. Reticulocyte hemoglobin content to diagnose iron deficiency in children. JAMA 1999;281:2225–30.
138. Shaker M, Jenkins P, Ulrich C, et al. An economic analysis of anemia prevention during infancy. J Pediatr 2009;154:44–9.
139. Ullrich C, Chen A, Armsby C, et al. Screening healthy infants for iron deficiency with reticulocyte hemoglobin content. JAMA 2005;294:924–30.
140. Stoffman N, Brugnara C, Woods ER. An algorithm using reticulocyte hemoglobin content (CHr) measurement in screening adolescents for iron deficiency. J Adolesc Health 2005;36:529.
141. d'Onofrio G, Zini G, Ricerca BM, et al. Automated measurement of red blood cell microcytosis and hypochromia in iron deficiency and beta-thalassemia trait. Arch Pathol Lab Med 1992;116:84–9.
142. Torsvik IK, Markestad T, Ueland PM, et al. Evaluating iron status and the risk of anemia in young infants using erythrocyte parameters. Pediatr Res 2013;73:214–20.
143. Ervasti M, Kotisaari S, Heinonen S, et al. Use of advanced red blood cell and reticulocyte indices improves the accuracy in diagnosing iron deficiency in pregnant women at term. Eur J Haematol 2007;79:539–45.
144. Radtke H, Meyer T, Kalus U, et al. Rapid identification of iron deficiency in blood donors with red cell indexes provided by Advia 120. Transfusion 2005;45:5–10.
145. Semmelrock MJ, Raggam RB, Amrein K, et al. Reticulocyte hemoglobin content allows early and reliable detection of functional iron deficiency in blood donors. Clin Chim Acta 2012;413:678–82.
146. Kiss JE, Steele WR, Wright DJ, NHLBI Retrovirus Epidemiology Donor Study-II. Laboratory variables for assessing iron deficiency in REDS-II Iron Status Evaluation (RISE) blood donors. Transfusion 2013;53:2766–75.
147. Karlsson T. Comparative evaluation of the reticulocyte hemoglobin content assay when screening for iron deficiency in elderly anemic patients. Anemia 2011;2011:925907.

148. Joosten E, Lioen P, Brusselmans C, et al. Is analysis of the reticulocyte haemo-globin equivalent a useful test for the diagnosis of iron deficiency anaemia in geriatric patients? Eur J Intern Med 2013;24:63–6.

149. Rutherford CJ, Schneider TJ, Dempsey H, et al. Efficacy of different dosing regimens for recombinant human erythropoietin in a simulated perisurgical setting: the impor-tance of iron availability in optimizing response. Am J Med 1994;96:139–45.

150. Brugnara C, Colella GM, Cremins J, et al. Effects of subcutaneous recombinant human erythropoietin in normal subjects: development of decreased reticulo-cyte hemoglobin content and iron-deficient erythropoiesis. J Lab Clin Med 1994;123:660–7.

151. Goodnough LT, Nemeth E, Ganz T. Detection, evaluation, and management of iron-restricted erythropoiesis. Blood 2010;116:4754–61.

152. Goodnough LT. Iron deficiency syndromes and iron-restricted erythropoiesis. Transfusion 2012;52:1584–92.

153. Roy CN. Anemia of inflammation. Hematol Am Soc Hematol Educ Program 2010;2010:276–80.

154. Sun CC, Vaja V, Babitt JL, et al. Targeting the hepcidin-ferroportin axis to develop new treatment strategies for anemia of chronic disease and anemia of inflammation. Am J Hematol 2012;87:392–400.

155. Wish JB. Assessing iron status: beyond serum ferritin and transferrin saturation. Clin J Am Soc Nephrol 2006;1(Suppl 1):S4–8.

156. KDOQI clinical practice guidelines and clinical practice recommendations for ane-mia in Chronic Kidney Disease, CKD. Kidney Int Suppl 2012;2:279–335. Available at: http://www2.kidney.org/professionals/KDOQI/guidelines_anemiaUP/.

157. Thomas DW, Hinchliffe RF, Briggs C, et al, British Committee for Standards in Haematology. Guideline for the laboratory diagnosis of functional iron defi-ciency. Br J Haematol 2013;161:639–48.

158. Fishbane S, Galgano C, Langley RC Jr, et al. Reticulocyte hemoglobin content in the evaluation of iron status of hemodialysis patients. Kidney Int 1997;52:217–22.

159. Mitsuiki K, Harada A, Miyata Y. Assessment of iron deficiency in chronic hemo-dialysis patients: investigation of cutoff values for reticulocyte haemoglobin con-tent. Clin Exp Nephrol 2003;7:52–7.

160. Fishbane S, Shapiro W, Dutka P, et al. A randomized trial of iron deficiency testing strategies in hemodialysis patients. Kidney Int 2001;60:2406–11.

161. Buttarello M, Pajola R, Novello E, et al. Diagnosis of iron deficiency in patients undergoing hemodialysis. Am J Clin Pathol 2010;133:949–54.

162. Tessitore N, Solero GP, Lippi G, et al. The role of iron status markers in predicting response to intravenous iron in haemodialysis patients on maintenance erythro-poietin. Nephrol Dial Transplant 2001;16:1416–23.

163. Kakimoto-Shino M, Toya Y, Kuji T, et al. Changes in hepcidin and reticulocyte hemoglobin equivalent levels in response to continuous erythropoietin receptor activator administration in hemodialysis patients: a randomized study. Ther Apher Dial 2014;18:421–6.

164. Chung M, Moorthy D, Hadar N, et al. Biomarkers for assessing and managing iron deficiency anemia in late-stage chronic kidney disease. Comparative Effective-ness Review No. 83. (Prepared by the Tufts Evidence-based Practice Center under Contract No. 290-2007-10055-I.) AHRQ Publication No. 12(13)-EHC140-EF. Rockville (MD): Agency for Healthcare Research and Quality; 2012. Available at: www.effectivehealthcare.ahrq.gov/reports/final.cfm.

165. Thomas C, Thomas L. Biochemical markers and hematologic indices in the diagnosis of functional iron deficiency. Clin Chem 2002;48:1066–76.

166. Thomas C, Kobold U, Balan S, et al. Serum hepcidin-25 may replace the ferritin index in the Thomas plot in assessing iron status in anemic patients. Int J Lab Hematol 2011;33:187–93.
167. van Santen S, van Dongen-Lases EC, de Vegt F, et al. Hepcidin and hemoglobin content parameters in the diagnosis of iron deficiency in rheumatoid arthritis patients with anemia. Arthritis Rheum 2011;63:3672–80.
168. Tessitore N, Girelli D, Campostrini N, et al. Hepcidin is not useful as a biomarker for iron needs in haemodialysis patients on maintenance erythropoiesis-stimulating agents. Nephrol Dial Transplant 2010;25:3996–4002.
169. Ford BA, Eby CS, Scott MG, et al. Intra-individual variability in serum hepcidin precludes its use as a marker of iron status in hemodialysis patients. Kidney Int 2010;78:769–73.
170. Cazzola M, Mercuriali F, Brugnara C. Use of recombinant human erythropoietin outside the setting of uremia. Blood 1997;89:4248–67.
171. Katodritou E, Zervas K, Terpos E, et al. Use of erythropoiesis stimulating agents and intravenous iron for cancer and treatment-related anaemia: the need for predictors and indicators of effectiveness has not abated. Br J Haematol 2008;142:3–10.
172. Nakanishi T, Kuragano T, Kaibe S, et al. Should we reconsider iron administration based on prevailing ferritin and hepcidin concentrations? Clin Exp Nephrol 2012;16:819–26.
173. Brugnara C, Mohandas N. Red cell indices in classification and treatment of anemias: from M.M. Wintrobes's original 1934 classification to the third millennium. Curr Opin Hematol 2013;20:222–30.
174. Goodnough LT, Shander A. Update on erythropoiesis-stimulating agents. Best Pract Res Clin Anaesthesiol 2013;27:121–9.
175. Brugnara C. Use of reticulocyte cellular indices in the diagnosis and treatment of hematological disorders. Int J Clin Lab Res 1998;28:1–11.
176. Buttarello M, Plebani M. Automated blood cell counts: state of the art. Am J Clin Pathol 2008;130:104–16.
177. Skarmoutsou C, Papassotiriou I, Traeger-Synodinos J, et al. Erythroid bone marrow activity and red cell hemoglobinization in iron sufficient beta-thalassemia heterozygotes as reflected by soluble transferrin receptor and reticulocyte hemoglobin in content. Correlation with genotypes and Hb A(2) levels. Haematologica 2003;88:631–6.
178. Brugnara C. Reticulocyte cellular indices: a new approach in the diagnosis of anemias and monitoring of erythropoietic function. Crit Rev Clin Lab Sci 2000;37:93–130.
179. Bridges KR, Barabino GD, Brugnara C, et al. A multiparameter analysis of sickle erythrocytes in patients undergoing hydroxyurea therapy. Blood 1996;88:4701–10.
180. Cappelletti P, Biasioli B, Buttarello M, et al. Mean reticulocyte volume (MCVr): reference intervals and the need for standardization [abstract]. Proceeding of the XIX International Symposium on Technological Innovation in Laboratory Hematology. ISLH. Lab Hematol 2006;12(3):169.
181. Parisotto R, Gore CJ, Emslie KR, et al. A novel method utilising markers of altered erythropoiesis for the detection of recombinant human erythropoietin abuse in athletes. Haematologica 2000;85:564–72.
182. De Franceschi L. Pathophysiology of sickle cell disease and new drugs for the treatment. Mediterr J Hematol Infect Dis 2009;1:e2009024.
183. Quarmyne MO, Risinger M, Linkugel A, et al. Volume regulation and KCl cotransport in reticulocyte populations of sickle and normal red blood cells. Blood Cells Mol Dis 2011;47:95–9.

184. Cappelletti P, Biasioli B, Bulian P, et al. Linee guida per il referto ematologico. 2002. Available at: http://www.simel.it/download/100124-documento.pdf.
185. Sandhaus LM, Meyer P. How useful are CBC and reticulocyte reports to clinicians? Am J Clin Pathol 2002;118:787–93.

Hematology Analyzers
Special Considerations for Pediatric Patients

Edward C.C. Wong, MD[a,b,*]

KEYWORDS

- Pediatrics • Hematology analyzers • Cell analysis

KEY POINTS

- There are many preanalytical issues that affect neonatal testing and interpretation; awareness of these preanalytical issues is necessary for proper interpretation of neonatal hematology testing and to accommodate logistical concerns.
- Current hematology analyzers offer alternative approaches to cellular analysis that may lead to greater insight in hematopoiesis, specifically in the areas of iron deficiency and thrombopoietic activity in patients recovering from chemotherapy or hematopoietic progenitor cell transplantation.
- The development of pediatric reference intervals, especially in neonates, is essential for proper interpretation of hematologic parameters in the context of disease and nondisease states.
- Clinical need for manual differential will likely decrease in the future with improvements in automated granulocyte enumeration and computerized cellular analysis technology.

HEMATOPOIETIC CHANGES DURING DEVELOPMENT

Dramatic hematologic changes occur after birth. These changes include qualitative and quantitative changes in the cellular content of blood and are influenced primarily by changes in α and β globin chain expression, hematopoietic activity, iron metabolism, and growth factor (eg, erythropoietin, thrombopoietin) responsiveness, and a developing cellular and humoral immune system, the latter of which has to respond to many infectious disease threats especially in the newborn period. Age-specific quantitative changes that parallel age-specific functional differences in cellular function exist from birth to adulthood. Normal full-term newborns, for example, have higher white blood cell (WBC), red blood cell (RBC), and platelets counts compared with

Disclosures: Speaker Honorarium, Sysmex USA.
a Division of Laboratory Medicine, Children's National Health System, 111 Michigan Avenue, Northwest Washington, DC 20010, USA; b Departments of Pediatrics and Pathology, George Washington School of Medicine and Health Sciences, Washington, DC, USA
* Division of Laboratory Medicine, Children's National Health System, 111 Michigan Avenue, Northwest Washington, DC 20010.
E-mail address: ewong@childrensnational.org

Clin Lab Med 35 (2015) 165–181
http://dx.doi.org/10.1016/j.cll.2014.10.010
0272-2712/15/$ – see front matter © 2015 Elsevier Inc. All rights reserved.

Abbreviations	
CBC	Complete blood count
IPF	Immature platelet fraction
MCH	Mean corpuscular hemoglobin
MCHC	Mean corpuscular hemoglobin concentration
MCV	Mean cell volume
NRBC	Nucleated RBC
RBC	Red blood cell
RET-He	Reticulocyte hemoglobin content
rHuEPO	Recombinant human erythropoietin
sTR	Soluble transferrin receptor
Tsat	Transferrin saturation
WBC	White blood cell

adults. Morphologically, peripheral smear examination shows age-specific differences in WBC nuclear to cytoplasmic ratio, cellular granularity, RBC anisocytosis/poikilocytosis, and differences in platelet size and granularity.[1–3] Theoretically, current hematology analyzers that possess advanced proprietary cellular analysis capabilities are well suited to capture such age-specific differences because analysis of many thousands of cells is performed.

PREANALYTICAL ISSUES IN HEMATOLOGIC TESTING
Limiting Blood Volume in Children

A major concern in hematologic testing in children is the amount of blood drawn for testing. Because of smaller blood volumes, especially in preterm infants, the risk of significant iatrogenic blood loss requiring additional blood transfusions is very high.[4] Term infants have total blood volumes ranging from 80 to 85 mL/kg, whereas preterm infants' blood volumes are approximately 105 mL/kg. Although this is much higher than the 60 to 65 mL/kg seen in women and men, respectively, the small blood volumes of neonates limit the amount of blood that can be drawn. In general, daily blood draws for testing should be no greater than 5% of a patient's blood volume. As a result, small EDTA whole blood microtainer tubes have been developed, allowing collection of less than 1 mL of whole blood.

Unfortunately, the small, nonstandard size of these tubes poses a challenge to clinical laboratories. These tubes must be manually handled because none of the current hematology analyzers can automatically process or adequately manipulate these tubes. In addition, these small tubes pose challenges for adequate labeling and identification. For example, often these tubes are inappropriately labeled with large labels by the clinical team, which frequently need to be adjusted or peeled back to get at the bar code label for identification by the hematology instrument. Other challenges include frequent incidence of hemolysis, clotting, and insufficient quantity for testing. These challenges may lead to delay in specimen processing and longer turnaround times and potentially result in the need for repeat phlebotomy, which can, in turn, lead to delays in reporting results. Although these microtainer tubes are frequently used in neonates in the neonatal intensive care unit, the use of these tubes is also frequent in older children. At the author's institution, for example, the use of microtainer tubes accounts for 40% to 50% of tubes used for hematology testing. Point-of-care devices that require only small sample volumes have been developed for the measurement of hemoglobin/hematocrit. However, these devices usually rely on conductivity measurements to determine hematocrit indirectly (with hemoglobin as a calculated ratio) and have well-known limitations in patients with electrolyte and protein disturbances.[5]

Variations of Blood Sampling Sites

Special neonatal concerns

There are several different approaches in obtaining blood from neonates and young children. Because of the difficulty of obtaining venous access in neonates, other approaches in obtaining blood are often used. These approaches include catheterization of umbilical vessels or peripheral veins, direct arterial puncture or arterial lines, central venous lines, and heel sticks.[6] In neonates, for example, a heel-stick sample is not considered to be equivalent to venous or arterial blood, and, in fact, contains a mixture of undetermined proportion of blood from both venous/arterial and interstitial fluids. In addition, the degree of perfusion and other factors may further affect the composition of the capillary blood. Microcirculatory disturbances, in particular, can significantly increase capillary hematocrit compared with venous hematocrit in neonates.[7]

There can be differences in WBC when simultaneous sampling of arterial, venous, and capillary blood is performed in neonates. In one study, the mean $\pm$ SD WBC count in venous blood was 82% $\pm$ 3.5% of the WBC count in capillary blood, and the count in arterial blood was even lower (77% $\pm$ 5.3%).[8] Gestational age, time elapsed since delivery, and other clinical conditions did not appear to influence these results. Thus, it is important to be aware of which site is used for phlebotomy because WBC counts from arterial blood may be lower and a neonate may be considered neutropenic, when the capillary WBC is actually normal. Total neutrophil counts, in contrast, are similar in different sample types.[9]

In regard to RBC indices, in a study of simultaneous venous and arterial sample, differences were found to be small, with mean hemoglobin concentration only slightly higher in venous blood.[10] Capillary mean cell volume (MCV) is lower than venous MCV, because of fluid loss from neonatal RBCs. In contrast, the mean corpuscular hemoglobin (MCH) and red cell distribution width is similar in capillary and venous blood, whereas mean corpuscular hemoglobin concentration (MCHC) is higher in capillary blood.[7]

The effect of sampling site on the platelet count is not clear, with some studies finding no difference in platelet count,[11,12] whereas other studies have found significantly decreased platelet counts, especially in capillary samples.[10] The latter findings may be the result of increased platelet activation/aggregation due to the heel puncture and massaging the area near the collection site. Supporting the concept that lower platelet counts may be the result of platelet activation is the finding that capillary platelets have a higher mean platelet volume compared with venous platelets. Activated platelets are associated with increased mean platelet volumes.[13]

Differences in the hemoglobin and neutrophil count values from capillary and arterial samples are even more pronounced in preterm infants. For example, Thurlbeck and McIntosh[12] found capillary hemoglobin values to be higher compared with arterial samples with a mean difference of 2.3 g/dL (0.6–4.9 g/dL). Similarly, capillary WBC count was also found to be significantly higher than the count from the arterial samples by an average difference of 1800/μL.[12]

Other preanalytical issues that can affect the white blood cell count

There are several preanalytical issues that can result in significant leukocytosis and/or neutrophilia. These issues include patient-related conditions, such as exertion, violent crying, circumcision, and physical therapy.[13] Total WBC count and neutrophil count can increase by 146% and 148%, respectively, after either circumcision or chest physical therapy.[11]

In neonates, the duration of umbilical cord clamping can significantly increase hemoglobin levels. In a recent meta-analysis, delaying cord clamping for 2 minutes or more after birth significantly increased hemoglobin levels, even resulting in asymptomatic polycythemia.[14] This increase in birth hemoglobin results in less severe physiologic anemia during the postneonatal period.[15] Interestingly, the mode of delivery also affects WBC counts. Neonates born by vaginal delivery also typically have higher WBC and band counts.

Because neonates have very immature immune systems, they are prone to a variety of viral and bacterial infections. Marked left shift is common. Many current analyzers now have the capability of enumerating immature granulocytes that would allow elimination of a manual differential.[16,17] However, the percentage and absolute immature granulocyte count must be interpreted with caution, because the initial studies for these analytes were performed in adults.[17] Adult immature granulocytes data cannot be extrapolated to children because granularity and size of immature granulocytes are different in children (especially neonates) versus adults.[18] Complicating this issue is the use of 100 cell differentials, which skews granulocyte counts toward 0, as observed by Nigro and colleagues.[19] An absolute band count has been shown to help in the determination of bacterial sepsis in children less than 3 months old.[20] It must be recognized that presently no hematology analyzer has the capability of distinguishing between segmented and band neutrophils, and therefore, use of the band count requires performing manual differentials that can be labor intensive and inaccurate. Use of other markers may be informative.[20]

An inadequate draw can result in WBC or platelet aggregates or fibrin precipitates and may result in spuriously decreased WBC and platelet counts, which may not be confirmed on repeat testing due to the limited blood available for testing.[21,22]

ANALYTICAL FACTORS AFFECTING HEMATOLOGY TESTING IN NEONATES AND YOUNG CHILDREN
Technological Differences Between Hematology Analyzers

There is very little literature regarding differences between hematology analyzers using different methodologies (aperture impedance vs laser optic technology) for pediatric blood samples. Hematology analyzers have different proprietary methodologies for performing the complete blood count (CBC) as well as nontraditional hematologic analysis. For example, with RBC analysis, Coulter and Advia technologies directly measure RBC count, hemoglobin, and MCV, whereas Sysmex technology directly measures RBC count, hemoglobin, and hematocrit. For further information on the technology of the analyzers, the reader is referred to several excellent reviews and to company Web sites for more information.[23–25] Although articles addressing the strengths of specific methods are found in the laboratory hematology literature, there is little discussion of the analytical aspects related to pediatric samples.[26,27] Although each individual instrument and method has its strengths and weaknesses, no one instrument or method has clear superiority in terms of overall usefulness in pediatric hematology. Furthermore, because of differences in cellular analysis, reference intervals for each hematologic parameter are not always interchangeable between instruments. For example, mean platelet volumes calculated using Sysmex technology are generally 2 to 3 fL higher than mean platelet volumes determined on Abbott, Siemens (Advia), or Coulter platforms.[28] On the other hand, the reticulocyte hemoglobin content as derived by Siemens (Advia) technology versus reticulocyte hemoglobin content (RET-He) on the Symex instrument is very similar, with R^2 ranging from 0.95 to 0.99.[29]

All current hematology analyzers can rapidly and accurately perform analysis of EDTA whole blood specimens. However, spurious results may be observed in a variety of conditions.[21,22] Samples from neonates can have unique interferences, such as hyperbilirubinemia, hyperlipidemia due to the use of total parenteral nutrition, resistance of neonatal RBCs to lysis, and the presence of nucleated RBCs. Current analyzers have appropriate flagging systems to indicate the possible presence of spurious results.

One well-known issue is neonatal RBC resistance to lysis, which can result in spurious increases in WBC counts. Manufacturers of hematology analyzers have solved this problem by (1) flagging the presence of RBCs resistant to lysis and allowing an extended mode with longer lysis, or (2) quantifying WBC nuclei after the use of a strong lysing solution, followed by use of a channel for a total WBC count and software adjustment of the WBC count after enumeration of the number of nucleated RBCs.[3]

Any cause of increased turbidity such as hyperlipidemia due to total parenteral nutrition, hyperbilirubinemia, or an elevated WBC count can lead to spuriously elevated hemoglobin levels and consequently cause incorrect calculated hemoglobin derivatives such as MCH and MCHC. Because of the low analytical sensitivity and high precision of current hematology instruments, correcting indices by adjusting results after dilution to decrease interference may be possible.

POSTANALYTICAL ISSUES: CHALLENGES IN INTERPRETATION OF HEMATOLOGIC TEST RESULTS IN TERM AND PRETERM NEWBORNS AND OTHER PEDIATRIC POPULATIONS

Test interpretation requires knowledge of normal hematologic values of newborns and young children; this is especially important in the neonatal period because of dynamic changes occurring at and shortly after birth. Knowledge of how analytical and postanalytical issues can influence test results is also important. A variety of instruments have been used to obtain blood counts in healthy children or children with disease; these instruments included Sysmex instruments (NE 8000, SE-9500, and XE-2100; Sysmex, Tokyo, Japan),[3,28,30–32] Coulter instruments (Beckman Coulter, Brea, CA, USA),[33–35] Abbott instruments (Cell-Dyn series; Abbott Diagnostics, Abbott Park, IL, USA),[9,36] and Siemens instruments (Advia series; Siemens Medical Solutions, Malvern, PA, USA).[3,28,30–32]

However, most of the reports have focused on measured or calculated hematologic indices and do not discuss strengths and limitations of the instruments when used in the evaluation of pediatric (especially neonatal) blood samples. One study compared automated differential counts on pediatric samples using the Coulter HmX hematology analyzer (Beckman Coulter) versus manual differential counts. This study demonstrated that automated counts using flow cytometry were superior to manual differential counts.[37]

Table 1 summarizes the preanalytical, analytical, and postanalytical issues associated with pediatric hematology specimen testing.

NEWER MARKERS OF HEMATOPOIETIC ACTIVITY
Reticulocyte Hemoglobin Content and Iron Deficiency

The gold standard for assessing iron deficiency is Prussian blue staining to detect the presence of iron in bone marrow aspirate preparations. Given the difficulty of performing this test, substitute markers of iron deficiency have been developed, including markers such as ferritin, soluble transferrin receptor, total iron binding capacity, and serum iron. These traditional markers are useful in determining whether iron deficiency is present; however, patients can have "subclinical" iron deficiency, whereby iron

Table 1
Preanalytical, analytical, and postanalytical issues with pediatric hematology specimens: age-specific considerations

| Testing Phase | Neonate | Age-Specific Issues with Hematology Analyzers | |
		Older Children	Adults
Preanalytical			
Small draw volumes	Insufficient or clotted sample, which may lead to repeat testing and iatrogenic blood and testing inefficiency	Less of an issue	Usually not an issue
Blood source	Heel stick: large proportion of samples	Less of an issue; heel stick usually not performed	Not an issue
Analytical			
Instrumentation	Differences in technologies usually not an issue with newer analyzers, need to account for NRBC interference with WBC count	Less of an issue with NRBC interference	Less of an issue with NRBC interference
	Very difficult to automate, given small tube sizes, manual manipulation often required	Less of an issue if standard adult size tubes are used	Automation often performed
Interferences	Lipemia or hyperbilirubin interference on hemoglobin analysis and other cellular components	Less of an issue except in rare patient populations	Less of an issue except in rare patient populations
	NRBC interference with WBC count	Less of an issue	Usually not an issue
Postanalytical			
Reference intervals	Important, extremely difficult to derive for logistical and ethnical reasons	Same as neonates except higher numbers of relatively well patients and higher blood volumes available for leftover testing	Relatively easy to derive
	Preterm and full-term reference intervals needed	Multiple age group intervals needed for older children	Generally one age interval needed, exception: geriatric group
	Ethnicity, blood source, gestational age (preterm vs full term) usually not taken into account	Less of an issue	Less of an issue
δ Checking	MCV unreliable	MCV more reliable	MCV more reliable

Abbreviation: NRBC, nucleated RBC.

stores are deficient, while erythopoiesis is still normal, or iron stores are normal but erythopoiesis is restrictive (also known as functional iron deficiency). In the situation wherein both iron stores and erythropoiesis are restrictive, true iron deficiency is evident. **Fig. 1** shows 4 possible iron deficiency states, based on reticulocyte hemoglobin content to assess erythropoiesis and the ratio of the soluble transferrin receptor to log ferritin to assess iron stores. The use of the soluble transferrin receptor to log ferritin ratio reduces the risk of inflammation which, if not accounted for, may mask decreased iron stores.

Many current hematology analyzers have the ability to enumerate reticulocytes and therefore determine the reticulocyte hemoglobin content. Measurements of reticulocyte hemoglobin content have been shown to provide useful information in diagnosing functional iron deficiency during recombinant human erythropoietin therapy,[38] iron-deficient states in infancy,[39] and response to iron therapy.[40–42] The use of reticulocyte hemoglobin content has been recently reviewed by Piva and colleagues.[43]

The major advantage of measuring reticulocyte hemoglobin content using a hematology analyzer (which can produce a result within minutes) is to minimize the need for additional iron studies (ie, ferritin, serum iron, total iron binding capacity). One major limitation of this approach had been the fact that these parameters were available only on Bayer (now Siemens) instruments. Recently, cellular hemoglobin content parameters have now become available also on the Sysmex instruments as a parameter called RET-He.[44,45] Receiver operating characteristic curve analysis for RET-He and the diagnosis of iron-deficiency anemia in hemodialysis patients was performed by Brugnara and colleagues[29] evaluating the ability of reticulocyte hemoglobin content to identify iron-deficient states. In this study, traditional parameters for iron deficiency (serum iron <40 g/dL, Transferrin saturation <20%, ferritin <100 ng/mL, and hemoglobin <11 g/dL) were used. Using a reticulocyte hemoglobin cutoff level of 27.2 pg, iron deficiency could be diagnosed with a sensitivity of 93.3% and a specificity of 83.2%.

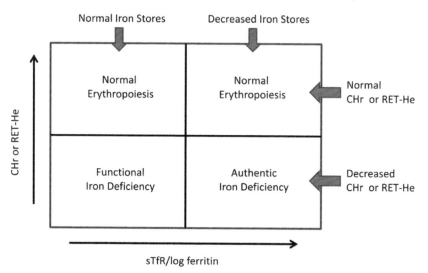

Fig. 1. Bivariate approach to iron status. Normal erythropoiesis is characterized by normal reticulocyte hemoglobin content (normal CHr or RET-He), whereas functional iron deficiency and true iron deficiency can be delineated by a decrease in CHr or RET-He and appropriate sTfR/log ferritin cutoffs to adjust for inflammation. CHr and RET-He represent Siemen (Advia series) and Sysmex names for reticulocyte hemoglobin content, respectively. sTfR, soluble transferrin receptor.

However, it should be noted that there are caveats in using reticulocyte hemoglobin content because α thalassemia minor (very common in patients) and β thalassemia trait have been associated with decreased hemoglobin content of reticulocytes.[46,47] These traits must be ruled out to appropriately interpret reticulocyte hemoglobin content for the diagnosis of iron deficiency.

Because soluble transferrin receptor level can be measured on automated chemistry analyzers, rapid assessment of iron deficiency can be determined by a combination of ferritin and reticulocyte hemoglobin content determinations.[48–50] However, future studies are needed to determine if this newer approach in assessing iron deficiency can lead to changes in treating and diagnosing pediatric patients with these disorders.

Immature Platelet Fraction and Thrombopoietic Activity

Reticulated platelets are increased in patients with thrombocytopenia. Methods such as flow cytometry, which have been used to accurately enumerate reticulated platelets, require specialized equipment and are labor intensive. Recent advances in reticulocyte enumeration by hematology analyzers have allowed identification of an immature platelet fraction (IPF) corresponding to a population of reticulated platelets determined by flow cytometry. Once this was realized, adult and pediatric patients with acute or chronic idiopathic thrombocytopenic purpura (acute idiopathic thrombocytopenic purpura or chronic idiopathic thrombocytopenic purpura) could easily be identified by their elevated IPF.[51] This elevated IPF was in contrast to pediatric patients with nonproliferative thrombocytopenia, who demonstrated a decreased IPF.[52] Several studies have now demonstrated the utility of the IPF as a marker for thrombopoietic activity after hematopoietic progenitor stem cell transplantation[53] or recovery from chemotherapy in children.[54] In an interesting study, platelet concentrates from donors with low (0.3%–3.5%) versus high IPF (3.6%–7.0%) were given to pediatric patients undergoing hematopoietic recovery following autologous hematopoietic progenitor stem cell transplantation. The pediatric patients who receive platelet concentrates with higher IPF% required significantly fewer platelet transfusions and had overall a decreased number of episodes of minor and major hemorrhage.[55] The use of absolute immature platelet count similar to the use of absolute reticulocyte count to follow erythropoiesis in severe aplastic anemia patients has been found useful in thrombocytopenic patients receiving platelet transfusion.[56,57] Critically important is the development of pediatric reference intervals, which can potentially improve evaluation of thrombopoiesis in patients with nonproliferative thrombocytopenia.[58]

Immature Granulocyte Count

Given the ability of current hematology analyzers to discriminate between different granulocyte populations, many studies performed in adults have supported the use of the immature granulocyte count as a substitute for a manual differential in the evaluation for sepsis.[17,59] Traditionally, the elevated band percentage in patients less than 3 months old has been found to be a useful diagnostic marker for neonatal sepsis[20]; this is of interest because no current hematology analyzer has the ability to discriminate between band and segmented neutrophils. In addition, band counting is very imprecise and labor intensive, involving manual differentials of typically only 100 cells. In a Q-Probe study by the College of American Pathologist, a wide variation on band percentage was reported by laboratories despite explicit definitions of band neutrophil appearance.[20] In contrast, the immature granulocyte count has been found in many adult studies to be comparable to manual enumeration with excellent reproducibility.[17,20,59] Several studies have shown that immature granulocyte count may aid in the detection of sepsis in both adults[60–63] and neonates.[16,19,64–66] However, recent studies have suggested that the use of the immature granulocyte count to detect sepsis in neonates or other immunocompromised children has low sensitivity.[19,64]

Table 2 summarizes the potential uses of these newer hematopoietic markers currently available on most hematology analyzers.

OTHER CHALLENGES AND OPPORTUNITIES
Peripheral Smear Review

There has been an increasing challenge to hematology laboratories to reduce laboratory staffing while continuing to provide laboratory testing, particularly smear review, in a timely and accurate manner. The increasing use of information technology has shifted the emphasis from laboratory testing to postanalytical processes of clinical laboratories.[67] However, reviewing peripheral smears is often required for hematologic consultation, which, if requested by hematologists in real-time, can interfere with laboratory operations. Thus, in hospitals with significant hematology and oncology pediatric populations, several laboratory technologists are often devoted to performing manual differentials and RBC and platelet morphology reviews.

Despite the observation that technological advances in automated peripheral smear differential have been in existence since the 1960s, it is only recently within the last 30 years that the technology has advanced sufficiently to become a routine part of hematology laboratories.[26,68–73] However, these early systems (Hematrak 590 and Micro 21) were problematic in terms of slower turn-around time (compared with technologists performing manual differentials), inability for easy integration into automated laboratory systems, and poor cell recognition algorithms. Often, these systems required intervention by medical technologists.[68] Two newer systems, the Cellavision Diffmaster Octavia and the Cellavision DM96, were introduced in 2001 and 2004, respectively, demonstrating good correlation with manual differentials of normal cells and blasts and better turn-around times.[70,71,74]

Regarding pediatric studies, one study compared conventional microscopy versus Cellavision DM96 in 521 newborn and infant slides. This study found that the Cellavision DM96 compared well versus conventional microscopy except for samples containing blasts, in which the percentage of leukemic cells was underestimated. Given the greater degree of morphologic variation in newborn smears compared with adult smears, it was not unexpected that this study found the lowest rates of overall accuracy and postclassification agreement with neonatal samples. The study also found that all red cell pathologies were identified and that this technology was helpful in identifying storage diseases. Overall time savings ranged from 1 to 10 minutes. The instrument was thus helpful in relatively uncomplicated pediatric peripheral smears. However, conventional microscopy continues to be essential in identifying malignant cells and in screening for platelet clumps, which can be a marker of pseudothrombocytopenia.[75] Advantages of using this automated cell identification system for peripheral smear review is the reduction of technologist time needed to perform manual differentials, improvement in consistency of RBC morphologic abnormalities, and the ability for clinicians to remotely review their patient's peripheral smear without having to review the glass smear in person. It also allows the possibility of virtual review of slides by other clinicians/laboratorians.

Handling of Small Blood Samples for Hematological Analysis

Handling of blood samples from newborns and infants is especially challenging because of the use of microtainer tubes due to the practice of minimizing

Table 2
Newer hematopoietic markers available on most current hematology analyzers

Hematopoietic Marker	Reference Intervals?	Potential Uses in Pediatric Patients	Comments	References
Immature granulocyte count	Yes	Neonatal sepsis Bacterial sepsis in older children	Possibly low sensitivity Limited retrospective reports, limitation in immunocompromised children	16,19,64–66 64
		Elimination of need to perform manual differential	Requires physician education; prospective studies needed to show advantage	17,19,59
Reticulocyte hemoglobin content	Yes	Definition of iron deficiency states with sTR/ferritin	Potentially useful, not widely used, although more so with automation of sTR. Future studies needed to determine if new approach can lead to improved changes in treatment. Often used without sTR/ferritin Caution in patients with other disease states that may lower values (eg, thalassemia)[48,49]	29,32,39,43–45,50
		Assessment of functional iron deficiency during recombinant human erythropoietin	Used in some centers	38
		Response to iron therapy	Used in some centers	40–42
IPF	Yes	Characterization of thrombopoietic activity in nonproliferative vs proliferative thrombocytopenia	Used in some centers	51,52
		Return of thrombopoietic activity after chemotherapy or hematopoietic progenitor cell transplantation	Not widely used, given other CBC parameters already being used	53,54
		Assessment of thrombopoietic activity in the presence of platelet transfusions (use of the absolute immature platelet count)	As above	56,57
		Selection of high IPF platelet donors for platelet transfusion in thrombocytopenic patients	Requires additional investigation	55

Abbreviation: sTR, soluble transferrin receptor.
Data from Refs.[16,17,19,29,32,38–45,50–57,59]

phlebotomy-associated blood loss. The currently available laboratory robotic systems and hematology analyzers do not readily process microtainer tubes automatically, including slide preparation and staining. In addition, automated slide maker and stainers require manual adjustment for pediatric specimens with variably high hematocrit. Tube holders for microtainer tubes are also not readily available. Thus, there is continued need for technological improvements to standardize processing, reduce turnaround time, and eliminate laboratory errors using an automated laboratory system. Current handling of pediatric specimens, especially from neonates, is very labor intensive with the potential for error.

In the future, technological improvements in imaging techniques and microfluidic technology may allow improved point-of-care testing, decreased blood use, and improved turn-around time in cellular analysis.[76,77]

Laboratory Interpretation: Accurate Reference Intervals Are Essential

Dramatic changes occur in pediatric hematologic indices, especially during the neonatal period; thus, establishment of pediatric reference ranges ranging from birth to adolescence is important for clinical interpretation. Although several studies have been published, many of these studies have been performed using older instrumentation and involving demographic populations that are unlikely to be representative today. In addition, performing pediatric reference interval studies is difficult for several reasons. One reason is the lack of a valid ethical rationale in performing a blood draw (which may be associated with pain and hematomas) in a healthy child. Drawing an extra sample may entail additional multiple sticks and result in additional pain and unjustified additional blood loss. For example, if an additional 1 mL of EDTA whole blood is drawn, this would constitute 0.33 mL/kg in a 3 kg neonate versus 0.014 mL/kg in a 70 kg adult man. In neonates, performing extra blood draws would be difficult without institutional review board approval. Thus, current ethical considerations make drawing blood from children, especially healthy neonates, for the development of reference intervals very difficult.

Many laboratories therefore use published reference intervals instead of developing pediatric reference intervals. In a recent College of American Pathologists Q-Probes study, 90% of laboratories relied on published sources to establish pediatric hematologic reference intervals.[78] One of the problems in using published reference intervals is that reference intervals are technology dependent. Many published reference intervals were developed using instrumentation that is no longer widely used. Another confounding factor is that many of the newer hematology analyzers have greater precision and accuracy than those in use 20 to 30 years ago. From an analytical standpoint, this would likely broaden the reference interval. Although many manufacturers have established their own reference intervals, most do not include reference intervals for children, especially neonates. Although hematology analyte harmonization would be useful, because reference intervals developed on one hematology analyzer platform could be translated to an equivalent analyte on an another hematology analyzer platform, different technologies for cellular analysis may prohibit complete translation from one platform to another. For example, a recent analysis of multiple hematology analyzers in platelet count enumeration on apheresis platelets found significant differences between instruments.[79]

One statistical approach in generating reference intervals uses the Hoffmann approximation, using leftover CBC samples from selected nonhematology/oncology, nonhospitalized children to generate reference intervals.[80] By using this approach, Soldin and colleagues[28] developed pediatric hematology reference intervals using a variety of hematology analyzers. However, the Hoffmann approximation has been criticized in that the reference intervals generated generally tend to be tighter than those obtained using standard population statistics.[81]

Another serious problem with most of the published pediatric reference intervals is the lack of information on sampling site (especially for neonates), gestational age/birth weight (especially for neonates), and ethnicity of subjects. Preterm infants, for example, have different hematology values compared with term infants. Preterm infants have lower hemoglobin and hematocrit values, higher MCV values, and lower WBC count (30%–50% lower) compared with term infants. Thus, caution should be used when using reference intervals for neonates because this may lead to error in diagnosing anemia, resulting in unnecessary laboratory evaluation, requiring additional blood samples that will, in turn, lead to worsening of the anemia. In addition, significant ethnic differences in hematologic values are well known. For example, hemoglobin, hematocrit, and MCV values are lower in African American infants and children than in Caucasian infants and children.[82,83] This finding is likely related to the greater prevalence of thalassemia in the African American population.[84]

In addition, as mentioned above, there is significant variability in blood source composition. For example, venous and arterial blood is significantly different in hematologic parameters compared with capillary blood. Current laboratory information systems often do not incorporate these preanalytical considerations when reporting reference intervals. Another challenge in using pediatric reference intervals is the need for age stratification. As many as 11 age-specific intervals may have to be used to adequately describe age-specific changes in hematologic parameters.[28] Furthermore, as mentioned previously, the lack of harmonization between hematology analyzers may not necessarily translate to adequate age-specific reference intervals from one analyzer to the next, given the continued divergence in hematology analyzer technology.[24]

Defining Critical Hematologic Tests and Values

There is no clear recommendation as to which hematology tests are critical or what value constitutes a critical result in pediatric patients. Critical tests are defined by the Joint Commission as assays that must be reported back to the clinician by the laboratory, irrespective of the result. Critical values are defined by each laboratory to ensure essential communication of important laboratory results back to the clinician. Timeliness of reporting critical values must be monitored. Performance improvement is required if quality thresholds are not achieved. Although critical values do exist for many hematologic analytes, there are no published pediatric guidelines for hematologic critical values. A College of American Pathologists Q-Probes analysis of 623 institutions found that only a few institutions have developed pediatric critical values for different age groups or for neonates.[85–87] Because many critical values for children have been derived from the adult literature, and, in general, are more conservative than adult values, many noncritical results are often reported as critical, resulting in an unnecessary workload for laboratory staff and increased burden to clinical staff for additional patient evaluation.

Challenges with Specimen Identification

Correct specimen identification can be problematic with pediatric hematology specimens. In adults and older children, the MCV is a very stable parameter and can be used to determine whether there is a problem with specimen identity. Unfortunately, there are significant and rapid hematologic changes that occur at birth and in the following weeks rendering using the MCV inadequate for specimen identification via delta checking in the neonatal period.[28] Thus, hematologic delta checking for very young children cannot be used reliably to identify errors in specimen processing, including specimen collection, handling, and labeling. The only adequate solutions have been the use of adequate procedures and techniques for proper identification and labeling of specimens.

REFERENCES

1. Palis J, Segel GB. Hematology of the fetus and newborn. In: Kaushansky K, Lichtman MA, Beutler E, et al, editors. Williams hematology. 8th edition. New York: McGraw-Hill; 2011. p. 87–104.
2. Wong EC, Luban NL. Hematology and oncology. In: Slonim AS, Pollack MM, editors. Pediatric critical care medicine. Philadelphia: Lippincott, Williams and Wilkins; 2006. p. 157–95.
3. Proytcheva MA. Issues in neonatal cellular analysis. Am J Clin Pathol 2009;131: 560–73.
4. Rosebraugh MR, Widness JA, Nalbant D, et al. A mathematical modeling approach to quantify the role of phlebotomy losses and need for transfusions in neonatal anemia. Transfusion 2013;53:1353–60.
5. Hopfer SM, Nadeau FL, Sundra M, et al. Effect of protein on hemoglobin and hematocrit assays with a conductivity-based point-of-care testing device: comparison with optical methods. Ann Clin Lab Sci 2004;34:75–82.
6. Paes B, Janes M, Vegh P, et al. A comparative study of heel-stick devices for infant blood collection. Am J Dis Child 1993;147:346–8.
7. Linderkamp O, Versmold HT, Strohhacker I, et al. Capillary-venous hematocrit differences in newborn infants, I: relationship to blood volume, peripheral blood flow, and acid base parameters. Eur J Pediatr 1977;127:9–14.
8. Christensen RD, Rothstein G. Pitfalls in the interpretation of leukocyte counts of newborn infants. Am J Clin Pathol 1979;72:608–11.
9. Ozyurek E, Cetinta S, Ceylan T, et al. Complete blood count parameters for healthy, small-for-gestational-age, full-term newborns. Clin Lab Haematol 2006; 28:97–104.
10. Kayiran SM, Ozbek N, Turan M, et al. Significant differences between capillary and venous complete blood counts in the neonatal period. Clin Lab Haematol 2003;25:9–16.
11. Christensen RD, editor. Hematologic problems of the neonate. Philadelphia: Saunders; 2000.
12. Thurlbeck SM, McIntosh N. Preterm blood counts vary with sampling site. Arch Dis Child 1987;62:74–5.
13. Bath PM, Butterworth RJ. Platelet size: measurement, physiology and vascular disease. Blood Coagul Fibrinolysis 1996;7:157–61.
14. Hutton EK, Hassan ES. Late vs early clamping of the umbilical cord in full-term neonates: systematic review and meta-analysis of controlled trials. JAMA 2007; 297:1241–52.
15. Ceriani Cernadas JM, Carroli G, Pellegrini L, et al. The effect of timing of cord clamping on neonatal venous hematocrit values and clinical outcome at term: a randomized, controlled trial. Pediatrics 2006;117:e779–86.
16. Celik IH, Demirel G, Aksoy HT, et al. Automated determination of neutrophil VCS parameters in diagnosis and treatment efficacy of neonatal sepsis. Pediatr Res 2012;71:121–5.
17. Fernandes B, Hamaguchi Y. Automated enumeration of immature granulocytes. Am J Clin Pathol 2007;128:454–63.

18. Beyrau M, Bodkin JV, Nourshargh S. Neutrophil heterogeneity in health and disease: a revitalized avenue in inflammation and immunity. Open Biol 2012;2: 120134. http://dx.doi.org/10.1098/rsob.120134.

19. Nigro KG, O'Riordan M, Molloy EJ, et al. Performance of an automated immature granulocyte count as a predictor of neonatal sepsis. Am J Clin Pathol 2005;123: 618–24.

20. Cornbleet PJ. Clinical utility of the band count. Clin Lab Med 2002;22:101–36.

21. Zandecki M, Genevieve F, Gerard J, et al. Spurious counts and spurious results on haematology analysers: a review. Part I: platelets. Int J Lab Hematol 2007;29:4–20.

22. Zandecki M, Genevieve F, Gerard J, et al. Spurious counts and spurious results on haematology analysers: a review. Part II: white blood cells, red blood cells, haemoglobin, red cell indices and reticulocytes. Int J Lab Hematol 2007;29:21–41.

23. Vajpayee N, Graham SS, Bem S. Basic examination of blood and bone marrow. In: McPherson RA, Pincus MR, editors. Henry's Clinical Diagnosis and Management by Laboratory Methods. 22nd edition. Philadelphia: WB Saunders; 2011. p. 509–35.

24. Buttarello M, Plebani M. Automated blood cell counts: state of the art. Am J Clin Pathol 2008;130:104–16.

25. Schoorl M, Schoorl M, Oomes J, et al. New fluorescent method (PLT-F) on Sysmex XN2000 hematology analyzer achieved higher accuracy in low platelet counting. Am J Clin Pathol 2013;140:495–9.

26. Bentley SA, Johnson A, Bishop CA. A parallel evaluation of four automated hematology analyzers. Am J Clin Pathol 1993;100:626–32.

27. Bourner G, Dhaliwal J, Sumner J. Performance evaluation of the latest fully automated hematology analyzers in a large, commercial laboratory setting: a 4-way, side-by-side study. Lab Hematol 2005;11:285–97.

28. Soldin SJ, Wong EC, Brugnara C, et al, editors. Pediatric reference intervals. 7th edition. Washington, DC: AACC Press; 2011.

29. Brugnara C, Schiller B, Moran J. Reticulocyte hemoglobin equivalent (Ret He) and assessment of iron-deficient states. Clin Lab Haematol 2006;28:303–8.

30. Mouzinho A, Rosenfeld CR, Sanchez PJ, et al. Revised reference ranges for circulating neutrophils in very-low-birth-weight neonates. Pediatrics 1994;94:76–82.

31. Maconi M, Rolfo A, Cardaropoli S, et al. Hematologic values in healthy and small for gestational age newborns. Lab Hematol 2005;11:152–6.

32. Osta V, Caldirola MS, Fernandez M, et al. Utility of new mature erythrocyte and reticulocyte indices in screening for iron-deficiency anemia in a pediatric population. Int J Lab Hematol 2013;35:400–5.

33. Forestier F, Daffos F, Catherine N, et al. Developmental hematopoiesis in normal human fetal blood. Blood 1991;77:2360–3.

34. Christensen RD, Jopling J, Henry E, et al. The erythrocyte indices of neonates, defined using data from over 12,000 patients in a multihospital health care system. J Perinatol 2008;28:24–8.

35. Schelonka RL, Yoder BA, desJardins SE, et al. Peripheral leukocyte count and leukocyte indexes in healthy newborn term infants. J Pediatr 1994;125:603–6.

36. Aldrimer M, Ridefelt P, Rödöö P, et al. Population-based pediatric reference intervals for hematology, iron and transferrin. Scand J Clin Lab Invest 2013;73: 253–61.

37. Finn LS, Hall J, Xu M, et al. Flow cytometric validation of automated differentials in pediatric patients. Lab Hematol 2004;10:112–8.

38. Brugnara C, Colella GM, Cremins J, et al. Effects of subcutaneous recombinant-human-erythropoietin in normal subjects – development of decreased

reticulocyte hemoglobin content and iron-deficient erythropoiesis. J Lab Clin Med 1994;123:660–7.

39. Ullrich C, Wu A, Armsby C, et al. Screening healthy infants for iron deficiency using reticulocyte hemoglobin content. JAMA 2005;294:924–30.

40. Brugnara C, Laufer MR, Friedman AI, et al. Reticulocyte hemoglobin content (Chr) – early indicator of response to iron therapy. Blood 1993;82:A93.

41. Brugnara C, Zelmanovic D, Sorette M, et al. Reticulocyte hemoglobin: an integrated parameter for evaluation of erythropoietic activity. Am J Clin Pathol 1997;108:133–42.

42. Thomas C, Thomas L. Biochemical markers and hematologic indices in the diagnosis of functional iron deficiency. Clin Chem 2002;48:1066–76.

43. Piva E, Brugnara C, Chiandetti L, et al. Automated reticulocyte counting: state of the art and clinical applications in the evaluation of erythropoiesis. Clin Chem Lab Med 2010;48:1369–80.

44. Canals C, Remacha AF, Sarda MP, et al. Clinical utility of the new Sysmex XE 2100 parameter – reticulocyte hemoglobin equivalent in the diagnosis of anemia. Haematologica 2005;90:1133–4.

45. Thomas L, Franck S, Messinger M, et al. Reticulocyte hemoglobin measurement – comparison of two methods in the diagnosis of iron-restricted erythropoiesis. Clin Chem Lab Med 2005;43:1193–202.

46. Mast AE, Blinder MA, Dietzen DJ. Reticulocyte hemoglobin content. Am J Hematol 2008;83:307–10.

47. Bartels PC, Schoorl M. Hemoglobinization and functional availability of iron for erythropoiesis in case of thalassemia and iron deficiency anemia. Clin Lab 2006;52:107–14.

48. Vernet M, Doyen C. Assessment of iron status with a new fully automated assay for transferrin receptor in human serum. Clin Chem Lab Med 2000;38: 437–42.

49. Pfeiffer CM, Cook JD, Mei Z, et al. Evaluation of an automated soluble transferrin receptor (sTfR) assay on the Roche Hitachi analyzer and its comparison to two ELISA assays. Clin Chim Acta 2007;382(1–2):112–6.

50. Skikne BS, Punnonen K, Caldron PH, et al. Improved differential diagnosis of anemia of chronic disease and iron deficiency anemia: a prospective multicenter evaluation of soluble transferrin receptor and the sTfR/log ferritin index. Am J Hematol 2011;86:923–7.

51. Kickler TS, Oguni S, Borowitz MJ. A clinical evaluation of high fluorescent platelet fraction percentage in thrombocytopenia. Am J Clin Pathol 2006;125:282–7.

52. Strauss G, Vollert C, von Stackelberg A, et al. Immature platelet count: a simple parameter for distinguishing thrombocytopenia in pediatric acute lymphocytic leukemia from immune thrombocytopenia. Pediatr Blood Cancer 2011;57:641–7.

53. Hennel E, Kentouche K, Beck J, et al. Immature platelet fraction as marker for platelet recovery after stem cell transplantation in children. Clin Biochem 2012; 45:749–52.

54. Have LW, Hasle H, Vestergaard EM, et al. Absolute immature platelet count may predict imminent platelet recovery in thrombocytopenic children following chemotherapy. Pediatr Blood Cancer 2013;60:1198–203.

55. Parco S, Vascotto F. Application of reticulated platelets to transfusion management during autologous stem cell transplantation. Onco Targets Ther 2012;5:1–5.

56. Bat T, Leitman SF, Calvo KR, et al. Measurement of the absolute immature platelet number reflects marrow production and is not impacted by platelet transfusion. Transfusion 2013;53:1201–4.

57. Saigo K, Sakota Y, Masuda Y, et al. Automatic detection of immature platelets for decision making regarding platelet transfusion indications for pediatric patients. Transfus Apher Sci 2008;38:127–32.
58. Seo A, Yuan D, Daniels S, et al. Reference intervals for immature platelet fraction and immature platelet count. Int J Lab Hematol 2014. http://dx.doi.org/10.1111/ijlh.12237.
59. Senthilnayagam B, Kumar T, Sukumaran J, et al. Automated measurement of immature granulocytes: performance characteristics and utility in routine clinical practice. Patholog Res Int 2012;2012:483670. http://dx.doi.org/10.1155/2012/483670.
60. Park DH, Park K, Park J, et al. Screening of sepsis using leukocyte cell population data from the Coulter automatic blood cell analyzer DxH800. Int J Lab Hematol 2011;33:391–9.
61. Ansari-Lari MA, Kickler TS, Borowitz MJ. Immature granulocyte measurement using the Sysmex XE-2100. Relationship to infection and sepsis. Am J Clin Pathol 2003;120:795–9.
62. Kim HW, Yoon JH, Jin SJ, et al. Delta neutrophil index as a prognostic marker of early mortality in gram negative bacteremia. Infect Chemother 2014;46(2):94–102.
63. Chaves F, Tierno B, Xu D. Quantitative determination of neutrophil VCS parameters by the Coulter automated hematology analyzer: new and reliable indicators for acute bacterial infection. Am J Clin Pathol 2005;124:440–4.
64. Ahn JG, Choi SY, Kim DS, et al. Limitation of the delta neutrophil index for assessing bacteraemia in immunocompromised children. Clin Chim Acta 2014;436:319–22.
65. Cimenti C, Erwa W, Herkner KR, et al. The predictive value of immature granulocyte count and immature myeloid information in the diagnosis of neonatal sepsis. Clin Chem Lab Med 2012;50:1429–32.
66. Hornik CP, Benjamin DK, Becker KC, et al. Use of the complete blood cell count in early-onset neonatal sepsis. Pediatr Infect Dis J 2012;31:799–802.
67. Bossuyt X, Verweire K, Blanckaert N. Laboratory medicine: challenges and opportunities. Clin Chem 2007;53:1730–3.
68. Tatsumi N, Pierre RV. Automated image processing. Past, present, and future of blood cell morphology identification. Clin Lab Med 2002;22:299–315, viii.
69. Houwen B. The differential cell count. Lab Hematol 2001;7:89–100.
70. Swolin B, Simonsson P, Backman S, et al. Differential counting of blood leukocytes using automated microscopy and a decision support system based on artificial neural networks–evaluation of DiffMaster Octavia. Clin Lab Haematol 2003;25:139–47.
71. Kratz A, Bengtsson H, Casey JE, et al. Performance evaluation of the CellaVisionDM96 system. WBC differentials by automated digital image analysis supported by an artificial neural network. Am J Clin Pathol 2005;124:770–81.
72. National Committee for Clinical Laboratory Standards. H20-A reference leukocyte differential count (proportional) and evaluation of instrumental methods; approved standard. Natl Committee Clin Lab Stand 1992;17:1–33.
73. Bland JM, Altman DG. Statistical methods for assessing agreement between two methods of clinical measurement. Lancet 1986;1:307–10.
74. Ceelie H, Dinkelaar RB, van Gelder W. Examination of peripheral blood films using automated microscopy; evaluation of Diffmaster Octavia and Cellavision DM96. J Clin Pathol 2006;60:72–9.

75. Billard M, Lainey E, Armoogum P, et al. Evaluation of the CellaVision DM automated microscope in pediatrics. Int J Lab Hematol 2010;32:530–8.
76. Smith ZJ, Gao T, Chu K, et al. Single-step preparation and image-based counting of minute volumes of human blood. Lab Chip 2014;14:3029–36.
77. Hollis VS, Holloway JA, Harris S, et al. Comparison of venous and capillary differential leukocyte counts using a standard hematology analyzer and a novel microfluidic impedance cytometer. PLoS One 2012;7:e43702.
78. Friedberg RC, Souers R, Wagar EA, et al. The origin of reference intervals. Arch Pathol Lab Med 2007;131:348–57.
79. Moroff G, Sowemimo-Coker SO, Finch S, et al. The influence of various hematology analyzers on component platelet counts. Transfus Med Rev 2005;19:155–66.
80. Hoffmann RG. Statistics in the practice of medicine. JAMA 1963;185:864–73.
81. Shaw JL, Cohen A, Konforte D, et al. Validity of establishing pediatric reference intervals based on hospital patient data: a comparison of the modified Hoffmann approach to CALIPER reference intervals obtained in healthy children. Clin Biochem 2014;47:166–72.
82. Alur P, Devapatla SS, Super DM, et al. Impact of race and gestational age on red blood cell indices in very low birth weight infants. Pediatrics 2000;106:306–10.
83. Cheng CK, Chan J, Cembrowski GS, et al. Complete blood count reference interval diagrams derived from NHANES III stratification by age, sex, and race. Lab Hematol 2004;10:42–53.
84. Modell B, Darlison M. Global epidemiology of haemoglobin disorders and derived service indicators. Bull World Health Organ 2008;86:480–7.
85. Howanitz PJ, Steindel SJ, Heard NV. Laboratory critical values policies and procedures: a College of American Pathologists Q-Probes study in 623 institutions. Arch Pathol Lab Med 2002;126:663–9.
86. Emancipator K. Critical values: ASCP practice parameter: American Society of Clinical Pathologists. Am J Clin Pathol 1997;108:247–53.
87. Kost GJ. Critical limits for emergency clinician notification at United States children's hospitals. Pediatrics 1991;88:597–603.

Verification and Standardization of Blood Cell Counters for Routine Clinical Laboratory Tests

Sue Ellen Verbrugge, PhD, Albert Huisman, PhD, PharmD*

KEYWORDS

- Validation • Verification • Standardization • Automated blood cell counter
- Hematology analyzers • Clinical hematology laboratory

KEY POINTS

- Verification of an automated blood cell counter (hematology analyzer) can be done according to the Clinical and Laboratory Standards Institute or the International Committee for Standardization in Haematology guidelines depending on the preference of the laboratory professional.
- For complete blood count parameters, a limited number of partially outdated reference methods is available; there is a need for updated methods for established parameters and reference methods for new parameters.
- International standardization of reporting units is desirable.

INTRODUCTION

Automated blood cell counters (or automated hematology analyzers [HAs]) belong to the standard inventory of most medical diagnostic laboratories worldwide and are a valuable tool in the laboratory diagnostic process. HAs are capable of measuring the concentration of hemoglobin (Hb) and of counting and identifying blood cells and blood cell characteristics. This measurement is frequently referred to as the complete blood count (CBC) and is often used as a screening tool in health and disease. In addition, the CBC is used to observe or monitor certain patient characteristics (ie, medical conditions or treatments) over time, and reported values that are related to these characteristics serve as a basis for interventions and treatments. A typical example of such a parameter is the level of Hb, which is the main determinant in blood

Financial disclosure/conflict of interest: The authors have nothing to disclose.
Department of Clinical Chemistry and Haematology, University Medical Center Utrecht, PO Box: 85500, Utrecht 3508 GA, The Netherlands
* Corresponding author.
E-mail address: a.huisman@umcutrecht.nl

Clin Lab Med 35 (2015) 183–196
http://dx.doi.org/10.1016/j.cll.2014.10.008
0272-2712/15/$ – see front matter © 2015 Elsevier Inc. All rights reserved.

Abbreviations	
µL	Microliter
AMI	Analytical measuring interval
CBC	Complete blood count
CD	Cluster of differentiation
CLSI	Clinical and Laboratory Standards Institute
CRI	Clinically reportable interval
dL	Deciliter
FDA	US Food and Drug Administration
g	Gram
HA	Automated hematology analyzers
Hb	Hemoglobin
ICSH	International Committee for Standardization in Haematology
ISLH	International Society for Laboratory Hematology
L	Liter
MCV	Mean cell volume
mmol	Millimole
MPV	Mean platelet volume
NRBC	Nucleated red blood cell
PCV	Packed cell volume
RBC	Red blood cell
RDW	Red cell distribution width
WBC	White blood cell

transfusions. In the production and design of an HA, it is standard procedure that an initial validation is performed by the manufacturer, and this is often also required by national (eg, the Food and Drug Administration [FDA] in the United States) or international regulations (eg, in the in vitro diagnostic device directives in the European Union). The objective of this validation process is to ensure that the manufacturer's claims on the performance of the HA are valid, and it includes a comparison of the current HA with a previous generation instrument. When a diagnostic laboratory acquires a new HA, or updates its current HA to a more modern model, a verification process (also referred to as a validation process) should be performed in which it is shown that the HA meets requirements and predefined criteria that are specifically set for this laboratory method. In addition to validation and verification, standardization also plays an important role in CBC parameters. Some of these parameters are based on a standard reference method that is universal and independent of the type of HA used, and other CBC parameters are reported by most manufacturers and are therefore considered more or less universal, whereas they may not officially be standardized. The latter group of parameters lead to an increased risk of interlaboratory differences. In addition, there are CBC parameters that are not universal or standardized but depend on the brand or type of HA, and these produce different results on different instruments.

Standards and Guidelines for Hematologic Laboratory Testing

There are several organizations that operate nationally or internationally to develop consensus standards and guidelines intended to prevent broad discrepancies in laboratory testing and documentation. These organizations include the World Health Organization, the International Organization for Standardization, the European and International Conference on Harmonization, and the FDA. In addition, The International Committee for Standardization in Haematology (ICSH) and the Clinical and Laboratory Standards Institute (CLSI), have recently developed and published guidelines and standards for validation and verification of HA, which are discussed in this article.[1,2] These guidelines are entitled "Validation, Verification, and Quality Assurance of Automated Hematology Analyzers," published by CLSI in 2010, and the "ICSH Guidelines for the Evaluation of Blood Cell Analyzers Including Those Used for Differential Leukocyte and Reticulocyte Counting," published by ICSH in 2014.[1,2] The use of a particular guideline is voluntary and puts the responsibility for performing these recommendations solely on the manufacturer and the end user. According to the ISO15189, a clinical laboratory accreditation program, a certain level of verification of any new HA has to be done according to a professional standard. It also stimulates laboratories to take patients' risk factors into consideration to meet these standards.[3]

This article provides an overview of the evaluation steps for HA that are important in a diagnostic laboratory, and discusses issues concerning standardization of various clinically important CBC parameters.

VALIDATION AND VERIFICATION

The CBC encompasses several parameters, including white blood cell (WBC) count, red blood cell (RBC) count, mean cell volume (MCV), hemoglobin (Hb) concentration, and platelet count (or thrombocyte count), amongst others. In addition, the nucleated red blood cells (NRBCs) and reticulocytes are also sometimes regarded as standard parameters of the CBC. **Table 1** provides an overview of parameters that are either measured or calculated in HA, including the units in which they are reported. These parameters are not discussed in full detail here but should, if applicable, all be included in a validation or verification process.

The Preanalytical Process

Preanalytical standardization and control are essential in generating and reporting accurate clinical and diagnostically relevant patient results. Therefore, the preanalytical part of CBC determination (ie, the blood-drawing process and all issues directly and indirectly related to this process) is also part of the validation and verification process. Venous or capillary blood subjected to a CBC should be drawn according to the available international guidelines (eg, CLSI document H03 and CLSI document H04) and furthermore in accordance with existing local agreements and procedures.[4,5] In specimen collection there are several items that need to be taken into account (**Table 2**). These items are requirements for blood samples used in the diagnostic process and also apply to a validation or verification protocol, because they could lead to different results when comparing two HAs.

In general, when performing a validation and verification process, essential components and results of the same blood samples are measured on different HAs and the results are compared. The most important preanalytical variable in this respect is time, because time-dependent alterations in CBC parameters may occur, because the CBC is measured on viable blood cells that undergo time-dependent degenerative processes. The most remarkable time-dependent changes include changes in blood cell volume (increase in MCV, mean platelet volume [MPV]) and WBC differential caused by morphologic alterations that can be observed by reference microscopy, but other time-dependent alterations may also be observed.[8–12] Therefore, the time between the drawing of blood and the measurement on the HAs should be monitored closely during a validation and verification process. Sample testing should occur within 4 to 8 hours after venipuncture and a comparison between two HAs should be made within a 4-hour time frame so that the compared samples are as similar as possible. Both the ICSH and the CLSI provide detailed guidelines on interfering

Table 1
CBC parameters determined by HA

Parameter	Description	Reporting Units
WBC count	Number of WBCs (or leucocytes) per volume blood	Number (usually $\times 10^9$)/L or number (usually $\times 10^3$)/μL
	WBC differential count: Usually 5-part differential[a]: Lymphocytes Monocytes Neutrophil granulocytes Eosinophil granulocytes Basophil granulocytes	Number (usually $\times 10^9$)/L or number (usually 10^3)/μL Or percentage of total WBC count
RBC count	Number of RBC (or erythrocytes) per volume blood	Number (usually $\times 10^{12}$)/L
MCV	Average volume of RBC	fL
MCH	Average amount of Hb per RBC	pg or fmol
MCHC	Average concentration of Hb in RBC	g/dL, g/L, or mmol/L
RDW	The variation of cellular volume of the RBC population	%CV or fL
Hematocrit	Fraction of whole blood that consists of RBC, sometimes also referred as PCV	% or L/L
Hb concentration	Hb concentration in blood	g/dL, g/L, or mmol/L
Platelet count	Number of platelets (or thrombocytes) per volume blood	Number (usually $\times 10^9$)/L or number (usually 10^3)/μL
MPV	Average volume of a platelet	fL
Reticulocyte count	Number of reticulocytes per volume blood	Number (usually $\times 10^9$)/L or as % of RBC count
NRBC	Number of NRBCs (also called erythroblasts or normoblasts) per volume blood	Number (usually $\times 10^9$)/L but may also be reported as number or % per 100 WBCs

Abbreviations: fL, femtoliter ($\times 10^{-15}$ L); fmol, femtomol ($\times 10^{-15}$ mol); MCH, mean cell Hb; MCHC, mean cell Hb concentration; MPV, mean platelet volume; pg, picogram ($\times 10^{-12}$ g); RDW, red cell distribution width; %CV, % coefficient of variation.

[a] Sometimes the WBC differential count consists of a 2-part WBC differential count (ie, monocytes and lymphocytes combined; sometimes referred to as mononuclear cells or agranulocytes) and granulocytes (combination of neutrophil granulocytes, eosinophil granulocytes, and basophil granulocytes). This combination is also called polymorphonuclear leukocytes/cells; a 3 part WBC differential count (lymphocytes, monocytes, and granulocytes); or an extra WBC differential category is added: immature granulocytes. There are numerous other parameters also reported by some HA, examples of these parameters include immature neutrophil granulocytes, hyperchromic RBCs and hypochromic RBCs, microcytic RBCs and macrocytic RBCs, fragmented RBCs, immature reticulocytes, reticulocyte Hb content, and reticulated (or immature) platelets. The nomenclature and definition may vary depending on the type of HA.

substances, ranging from lipid to clot interference; these are beyond the scope of this article (exclusion criteria, intrinsic interferences). For an extensive review on spurious CBC results caused by interference, the reader is referred to Zandecki and colleagues.[13,14] The measurements are performed in de-identified surplus blood that remains after all other laboratory testing has been conducted. Specifically, on material which would otherwise have been discarded.

Table 2
Standard procedures and considerations in specimen collection

Item	Description
Tourniquet technique	Tourniquet should be applied immediately before venipuncture and released instantly after puncture (within 1 min) after blood flow to prevent hemoconcentration[6]
Anticoagulant	K-EDTA should be used; either K2-EDTA (preference of CLSI guideline) or K2-EDTA or K3-EDTA (ICSH guideline). The anticoagulant should remain the same throughout the full validation/verification process and routine use thereafter because changes in anticoagulant may lead to changes in reported CBC results[7]
Mixing of tubes	Collection tubes should be mixed immediately after filling; at least 8–10 complete inversions, to prevent clotting
Order of tube draw	The EDTA tube usually is one of the last tubes that is drawn, depending on local guidelines
IV lines	Dilution of the sample with IV fluids should be avoided when drawing blood from an IV line, and fluid should be completely discarded
Short draw	This may cause dilution when the EDTA anticoagulant is in liquid form, and alteration of reported CBC parameters may occur because of high EDTA concentration
Blood source	Capillary, arterial, and venous samples may have different concentrations of various CBC parameters
Patient fasting	Food (especially a fatty meal) may interfere with some CBC measurements because of lipemia and chylomicron interference
Specimen identification	Proper patient and positive specimen identification are necessary to prevent CBC reporting errors
Storage and transport	Blood samples should be stored at room temperature and analyzed within 4–8 h after venipuncture

Abbreviations: EDTA, ethylene diamine tetraacetic acid; IV, intravenous.
Data from Refs.[1,4,5]

Instrument Validation by the Manufacturer

The World Health Organization defines validation as "the action or process of proving that a procedure, process, system, equipment, or method used works as expected and achieves the intended results."[15] According to the CLSI standards, the manufacturer of an HA is responsible for setting objectives for the analytical application of an instrument and its performance.[1] These objectives should be investigated, using well-defined testing protocols, and their performance validated against either an accepted reference method or an on-market analyzer if there is no reference methodology. General parameters assessed and included in specimen overview include:

- Limit of blank or background
- Carryover
- Imprecision (reproducibility)
- Analytical measuring interval (AMI) (linearity)
- Lower limit of detection
- Comparability
- Interferences

The CLSI guideline gives a detailed description of the number of measurements and goals that should be achievable.[1] National ethics and standard evaluation organizations determine whether validation studies require patients' consent and an extensive risk analysis should be stipulated with registration of adverse events, if applicable.

Instrument Evaluation by an Independent Organization

There are several stages of evaluation before the implementation of an analyzer by a laboratory. According to the ICSH standards, new instruments could also be evaluated by an independent national organization following the ICSH guidelines, after which the end user has to perform a less extensive evaluation.[2] In countries lacking these official organizations, the end-user laboratory is expected to seek counsel in evaluations published in peer-reviewed journals and to determine its own extent of validation and or verification strategy, depending on its own objectives. Evaluation should include instrument installation, user application, blood samples, and instrumentation evaluation.[2]

Instrument Validation and/or Verification by the End-user Laboratory

ICSH and CLSI guidelines as well as ISO (International Organization for Standardization) 15189 accreditation regulations state that the responsibility for instrument installation, setup, and initial calibration using specified methods lies with the manufacturer. Once this is achieved, the end user should assess whether the manufacturer's claims on performance of the specific instrument also apply to intended-use criteria by the laboratory.[3] This process is usually called verification, but is sometimes also referred to as validation, which may be confusing. The verification includes performance analysis of an HA on:

- Accuracy
- Precision
- Reportable range of test results and reference intervals (normal ranges)
- Background (limit of blank)
- Carryover (sample)
- Lower limits of detection
- Quantitation
- Clinically reportable intervals (CRIs)
- AMI

In general, these items should all be verified by the same procedures as used for validation. Anonymous surplus samples that are available in laboratories can be used to determine short-term and long-term imprecision (reproducibility) verification in which the medical decision levels are eminent. Samples should be selected to ensure that extensive variation of pathologic samples is included in the analysis and samples may be manipulated (eg, diluted) to acquire a broad range of results. **Table 3** provides a condensed overview of the CLSI and ICSH guidelines on verification of HA. The type of laboratory (physician's office laboratory or academic hospital laboratory), its clinical affiliations, and its patient-related population is the primary focus in verification of comparability (correlation). When adopting a new HA it is important to compare this with the existing HA to ensure that patient results are not affected. CLSI standards list a minimum of validation points for mode-to-mode verification comparison with manufacturer's specifications.[1] In terms of interferences, similar rules apply as mentioned before: the user should validate the instrument on interferences that are encountered in practice. For ISO15189 accreditation a laboratory should define the importance of such occurrences based on prior risk analysis. The ISO15189 promotes a "Verification if possible, validation if

Table 3
Comparison of CLSI and ICSH protocols regarding performance evaluation

	CLSI	ICSH
Verification	The laboratory (end user) should follow the procedures of manufacturer validation, but the verification may be abbreviated; the goal is to verify that the manufacturer's stated performance is correct	Verification is conformation of the evaluation performed by the manufacturer or published in the literature; the verification may be abbreviated (ie, focused to meet specific requirements at the test site)
Precision/imprecision (within-run reproducibility; closeness of agreement between test results)	Should be performed with normal samples and samples at medical decision levels available in clinical laboratories. No specifications for number of measurements and reporting	Single run of 10 measurements on the same sample (all reported parameters). 3 levels (normal, abnormal low, and abnormal high, around clinical decision points). Reported as SD and %CV
Precision (between batch, long term)	Should be performed with normal samples and samples at medical decision levels available in clinical laboratories. No specifications for time period and number of measurements	Single sample, repeated daily, for a period of 20–30 d. Three levels (all parameters, abnormal low and abnormal high, around clinical decision points). Fixed blood (control material) may be required
Carryover (contamination by a preceding sample)	For WBC, RBC, Hb, and platelets, 3 high samples followed by 3 low samples	For WBC, Hb, platelets, reticulocytes, and NRBC, 3 high samples followed by 3 low samples
Linearity (linear relationship at various dilutions)	The reportable range (ie, the CRIs) should be established, including a background (LoB) and LoD and AMI	The reportable range (ie, the CRI) should be established, including a background (LoB), LoD, and AMI
Comparability (comparison between evaluation HA and current HA)	Should be performed but not specified, if different modes are available, whether an extensive mode-to-mode comparability should be performed	At least 250–300 samples, measured on both HA with samples with various disorders and with interfering substances
Accuracy (closeness of agreement between measurement and true value)	Should be performed; not otherwise specified	Depending on availability of reference method, often not applicable; in practice often compared with current HA
Reference intervals	Must be established or verified for all reportable parameters	Should be calculated for all components of the CBC; at least 120 samples from apparently healthy individuals (60 male, 60 female)

Abbreviations: LoB, limit of blank; LoD, limit of detection; SD, standard deviation.

Data from Rabinovitch A, Barnes P, Curcio KM, et al. H26-A2: validation, verification, and quality assurance of automated hematology analyzers; approved standard - second edition. CLSI document H26-A2. Wayne (PA): Clinical and Laboratory Standards Institute; 2010; and International Council for Standardization in Haematology. Writing Group, Briggs C, Culp N, Davis B, et al. ICSH guidelines for the evaluation of blood cell analysers including those used for differential leucocyte and reticulocyte counting. Int J Lab Hematol 2014;36:613–27.

necessary" policy.[3] This policy allows end users to determine their own objectives as to the extent of verification or the need for a suitable validation. The 2 guidelines discussed in this article are comparable, not identical, but differences are generally limited. There are differences in terminology and nomenclature. The CLSI directive generally adheres strictly to official nomenclature (eg, measurand instead of parameter, as used by the ICSH guideline and in daily practice) but existing deviations in definitions are also minor. The CLSI guideline is intended for use by HA manufacturers and laboratories (end users), whereas the ICSH guideline is intended for laboratories only.[1,2]

The ICSH guideline is available free via the Web site of the International Journal of Laboratory Hematology (the official journal of the International Society for Laboratory Hematology [ISLH], www.ISLH.org) and via the ICSH Web site (www.ICSH.org). A subscription is needed for the CLSI guideline. The final choice for 1 of 2 guidelines depends on local circumstances and preferences. In addition, it is always possible for a laboratory to deviate from the guidelines for professional reasons.

STANDARDIZATION

Current globalization calls for clinical laboratories across the world to produce standardized results. Worldwide, clinical laboratories operate under different conditions, use different procedures for specimen collection, and run tests using analyzers from different manufacturers. Standardization can only be attained when this is done using the same high level of accuracy, precision, and reproducibility. It depends on reference materials and reference methods/procedures (gold standard) and involves validation, verification, quality assurance, and quality control. Guidelines on standardization of laboratory procedures and analyzers are based on reference materials and methods and are often created by field specialists after careful evaluation.

Current Reference Methods for Automated Hematology Analyzers

For an HA there are only a few reference methods available (**Box 1**). Most reference methods are cumbersome and impractical in daily practice and they can only be used during a verification process.

- For Hb, the reference method is the hemiglobincyanide method.[16,17] Cyanide-containing reagents are no longer in use for various reasons (eg, cyanide toxicity) and have been replaced by alternate methods; therefore, manufacturers must carefully validate their noncyanide methods. Hb is the only parameter of the

---

Box 1
Reference methods available for HA

Available reference methods:

Hemoglobin

PCV

Reticulocyte count

RBC count

WBC count

WBC differential count

Platelet count

CBC for which a reference standard exists and an international Hb standard is available for laboratories, which can be used as a reference in a verification protocol.[18]

- For packed cell volume (PCV), a microhematocrit method is available in which a sample is centrifuged in a glass capillary and then the height of the packed RBC column is measured in relation to the height of the total blood column. The PCV method has some disadvantages (there is a biohazard risk [broken glass capillaries]) and the time since draw can influence the PCV, because the MCV increases with time. In addition, the PCV may be erroneous in cases of aberrant RBC morphology (eg, in sickle cell anemia when the RBC packing of the capillary is unfavorable and may contain a relative large amount of trapped plasma). When using the microhematocrit as a reference method for PCV validation care should be taken to include samples with abnormal MCV and RBC counts.[19,20]
- For the reticulocyte count, a flow cytometric method is described in which the reticulocytes are separated from mature RBCs based on distinct cellular properties, which is more precise than a microscopic method in which the reticulocytes are counted using a vital staining using new methylene blue.[21,22]
- For RBC count and WBC count, a reference method was published in 1994 by an Expert Panel on Cytometry of the ICSH Standards Committee and has been maintained to this day.[23] The method is based on automated cell counting using the impedance principle and this method replaced earlier techniques using a counting chamber in combination with a microscope.
- For WBC differential count, a microscopic manual method is used in which 400 cells are classified, produced from the average of two 200-cell differentials by different experienced and qualified microscopists using a Romanowsky staining method.[24]
- For platelet count, a flow cytometric reference method has been published, based on recognition of platelets by specific monoclonal antibodies. The current reference method for platelet counts, especially in thrombocytopenia, is the use of a selective platelet monoclonal antibody (eg, anti-CD61, anti-CD41a).[25]

Some of the reference methods described earlier are more or less outdated; this is especially true for the RBC and WBC counts and the WBC differential count. For the RBC and WBC counts, the current reference technique is based on the impedance principle and better alternatives for this method are available. A new reference method could be based on optical counting (flow cytometry) in combination with specific fluorescent cluster of differentiation (CD) markers for RBC and WBC. Such a method would have fewer interferences and improved specificity. For the WBC differential, flow cytometry is now a candidate reference method because its accuracy and statistical precision seem to be higher than those of the manual method, but there are still many points to consider.[26] One of the issues regarding this suggested method is the paradigm shift in WBC differential nomenclature from a microscopy-based nomenclature to a CD marker–based nomenclature. Therefore, no definitive reference method has been published to date.

Apart from the parameters discussed here, a schistocyte count (fragmented RBCs, fragmentocytes) has recently been introduced as an HA parameter; however, this parameter is only available on a limited number of HAs.[27,28] Schistocytes are a valuable parameter in the differential diagnosis of thrombotic thrombocytopenic purpura and other pathologic states. The ICSH recently published a guideline on schistocyte enumeration that supports further development of automated schistocyte measurements.[29–31]

Complete Blood Count Parameters for Which No Reference Method Is Available, but for Which This Would Be Desirable

Except for the methods mentioned earlier, no other reference methods are published. Many CBC parameters are clinically relevant and also widely used in scientific research, but there are no reference methods, which can cause differences in clinical interpretation and this may prevent wider use and valid comparison or aggregation of clinical and scientific data. Many clinicians and researchers are not even aware that differences in reported results (eg, between different hospitals) may be caused by different HAs being used. Therefore there is a need for more internationally accepted reference methods, especially for the following clinically relevant parameters:

- The MCV has been widely used clinically since its introduction by Wintrobe[32]; for example, in diagnostic algorithms for anemia, and as a compliance marker for various drugs.[32–34] Differences in MCV can occur because of various analytical interferences.[35] So far, no internationally accepted reference method has been published. However, various manufacturers offer calibration materials, often based on latex particles or fixed RBCs of which the exact volume is known, which have their own disadvantages because they behave differently in an HA in comparison with viable RBCs. The MCV also serves as a source for other (calculated) parameters like the red cell distribution width (RDW). An increase in RDW has been linked to various pathologic states.[36–38] Therefore a reference method would be a step forward.
- Various HAs report derived RBC parameters such as microcytic RBCs and hyperchromic RBCs.[39,40] These extended RBC parameters may be helpful in the work-up of some specific RBC-related disorders. For example, microcytic RBCs may be used in the differential diagnosis of microcytic anemia to distinguish iron deficiency from thalassemia, and hyperchromic RBCs can be used in the diagnosis of hereditary spherocytosis.[41,42] However, the specific nomenclature for the extended RBC parameters, cutoff levels, and measurement method may differ depending on the type of HA used, which may lead to confusion and misclassification when interpreting reported data.
- Reticulocyte Hb content is a parameter generated by some HAs, and this parameter has added value in the diagnosis of functional iron deficiency and other pathologic states, and it even has a place in clinical guidelines on the diagnosis and treatment of iron deficiency in patients on dialysis.[39,40,43–46] However, as with some other reported CBC parameters, the reticulocyte Hb content lacks standardization and has differences in nomenclature, limiting its clinical use.
- The MPV has clinical value in various pathologic states of platelet count and platelet function[39,47,48]; however, the clinical use of MPV (and derived parameters such as platelet distribution width and plateletcrit) is limited by the lack of standardization. At present, the ICSH is working on a guideline for MPV standardization.
- Reticulated platelets are young platelets that still contain some RNA and their levels increase with increasing platelet production by the bone marrow, which makes this parameters usable in thrombocytopenic patients to distinguish peripheral platelet destruction from bone marrow failure syndromes or as a guide in platelet transfusion therapy.[39,48–50] As with the other discussed parameters, the nomenclature may differ depending on the type of HA used, and differences may occur because of different cutoff levels and measurement methods.

Standardization of Reporting Units

The expression of results (reporting units) for CBC parameters is currently not internationally standardized. The ICSH is working on a guideline dealing with the standardization of hematology reporting units but this has to date not been published. Standardization would greatly increase the interchangeability and standardization of CBC results, with many apparent advantages, for example in international exchange of patient results and research data. However, standardization of reporting units is a complex matter involving national and international scientific organizations and regulatory bodies, governmental agencies, clinical practice protocols, studies and trials, medical decisions, and changes in laboratory information systems, among others. Therefore, reaching an agreement on reporting units, even on a national level, is a challenging task that requires compromise. In **Table 1**, different reporting units for the CBC parameters are listed. In the opinion of the authors, for the unit of volume in the reporting of Hb concentration, RBC count, WBC count, and WBC differential count, there is a preference for liters (L) because this is the most universal unit of volume, although it is not an official SI (International System of Units) unit. Other units of volume currently in use, like microliter (μL) or deciliter (dL), are less acceptable. The Hb concentration is currently reported in either millimoles per liter, grams per liter, or grams per deciliter; both gram (g) and millimole (mmol) are official SI units. However, because Hb in the human circulation consists of different molecules (HbA, HbA_2, HbF, pathologic Hb), the relative concentrations of which can vary in different age groups and in various pathologic states, assigning an exact molecular weight to Hb is not possible, although the differences are probably negligible. Therefore, it could be argued that gram is more accurate than mole. It is the expectation of the authors that it will take a long time before a consensus is reached and implemented with respect to this complex issue.

SUMMARY

The validation or verification process of an HA by an end-user laboratory involves issues with regard to the preanalytical and analytical phase, which should be standardized and controlled. There are 2 published guidelines on this subject, both of which contain procedures describing the essential parts of this process. They contain matters that overlap and descriptions of protocols in which deviations for professional reasons are allowed. Regardless, the final choice for one of both guidelines is at the discretion of the laboratory professional. Key points of standardization of HAs are discussed in this article with regard to their importance in a diagnostic setting and the current reference methods, existing only for a few selected CBC parameters, are described. CBC parameters that show potential in the diagnosis of specific diseases may not be standardized in the near future. Nonetheless, reference methods and standardization of current CBC parameters and of reporting units are desirable and would facilitate the use of these clinically relevant parameters.

REFERENCES

1. Rabinovitch A, Barnes P, Curcio KM, et al. H26–A2: Validation, verification, and quality assurance of automated hematology analyzers; approved standard - second edition. CLSI document H26-A2. Wayne (PA): Clinical and Laboratory Standards Institute; 2010.
2. International Council for Standardization in Haematology, Writing Group, Briggs C, Culp N, Davis B, et al. ICSH guidelines for the evaluation of blood

cell analysers including those used for differential leucocyte and reticulocyte counting. Int J Lab Hematol 2014;36:613–27.

3. International Organization for Standardization. Medical laboratories - particular requirements for quality and competence ISO document 15189. 2nd edition. Geneva (Switzerland): International Organization for Standardization; 2007.

4. Clinical Laboratory Standards Institute. Procedures for the collection of diagnostic blood specimens by venipuncture. CLSI H3-A6 document. 6th edition. Wayne (PA): Clinical Laboratory Standards Institute; 2007.

5. Clinical Laboratory Standards Institute. Procedures and devices for the collection of diagnostic capillary blood specimens; approved standard—sixth edition. CLSI document H04–A6. Wayne (PA): Clinical Laboratory Standards Institute; 2008.

6. Lippi G, Salvagno GL, Montagnana M, et al. Venous stasis and routine hematologic testing. Clin Lab Haematol 2006;28:332–7.

7. Lima-Oliveira G, Lippi G, Salvagno GL, et al. Brand of dipotassium EDTA vacuum tube as a new source of pre-analytical variability in routine haematology testing. Br J Biomed Sci 2013;70:6–9.

8. Hedberg P, Lehto T. Aging stability of complete blood count and white blood cell differential parameters analyzed by Abbott CELL-DYN Sapphire hematology analyzer. Int J Lab Hematol 2009;31:87–96 [Erratum appears in Int J Lab Hematol 2009;31:118].

9. Cornet E, Behier C, Troussard X. Guidance for storing blood samples in laboratories performing complete blood count with differential. Int J Lab Hematol 2012;34:655–60.

10. Huisman A, Stokwielder R, van Solinge WW. Mathematical correction of the invitro storage–related increase in erythrocyte mean cell volume of an automated hematology analyzer–the Cell-Dyn 4000. Lab Hematol 2004;10:68–73.

11. Imeri F, Herklotz R, Risch L, et al. Stability of hematological analytes depends on the hematology analyser used: a stability study with Bayer Advia 120, Beckman Coulter LH 750 and Sysmex XE 2100. Clin Chim Acta 2008;397:68–71.

12. Zini G, International Council for Standardization in Haematology (ICSH). Stability of complete blood count parameters with storage: toward defined specifications for different diagnostic applications. Int J Lab Hematol 2014;36:111–3.

13. Zandecki M, Genevieve F, Gerard J, et al. Spurious counts and spurious results on haematology analysers: a review. Part I: platelets. Int J Lab Hematol 2007;29:4–20.

14. Zandecki M, Genevieve F, Gerard J, et al. Spurious counts and spurious results on haematology analysers: a review. Part II: white blood cells, red blood cells, haemoglobin, red cell indices and reticulocytes. Int J Lab Hematol 2007;29:21–41.

15. World Health Organization. Glossary of terms for biological substances used for texts of the requirements. Expert committee on biological standardization. WHO unpublished document BS/95.1793. Geneva (Switzerland): World Health Organization; 1995.

16. Zwart A, van Assendelft OW, Bull BS, et al. Recommendations for reference method for haemoglobinometry in human blood (ICSH standard 1995) and specifications for international haemoglobin cyanide standard (4th edition). J Clin Pathol 1996;49:271–4.

17. Clinical and Laboratory Standards Institute. Reference and selected procedures for the quantitative determination of hemoglobin in blood. H15–A3. Wayne (PA): Clinical and Laboratory Standards Institute; 2000.

18. Davis BH, Jungerius B. International Council for Standardization in Haematology technical report 1-2009: new reference material for haemiglobincyanide for use in

standardization of blood haemoglobin measurements. Int J Lab Hematol 2010; 32:139–41.

19. Bull BS, Fujimoto K, Houwen B, et al. International Council for Standardization in Haematology (ICSH) recommendations for "surrogate reference" method for the packed cell volume. Lab Hematol 2003;9:1–9.

20. Clinical and Laboratory Standards Institute. Procedure for determining packed cell volume by the microhematocrit method. Approved standard – third edition. H07–A3. Wayne (PA): Clinical and Laboratory Standards Institute; 2000.

21. Clinical and Laboratory Standards Institute. no.15. Methods for reticulocyte counting (automated blood cell counters, flow cytometry, and supravital dyes). Approved Guideline, H44-A2. Wayne (PA): Clinical and Laboratory Institute; 2004.

22. ICSH Expert Panel on Cytometry. Proposed reference method for reticulocyte counting based on the determination of the reticulocyte to red cell ratio. Clin Lab Haematol 1998;20:77–9.

23. ICSH. Reference method for the enumeration of erythrocytes and leucocytes. Prepared by the Expert Panel on Cytometry. Clin Lab Haematol 1994;16:131–8.

24. CLSI. Reference leukocyte (WBC) differential count (Proportional) and evaluation of instrumental methods. H20–A2. Wayne (PA): Clinical and Laboratory Standards Institute; 2007.

25. International Council for Standardization in Haematology Expert Panel on Cytometry, International Society of Laboratory Hematology Task Force on Platelet Counting. Platelet counting by the RBC/platelet ratio method: a reference method. Am J Clin Pathol 2001;115:460–4.

26. Roussel M, Davis BH, Fest T, et al, International Council for Standardization in Hematology (ICSH). Toward a reference method for leukocyte differential counts in blood: comparison of three flow cytometric candidate methods. Cytometry A 2012;81(11):973–82.

27. Lesesve JF, Asnafi V, Braun F, et al. Fragmented red blood cells automated measurement is a useful parameter to exclude schistocytes on the blood film. Int J Lab Hematol 2012. [Epub ahead of print].

28. Chalvatzi K, Spiroglou S, Nikolaidou A, et al. Evaluation of fragmented red cell (FRC) counting using Sysmex XE-5000-does hypochromia play a role? Int J Lab Hematol 2013;35:193–9.

29. Zini G, d'Onofrio G, Briggs C, et al, International Council for Standardization in Haematology (ICSH). ICSH recommendations for identification, diagnostic value, and quantitation of schistocytes. Int J Lab Hematol 2012;34:107–16.

30. Huh HJ, Chung JW, Chae SL. Microscopic schistocyte determination according to International Council for Standardization in Hematology recommendations in various diseases. Int J Lab Hematol 2013;35:542–7.

31. Lesesve JF, El Adssi H, Watine J, et al. Evaluation of ICSH schistocyte measurement guidelines in France. Int J Lab Hematol 2013;35:601–7.

32. Wintrobe MM. The size and hemoglobin content of the erythrocyte. Methods of determination and clinical application. J Lab Clin Med 1932;115:374–87.

33. Ford J. Red blood cell morphology. Int J Lab Hematol 2013;35(3):351.

34. Romanelli F, Empey K, Pomeroy C. Macrocytosis as an indicator of medication (zidovudine) adherence in patients with HIV infection. AIDS Patient Care STDS 2002;16:405–11.

35. De la Salle BJ, Briggs C, Bleby J, et al. Mean cell volume measurement on Sysmex XE series instruments using the RPU-2100 diluent system: how external quality assessment works to provide more accurate MCV results and potentially benefit patient management. J Clin Pathol 2013;66:449–50.

36. Huang YL, Hu ZD, Liu SJ, et al. Prognostic value of red blood cell distribution width for patients with heart failure: a systematic review and meta-analysis of cohort studies. PLoS One 2014;9:e104861.
37. Patel KV, Semba RD, Ferrucci L, et al. Red cell distribution width and mortality in older adults: a meta-analysis. J Gerontol A Biol Sci Med Sci 2010;65(3):258–65.
38. Clarke K, Sagunarthy R, Kansal S. RDW as an additional marker in inflammatory bowel disease/undifferentiated colitis. Dig Dis Sci 2008;53:2521–3.
39. Briggs C. Quality counts: new parameters in blood cell counting. Int J Lab Hematol 2009;31:277–97.
40. Ermens AA, Hoffmann JJ, Krockenberger M, et al. New erythrocyte and reticulocyte parameters on CELL-DYN Sapphire: analytical and preanalytical aspects. Int J Lab Hematol 2012;34:274–82.
41. Urrechaga E, Hoffmann JJ, Izquierdo S, et al. Differential diagnosis of microcytic anemia: the role of microcytic and hypochromic erythrocytes. Int J Lab Hematol 2014. http://dx.doi.org/10.1111/ijlh.12290.
42. Rooney S, Hoffmann JJ, Cormack OM, et al. Screening and confirmation of hereditary spherocytosis in children using a CELL-DYN Sapphire haematology analyser. Int J Lab Hematol 2014. [Epub ahead of print].
43. Jonckheere S, Dierick J, Vanhouteghem H, et al. Erythrocyte indices in the assessment of iron status in dialysis-dependent patients with end-stage renal disease on continuous erythropoietin receptor activator versus epoetin beta therapy. Acta Haematol 2010;124:27–33.
44. Brugnara C, Laufer MR, Friedman AJ, et al. Reticulocyte hemoglobin content (CHr): early indicator of iron deficiency and response to therapy. Blood 1994; 83:3100–1.
45. Locatelli F, Aljama P, Bárány P, et al, European Best Practice Guidelines Working Group. Revised European best practice guidelines for the management of anaemia in patients with chronic renal failure. Nephrol Dial Transplant 2004; 19(Suppl 2):ii1–47.
46. KDOQI. KDOQI clinical practice guideline and clinical practice recommendations for anemia in chronic kidney disease: 2007 update of hemoglobin target. Am J Kidney Dis 2007;50:471–530.
47. Briggs C, Harrison P, Machin SJ. Continuing developments with the automated platelet count. Int J Lab Hematol 2007;29:77–91.
48. Vinholt PJ, Hvas AM, Nybo M. An overview of platelet indices and methods for evaluating platelet function in thrombocytopenic patients. Eur J Haematol 2014; 92:367–76.
49. Parco S, Vascotto F. Application of reticulated platelets to transfusion management during autologous stem cell transplantation. Onco Targets Ther 2012;5:1–5.
50. Hennel E, Kentouche K, Beck J, et al. Immature platelet fraction as marker for platelet recovery after stem cell transplantation in children. Clin Biochem 2012; 45:749–52.

Hematology Testing in Urgent Care and Resource-Poor Settings

An Overview of Point of Care and Satellite Testing

Anthony N. Sireci, MD, MSc

KEYWORDS

- Point of care hemoglobin • Satellite hematology laboratories
- Noninvasive hemoglobin monitoring • Point-of-care complete blood count
- Point-of-care CD4+ enumeration • Hematology in resource-poor settings

KEY POINTS

- In the United States, Point-of-care instruments are categorized as "Waived" under the Clinical Laboratory Improvements Amendments of 1988 (CLIA 88).

- In the hematology category, only instruments measuring hemoglobin and hematocrit are CLIA-waived. Devices that noninvasively measure hemoglobin, or that measure white blood cell counts, provide white cell differentials, or enumerate CD4+ T-cells are not yet waived.

- The advantages of point-of-care (POC) testing include decreased turnaround times, small sample volume requirements, and minimal training requirements, whereas concerns include limited test menus, questionable accuracy and reproducibility because of limited regulatory requirements, and high costs.

- Satellite laboratories function as branches of the main laboratory, are staffed by laboratory professionals, and offer a wider variety of testing than POC devices while still decreasing turnaround times.

INTRODUCTION

The complete blood count (CBC) is a commonly ordered test that is routinely performed in central laboratories on large, automated hematology analyzers. Information from the CBC drives urgent clinical decisions, such as whether to transfuse, administer chemotherapy, or administer antibiotics. Today, the increasing requirement for

Disclosure: The author has no conflicts of interest to disclose.
Laboratory of Personalized Genomic Medicine, Department of Pathology and Cell Biology, Columbia University, College of Physicians and Surgeons, 630 West 168th Street, PS17-401, New York, NY 10032, USA
E-mail address: ans2133@columbia.edu

Clin Lab Med 35 (2015) 197–207
http://dx.doi.org/10.1016/j.cll.2014.10.009

Abbreviations	
CBC	Complete blood count
CLIA	Clinical Laboratory Improvement Amendments
HCS	Hemoglobin Colour Scale
ICSH	International Council for Standardization in Haematology
POC	Point of care
WBC	White blood cell

rapid turnaround times coinciding with advances in biomedical technology has brought the CBC closer to the point of patient care. Whether in the form of handheld devices providing hemoglobin measurements, or small, portable benchtop analyzers stationed in satellite laboratories providing additional parameters, devices and platforms exist to meet the developing requirements for rapid diagnostics. This article provides an overview of the use of point-of-care (POC) testing and satellite laboratories in hematology. The section on POC testing is based on methods and devices operated at the bedside and provides an overview of the risks and benefits of this testing, regulatory considerations, methodologies available, and guidance on platform selection. The section on satellite laboratories focuses on the use of benchtop hematology analyzers and their advantages over core laboratories or handheld platforms.

POINT-OF-CARE TESTING IN HEMATOLOGY

POC testing is defined as the testing of patient samples at the point of patient contact. For the purposes of this article, POC tests are those that are performed at the patient's bedside. The need for rapid turnaround times to facilitate real-time clinical decision making in emergency and operating rooms or in areas of destruction and devastation have driven the development of POC hematology platforms. Additionally, the ease of use, low maintenance, and portability of these methods has made them popular in resource-poor settings where basic laboratory testing would otherwise not be available. Examples of applications for POC hematology testing platforms measuring hemoglobin or hematocrit include population screening for anemia, assessment of the adequacy of potential blood donors, triage of trauma victims, and perioperative assessment of a patient's transfusion needs. More detailed information on white blood cell (WBC) counts and differentials is helpful in the triage of oncology patients before chemotherapy, the diagnosis of neonatal sepsis, and the diagnosis of immunodeficiency or marrow failure. These applications are outlined in **Box 1**. This section reviews POC testing in hematology by discussing the risks and benefits of introducing POC testing, the potential methodologies available for use in various clinical settings, and the considerations to be weighed in choosing the optimal platform.

Potential Benefits and Risks of Point-of-Care Testing

The potential benefits and risks of using POC platforms in a hospital or clinic setting are summarized in **Box 2**. POC testing platforms have several benefits in hematology. First, most platforms require a fraction of the sample volume used by instruments in use in the central laboratory, reducing the occurrence of iatrogenic anemia in patient populations in whom blood loss is a major consideration, such as neonates or the critically ill.[1]

Additionally, many platforms can be run on capillary blood samples obtained from a fingerstick rather than requiring venous or arterial blood samples, which can only be

---

Box 1
Potential applications for point-of-care platforms

Hemoglobin and/or hematocrit

- Population screening for anemia
- Blood donor assessment
- Assessing transfusion needs of critically ill patients

White blood cell count with/without differential

- Screening for neonatal sepsis
- Triage of oncology patients before chemotherapy
- Diagnosis of immunodeficiency or marrow failure

---

obtained via venipuncture and are commonly required by central laboratories. This ability is particularly helpful in patients with poor vascular access such as the elderly, neonates, and those who are critically ill.

The readout of results within minutes at the patient's bedside can have a potentially large impact on turnaround times compared with sending samples to central core laboratories. This function not only facilitates real-time clinical decision making but has been shown to decrease length of hospital stay and in-clinic wait times.[2,3]

Introduction of POC testing is not without risks. The less-stringent regulatory oversight of POC testing means that the staff performing the testing is often nonlaboratory personnel. Training and competency of staff must be monitored to produce reproducibly accurate results. The lack of performance and documentation of quality control and accuracy checks can increase the possibility of unreliable results. Procedures addressing these issues must be implemented to ensure quality. Concerns about comparability of results to those obtained in the central laboratory must be rigorously addressed before any platform is implemented. The hematology test menu currently

---

Box 2
Potential benefits and risks of adopting point-of-care testing

Benefits

- Small sample volume requirements
- Decreased turnaround times
- Decreased in-hospital length of stay
- Decreased in-clinic wait times

Risks

- Operated by nonlaboratory personnel
- Less stringent control on result quality
- Potential cost
- Comparison of results to central laboratory results
- Limited test menu limits utility

Although this list is generated considering hematology POC testing, the same issues might apply to POC testing of any analyte.

---

amenable to and available on POC platforms is limited and can restrict the utility of this testing in certain clinical settings. Finally, the low volume and disposable nature of POC platforms makes them often more costly than standard testing and may be a barrier to adoption.

Regulatory Considerations

In the United States, most POC testing falls under the waived category established by the Clinical Laboratory Improvement Amendments of 1988 (CLIA '88), which classifies laboratory testing into waived, moderate complexity, and high complexity based on the level of technical expertise required to perform the assay. This classification schema serves as the regulatory framework for establishing tiered compliance standards. Laboratories performing waived testing under a certificate of waiver follow the least stringent regulatory criteria. When compared with moderate- and high-complexity testing, waived tests performed under a certificate of waiver do not need to comply with personnel requirements, proficiency testing, quality control, quality assurance, and patient test management.[4]

Tests can be performed by a laboratory under a certificate of waiver if they pose "an insignificant risk of an erroneous result, including those that (a) employ methodologies that are so simple and accurate as to render the likelihood of erroneous results by the user negligible, or (b) the Secretary [of Health and Human Services] has determined pose no unreasonable risk of harm to the patient if performed incorrectly."[4]

In order for a POC instrument to qualify as "simple" it must automatically perform the test on an unprocessed sample and provide a direct readout of results, with clear instructions for confirmatory testing when appropriate. Additionally, to demonstrate an "insignificant risk of erroneous results," the instrument must have in place fail-safe mechanisms that prevent results from showing inappropriate values (ie, values obtained when the instrument is not optimally operating).

At the time of writing, the only CLIA-waived POC tests available in the field of hematology are those used to measure hemoglobin and hematocrit.

Point-of-Care Platforms in Hematology

The following section provide an overview of the platforms currently available for the measurement of hemoglobin and hematocrit, WBC count and differential, and, finally, CD4+ lymphocyte counts. The various methods used are reviewed, example platforms presented, and, whenever possible, comparison of performance to standard laboratory testing discussed.

Visual methods

The Hemoglobin Colour Scale (HCS) was developed by the World Health Organization for use in the developing world.[5] It is simple, rapid, and easy to use.[6] The method is based on comparing the color of a drop of blood absorbed onto filter paper against a standardized color scale provided on a laminated card. The colors on the scale are divided by units of 2 g/dL of hemoglobin and range from 4 to 14 g/dL. Interpretation is subjective. A meta-analysis published in 2005 estimated the sensitivity of the HCS, when performed in a laboratory setting, to be 87% for the detection of anemia, with a specificity of 97% using a cutoff of 12 g/dL.[6] Because of the heterogeneity in study design in studies estimating the performance of HCS in "real life," a pooled analysis could not be performed. However, the sensitivity and specificity were found to be significantly lower in these studies, ranging from 76% to 88% for sensitivity and 40% to 80% for specificity. Interference caused by high WBC counts, hyperproteinemia, and hyperlipidemia has been reported.[7] This technology is most appropriately used for anemia screening in resource poor settings where laboratory facilities are not available.

Another method that is easily adaptable to resource-poor settings for the measurement of hemoglobin is the so-called Sahli method. A predefined volume of hydrochloric acid is mixed with 20 μL of blood, creating acid hematin, which has a brown color. Water is added until the color of the solution matches the color of standard test rods. Results are read in 3 minutes. The method was compared with the HCS and shown to perform similarly in the detection of anemia.[8]

Optical methods: HemoCue

The gold standard method for measuring hemoglobin is the spectrophotometric analysis of hemoglobin derivatives at 1 or more wavelengths of light. Hemoglobin is exposed to a cyanide-containing reagent that converts it to cyanmethemoglobin, which is measured spectrophotometrically. Although this is the reference standard (the International Council for Standardization in Haematology [ICSH] provides a cyanmethemoglobin standard for calibration of instruments), it is technique-dependent, time and labor-intensive, and expensive. However, the basic concept of optical methods for measuring hemoglobin has been adapted to the POC.

The most commonly used and extensively studied POC hemoglobin system is the HemoCue series of portable hemoglobinometers. These instruments can be operated using battery power; can use capillary, venous, or arterial blood as matrices for analysis; and yield results in less than 60 seconds. Blood is introduced into the analytical cuvette via capillary action either from a fingerstick or from a sample obtained by phlebotomy. Older versions of this technology house reagents that lyse red cells within the cuvette and derivatize the endogenous hemoglobin into azide-methemoglobin. The derivative is then spectrophotometrically measured. The HemoCue 201+ and 201DM use this method.[9] Newer versions, such as the HB301 and DonorHb Checker, are based on the absorbance of hemoglobin and oxygenated hemoglobin (Hb/HbO_2) at an isosbestic point.[10] Overall, studies comparing hemoglobin measurements using the suite of HemoCue products have shown acceptable concordance with laboratory-based hemoglobin measurements in a variety of clinical settings, including perioperative,[11,12] pediatrics/neonatal,[13] gastrointestinal bleeds,[14] and blood donor screening.[15] However, some studies have shown significant bias of measurements when compared with standard laboratory methods.[16–18] Although the system is cleared for use on whole blood capillary samples obtained from a fingerstick, these results have been suggested to be less accurate than those from venous or arterial blood when compared with results obtained from traditional laboratory instrumentation. Additionally, introduction of air into the microcuvettes has been shown to cause significant error.[19]

Conductivity-based methods: i-STAT system

The conductivity method is based on the fact that the electrical conductivity of a whole blood sample is reduced with increasing numbers of cellular elements (ie, red cells) in the blood.[20,21] In other words, conductivity is inversely proportional to hematocrit. These devices then calculate hemoglobin based on physiologic assumptions. The most commonly used POC instrument employing this technology is the i-STAT instrument (Abbot Point of Care, Princeton, NJ, USA). Venous, arterial, or capillary whole blood samples are placed in a biosensor cartridge equipped with reference electrodes and analyte-specific sensors. The device is compact and requires low sample volume. However, elevated WBC count, hyperlipidemia, hyperproteinemia, changes in sodium concentrations, and use of volume expanders will impact the accuracy of this method.[22–24]

Noninvasive methods

Despite the low small-volume requirements of most POC devices (ie, 10 μL), they still require either fingerstick or venipuncture. A noninvasive device would save patients the discomfort of a blood draw and make hemoglobin assessment in cases of limited vascular access more feasible. Additionally, these methods allow for the continuous monitoring of hemoglobin at the bedside, in real time, which is particularly useful for the unstable patient. Spectrophotometry-based methods of monitoring hemoglobin concentrations based on the differential optical density of wavelengths of light passed through the finger, similar to pulse oximetry, have been developed and tested in steady state[25–28] and in the critically ill.[29–33] The accuracy of this method is reported to be affected by low arterial profusion, low oxygen saturation, high bilirubin, and severe anemia. The model instrument using this methodology is the Masimo Radical 7 (Masimo, Irvine, CA, USA), and the clinical utility of using this technology to make transfusion decisions at the critical cutoffs remains in question.[34]

Additional methods for noninvasive hemoglobin determination are in development and have shown promise. These techniques include optoacoustic spectroscopy and electrical admittance plethysmography and photoplethysmography.[35]

White Blood Cell Measurement

Hemoglobin and hematocrit are the only measurements currently available on CLIA-waived POC instruments. However, outside of the United States, advances in technology have made other CBC parameters available at the point of patient contact.

Coulter method

The Coulter principle is based on interruption of an electrical current as cellular components of blood pass through a fixed aperture. The size and shape of a cell can be determined based on the length of the electrical interruption, and the identity of the cell can be deduced based on these parameters. This technology has been used in the POC setting to provide differentials on fingerstick samples. An example is the Chempaq XBC analyzer (Chempaq A/S, Denmark), which measures hemoglobin and WBC count and provides a 3-part differential including lymphocytes, monocytes, and granulocytes. The system consists of a reader and a single-use cassette called a *PAQ* (particle analyzer and quantifier). These cassettes are preloaded with all required reagents, and a fingerstick or sample of blood from an ethylenediaminetetraacetic acid (EDTA) tube is applied to it directly. Results are ready to read in 3 minutes. Clinical testing of this type of POC approach has shown reasonable correlation to laboratory-based results.[36]

Image analysis technology

The gold standard for measuring WBC count is microscopic examination of a diluted blood sample in a counting chamber by a trained technologist, with subsequent enumeration of white cells. With developments in image analysis software, microscopic examination has become automated. The HemoCue AB (HemoCue, Brea, CA, US) is a portable device that uses image analysis technology to obtain the WBC count in peripheral capillary or venous blood. The system consists of a microscopic image detector, a cuvette holder, and an LCD-display and is powered by 6 AA batteries; 10 μL of blood enter the cuvette, where red blood cells are lysed and white cell nuclei are stained with methylene blue. An image is taken and the image analysis software counts the stained nuclei within 2 minutes, while correcting for platelets. Inaccuracy of WBC counts caused by increased numbers of circulating normoblasts and/or reticulocytes has been reported using this methodology. However, studies using both capillary and venous samples have shown good correlation with reference laboratory methods.[37,38]

Enumeration of CD4+ T Cells

The current gold standard for measuring CD4+ T cells is flow cytometry. This technique requires expensive instrumentation, reagents, and skilled laboratory technologists. Additionally, turnaround times can be long, which can result in losing patients to follow-up. POC devices that measure CD4+ T-cell counts are of great utility in HIV-testing sites, where this information is used to make several important clinical decisions, including whether to initiate antiretroviral therapies or prophylactic therapies against opportunistic infections. The Alere Pima CD4 Analyser (Alere, Orlando, FL, USA) is an example of a POC device that can be used for these purposes. Using 25 μL of capillary blood obtained by fingerstick and introduced into a sample cartridge containing all required reagents, the result is provided in 20 minutes. A fixed volume of blood introduced into the cartridge is exposed to fluorescently labeled monoclonal antibodies against CD3 and CD4. The labeled cells are then imaged and the cells containing the colocalized labels are counted and reported. Importantly, the system provides an estimate of absolute numbers of CD4+ T cells per unit volume as opposed to a percentage of total T cells. Although the system yields results comparable to traditional flow cytometric assays when venous blood is pipetted into the test cartridge, the performance in the field, where capillary samples are used, showed poor correlation in one study.[39] Despite this, the platform and others like it remain promising in the field of HIV treatment.

Choosing a Point-of-Care Platform

After weighing the risks and benefits described earlier, selecting the best platform is the next important step. Although the weight attributed to each factor influencing test selection will be unique to each individual laboratory or health care setting, some common considerations exist and are summarized in **Table 1**.

In resource-poor settings, where electricity and other amenities may be limited, the power source used by the POC platform may play a major role in selecting an instrument. Battery-powered instruments might be preferred in these settings. Additionally, the stability of reagents at ambient conditions, particularly in heat and humidity, is a major concern in areas where access to refrigeration and climate control is limited.

In the hospital or advanced clinical setting, result interfacing with the locally used electronic medical record and compatibility with central laboratory results for continuity of clinical care often play a larger role in deciding between platforms. In the United States, whether a device is CLIA-waived dictates whether the platform can be administered by nonlicensed personnel at the point of patient contact.

Table 1	
Factors influencing which point-of-care platform to select	
Care Setting	**Factor**
Resource-poor setting	Power supply required Reagent/control stability
Hospital or advanced care setting	Interfacing of results to EMR Correlation of results with central laboratory
US health care setting	CLIA-waived status
Setting agnostic	Cost of capital equipment and consumables Available test menu Ease of use (eg, operator skill requires, reagent/sample preparation, quality control protocol)

Ease of use is a universal factor that is weighed in selecting a platform. This category includes the level of operator skill required to operate the equipment, the reagent/sample preparation involved in testing, and the protocol for quality control. Additionally, assessing whether the platform offers a test menu and covers the analytical ranges that address the clinical needs of the patient population being served is a universal requirement. Finally, consideration of the capital cost required and the cost of consumables will play a big role in decision making. Although the per-test cost of a POC test may be higher than the cost of analysis in a central laboratory because of the lower cost-efficiency of low-volume testing, this additional cost must be weighed against the benefits, previously enumerated, of POC testing.

A score card was developed using these and several other factors. Each factor was uniquely weighted and used to evaluate various CD4 T-lymphocyte cell counting systems for use in caring for patients with HIV in rural settings. This analysis demonstrated the utility of a rigorous assessment before selection of a platform.[40] Additionally, guidelines published by the ICSH provide a framework for selecting, implementing, and managing POC testing locally to help ensure quality results and patient care.[7]

SATELLITE LABORATORIES

A satellite laboratory is a branch of the central or core laboratory located close to the point of patient care delivery. The satellite laboratory remains under the management and leadership of the central laboratory. The satellite laboratory is sometimes also referred to as an *STAT laboratory* and is generally situated near units requiring more rapid turnaround times than those available from the central laboratory. These areas might include emergency rooms, operating suites, hemodialysis units, intensive care units, and outpatient clinics.

Like POC platforms, the proximity to the site of care delivery of satellite laboratories helps alleviate delays in turnaround time that occur from sample delivery to the central laboratory via courier, transport system, or pneumatic tube systems. Also, because the satellite laboratory focuses on testing for a smaller fraction of the patient population than covered by the central laboratory, delays in sample receipt, accessioning, and processing are minimized. In one study, introducing a hematology satellite laboratory in an emergency room setting helped reduce the time to hematology results when compared with sending samples to the central laboratory. Additionally, the decision to discharge the patient was made much faster after the satellite laboratory was opened.[41]

Satellites are staffed by trained laboratory personnel and can therefore offer moderate or high complexity testing and use more traditional laboratory instrumentation. These 2 features of satellite laboratories, the personnel employed and the instrumentation used, address and mitigate some of the risks of POC testing outlined in the previous section. In particular, they address the limited test menu that is currently available on CLIA-waived POC platforms. For example, no CLIA-waived platform currently exists for the determination of white cell differentials. Satellite laboratories can operate more traditional, benchtop hematology analyzers found in clinical laboratories, thereby allowing for a 3- or 5-part differential in less time and meeting needs not covered by POC platforms. One study showed that introduction of a mobile benchtop analyzer to a hematology clinic enabled the facility to reach benchmark in-clinic wait times for their patients. The prior introduction of a pneumatic tube system did not achieve this goal.[3]

Finally, the per-test cost is usually lower in satellite laboratories than that incurred using POC platforms. Because benchtop instruments used in satellite laboratories are generally not required to handle large sample throughput per hour, they can be smaller and less automated, and are therefore also less expensive than those used in the central laboratory. Eradicating disposable, one-use cartridges also decreases consumable costs.

SUMMARY

The need for rapid turnaround times in the urgent care setting has inspired the development of various devices and platforms either housed in satellite laboratories or operated at the patient's bedside. The use of POC testing will continue to expand as the model of health care provision moves away from inpatient medicine. As more POC platforms are adopted, quality control and quality management systems must be established, either locally or nationally, to oversee possible issues of accuracy and reproducibility. Specific to the field of hematology, a great need exists in the United States for a POC device to measure WBC counts and provide WBC differentials.

REFERENCES

1. Widness JA, Madan A, Grindeanu LA, et al. Reduction in red blood cell transfusions among preterm infants: results of a randomized trial with an in-line blood gas and chemistry monitor. Pediatrics 2005;115:1299–306.
2. Holland LL, Smith LL, Blick KE. Reducing laboratory turnaround time outliers can reduce emergency department patient length of stay: an 11-hospital study. Am J Clin Pathol 2005;124:672–4.
3. Galloway MJ, Woods RS, Nicholson SL, et al. An audit of waiting times in a haematology clinic before and after the introduction of point-of-care testing. Clin Lab Haematol 1999;21:201–5.
4. Recommendations: Clinical Laboratory Improvement Amendments of 1988 (CLIA) waiver applications for manufacturers of in vitro diagnostic devices. U.S. Food and Drug Administration Web site. Available at: http://www.fda.gov/medicaldevices/Deviceregulationandguidance/guidancedocuments/ucm079632. Accessed October 1, 2012.
5. Stott GJ, Lewis SM. A simple and reliable method for estimating haemoglobin. Bull World Health Organ 1995;73:369–73.
6. Critchley J, Bates I. Haemoglobin colour scale for anaemia diagnosis where there is no laboratory: a systematic review. Int J Epidemiol 2005;34:1425–34.
7. Briggs C, Kimber S, Green L. Where are we at with point-of-care testing in haematology? Br J Haematol 2012;158:679–90.
8. Barduagni P, Ahmed AS, Curtale F, et al. Performance of Sahli and colour scale methods in diagnosing anaemia among school children in low prevalence areas. Trop Med Int Health 2003;8:615–8.
9. Vanzetti G. An azide-methemoglobin method for hemoglobin determination in blood. J Lab Clin Med 1966;67:116–26.
10. van Kampen EJ, Zijlstra WG. Spectrophotometry of hemoglobin and hemoglobin derivatives. Adv Clin Chem 1983;23:199–257.
11. Lardi AM, Hirst C, Mortimer AJ, et al. Evaluation of the HemoCue for measuring intra-operative haemoglobin concentrations: a comparison with the Coulter Max-M. Anaesthesia 1998;53:349–52.
12. Spielmann N, Mauch J, Madjdpour C, et al. Accuracy and precision of hemoglobin point-of-care testing during major pediatric surgery. Int J Lab Hematol 2012;34:86–90.

13. Rechner IJ, Twigg A, Davies AF, et al. Evaluation of the HemoCue compared with the Coulter STKS for measurement of neonatal haemoglobin. Arch Dis Child Fetal Neonatal Ed 2002;86:F188–9.
14. Gomez-Escolar Viejo L, Sala GS, Azorin JM, et al. Reliability of hemoglobin measurement by HemoCue in patients with gastrointestinal bleeding. Gastroenterol Hepatol 2009;32:334–8.
15. Morris LD, Osei-Bimpong A, McKeown D, et al. Evaluation of the utility of the HemoCue 301 haemoglobinometer for blood donor screening. Vox Sang 2007; 93:64–9.
16. Van de Louw A, Lasserre N, Drouhin F, et al. Reliability of HemoCue in patients with gastrointestinal bleeding. Intensive Care Med 2007;33:355–8.
17. Gomez-Simon A, Navarro-Nunez L, Perez-Ceballos E, et al. Evaluation of four rapid methods for hemoglobin screening of whole blood donors in mobile collection settings. Transfus Apheresis Sci 2007;36:235–42.
18. Mendrone A Jr, Sabino EC, Sampaio L, et al. Anemia screening in potential female blood donors: comparison of two different quantitative methods. Transfusion 2009;49:662–8.
19. Agarwal R, Heinz T. Bedside hemoglobinometry in hemodialysis patients: lessons from point-of-care testing. ASAIO J 2001;47:240–3.
20. Myers GJ, Browne J. Point of care hematocrit and hemoglobin in cardiac surgery: a review. Perfusion 2007;22:179–83.
21. Patel KP, Hay GW, Cheteri MK, et al. Hemoglobin test result variability and cost analysis of eight different analyzers during open heart surgery. J Extra Corpor Technol 2007;39:10–7.
22. Papadea C, Foster J, Grant S, et al. Evaluation of the i-STAT Portable Clinical Analyzer for point-of-care blood testing in the intensive care units of a university children's hospital. Ann Clin Lab Sci 2002;32:231–43.
23. Hopfer SM, Nadeau FL, Sundra M, et al. Effect of protein on hemoglobin and hematocrit assays with a conductivity-based point-of-care testing device: comparison with optical methods. Ann Clin Lab Sci 2004;34:75–82.
24. Steinfelder-Visscher J, Teerenstra S, Gunnewiek JM, et al. Evaluation of the i-STAT point-of-care analyzer in critically ill adult patients. J Extra Corpor Technol 2008; 40:57–60.
25. Dewhirst E, Naguib A, Winch P, et al. Accuracy of noninvasive and continuous hemoglobin measurement by pulse co-oximetry during preoperative phlebotomy. J Intensive Care Med 2013;29:238–42.
26. Myers D, McGraw M, George M, et al. Tissue hemoglobin index: a non-invasive optical measure of total tissue hemoglobin. Crit Care 2009;13(Suppl 5):S2.
27. Frasca D, Dahyot-Fizelier C, Catherine K, et al. Accuracy of a continuous noninvasive hemoglobin monitor in intensive care unit patients. Crit Care Med 2011;39: 2277–82.
28. Gayat E, Bodin A, Sportiello C, et al. Performance evaluation of a noninvasive hemoglobin monitoring device. Ann Emerg Med 2011;57:330–3.
29. Butwick A, Hilton G, Carvalho B. Non-invasive haemoglobin measurement in patients undergoing elective Caesarean section. Br J Anaesth 2012;108: 271–7.
30. Causey MW, Miller S, Foster A, et al. Validation of noninvasive hemoglobin measurements using the Masimo Radical-7 SpHb Station. Am J Surg 2011;201: 592–8.
31. Joseph B, Hadjizacharia P, Aziz H, et al. Continuous noninvasive hemoglobin monitor from pulse ox: ready for prime time? World J Surg 2013;37:525–9.

32. Applegate RL 2nd, Barr SJ, Collier CE, et al. Evaluation of pulse cooximetry in patients undergoing abdominal or pelvic surgery. Anesthesiology 2012;116: 65–72.
33. Bland JM, Altman DG. Agreement between methods of measurement with multiple observations per individual. J Biopharm Stat 2007;17:571–82.
34. Rice MJ, Gravenstein N, Morey TE. Noninvasive hemoglobin monitoring: how accurate is enough? Anesth Analg 2013;117:902–7.
35. McMurdy JW, Jay GD, Suner S, et al. Noninvasive optical, electrical, and acoustic methods of total hemoglobin determination. Clin Chem 2008;54:264–72.
36. Rao LV, Ekberg BA, Connor D, et al. Evaluation of a new point of care automated complete blood count (CBC) analyzer in various clinical settings. Clin Chim Acta 2008;389:120–5.
37. Yang ZW, Yang SH, Chen L, et al. Comparison of blood counts in venous, fingertip and arterial blood and their measurement variation. Clin Lab Haematol 2001;23:155–9.
38. Osei-Bimpong A, Jury C, McLean R, et al. Point-of-care method for total white cell count: an evaluation of the HemoCue WBC device. Int J Lab Hematol 2009;31: 657–64.
39. Glencross DK, Coetzee LM, Faal M, et al. Performance evaluation of the Pima point-of-care CD4 analyser using capillary blood sampling in field tests in South Africa. J Int AIDS Soc 2012;15:3.
40. Lehe JD, Sitoe NE, Tobaiwa O, et al. Evaluating operational specifications of point-of-care diagnostic tests: a standardized scorecard. PLoS One 2012;7: e47459.
41. Leman P, Guthrie D, Simpson R, et al. Improving access to diagnostics: an evaluation of a satellite laboratory service in the emergency department. Emerg Med J 2004;21:452–6.

Novel Parameters in Blood Cell Counters

Thomas Pierre Lecompte, MD*, Michael Pierre Bernimoulin, MD

KEYWORDS

- Complete blood cell count • Hematology analyzers • Schistocytes • Anemia
- Thrombocytopenia • New parameters

KEY POINTS

- Recently developed automated hematology analyzers (HA) incorporate technological improvements that provide more accurate complete blood cell counts and novel parameters.
- Several new red blood cell parameters are potentially useful in the differential diagnosis of anemias with abnormal hemoglobinization, especially of iron-restricted erythropoiesis.
- Schistocytes, a hallmark of thrombotic microangiopathies, can be identified or at least suspected by modern HA: the fragmented red cell flag has a low specificity, but the negative predictive value of its absence is good.
- The proposed new platelet parameters are mainly intended to help in the diagnosis and management of thrombocytopenias; they include the immature platelet fraction, new methods for the assessment of the platelet volume, provide insights on the contents of platelets.
- Careful examination of platelet volumes (results of HAs and of microscopic examination) is important to suspect and diagnose inherited thrombocytopenias.

Recently developed automated hematology analyzers (HA) incorporate technologic improvements yielding novel parameters or determining those of the complete blood count with better accuracy. These newer instruments are, in alphabetical order of the manufacturers,[1] Sapphire (Abbot Diagnostics Cell Dyn),[2] LH750 and UniCel DxH 800 (Beckman Coulter), Pentra (Horiba Medical),[3] BC 6800 (Mindray),[4] Advia (Siemens),[5] and XE and now XN series (Sysmex).

Most of the recently introduced or improved parameters are listed in **Table 1**. The determination of what can be considered to be recent is rather arbitrary, and new does not necessarily mean novel. Many of these parameters are often derived from established technologies using new algorithms with improved data processing.

Disclosure: None.
Haematology Division, Faculty of Medicine, Hôpitaux Universitaires de Genève, Geneva University, Rue Gabrielle-Perret-Gentil 4, Geneva 14 CH-1211, Switzerland
* Corresponding author.
E-mail address: ThomasPierre.Lecompte@hcuge.ch

Clin Lab Med 35 (2015) 209–224
http://dx.doi.org/10.1016/j.cll.2014.11.001
0272-2712/15/$ – see front matter © 2015 Elsevier Inc. All rights reserved.
labmed.theclinics.com

Abbreviations	
BSS	Bernard-Soulier syndrome
CKD	Chronic kidney disease
HA	Automated hematology analyzers
HSC	Hematopoietic stem cells
IDA	Iron deficiency anemia
IRE	Iron-restricted erythropoiesis
ITP	Immune thrombocytopenia
MPV	Mean platelet volume
MYH9-RD	MYH9-related diseases
PDW	Platelet distribution width
RBC	Red blood cell
RDW	Red cells distribution width
TMA	Thrombotic microangiopathies
WBC	White blood cell

Only a few are the result of actual improvements of the testing procedure, such as the use of new fluorescent dyes. Not all new parameters are already available for clinical use; many are designated by the manufacturer as "for research use only." Many new parameters seem theoretically useful, but their clinical utility sometimes remains poorly documented. External quality control is not always possible, and even internal quality control may not be available. The reproducibility among the same kind of instruments used in every day practice and in different sites is known only for well-established parameters, such as cell counts through external quality assurance scheme exercises; the external control of volumetric parameters remains a worrisome problem.

It is important to remember that parameters with the same name, or with closely resembling names, or with different names but the same aim, are often not interchangeable because of marked differences in measurement principles, calibration, and algorithms. The most conspicuous example is the mean platelet volume (MPV), which has been available for years, but the clinical use of which remains problematic. Clinical guidelines that rely on a parameter that can be obtained only with one kind of instrument from one manufacturer cannot be implemented by most laboratories that do not use those instruments.

Formal validation of a laboratory parameter should include the following steps: metrologic characteristics, diagnostic performance, and clinical utility in daily practice. In addition, the preanalytical aspects should have been properly addressed. Only very few new parameters have successfully fulfilled all these steps during the past years. Moreover, the assessment of diagnostic performance can be challenging when the reference method is cumbersome, barely reproducible, and sometimes even notoriously prone to inaccuracy, or even obsolete. Regarding the clinical usefulness, the challenge can be even greater, for instance when it is difficult to adequately classify patients with complex disorders, such as "anemia of chronic disease" associated with iron-restricted erythropoiesis (IRE), or a disease for which there is no gold-standard laboratory test, such as autoimmune thrombocytopenia.

Generally speaking, the improvements of the instruments and methods aim at lowering false-positive alarms for fragmented red blood cells (RBCs), abnormal white blood cells (WBCs), and platelet clumps, thus limiting unnecessary and time consuming blood film examinations; providing sensitive detection and accurate enumeration of abnormal cells or cells not normally present in peripheral blood; and providing genuinely novel parameters of potential clinical relevance.

Table 1
Overview of recently introduced red cell parameters of hematology analyzers and their potential clinical use distinguishing parameters with certain, uncertain, or no clinical usefulness

Cell Line	Parameter	Manufacturer/Machine	Reportable	Measures	Clinical Use (Yes or No or Unknown)	IQC
A. Abnormal elements						
Progenitor cells	Hematogenic progenitor cells	Sysmex XE series	Y	Very immature WBC	N: CD34 and not hematogenic progenitor cells used for stem cell collections	Y
Erythroblasts	Nucleated red blood cells	Abott/Sapphire	Y	Erythroblast quantification	Y: correction of WBC	Y
		Beckman Coulter/LH 750	Y			Y
		Horiba Medical/Pentra	Y			Y
		Siemens/Advia	Y			Y
		Sysmex XE series	Y			Y
Schistocytes	Fragmented red cells	Siemens/Advia	N (research)	Fragmentocytes	Y: automated screening for fragmentocytes, flagging	N
		Sysmex XE series	N (research)			N
B. Specifications of elements						
White blood cells	Immature granulocyte	Horiba Medical/Pentra	N (research)	WBC impedance	U: some infections	N
		Sysmex XE series	Y	Neutrophil scatter and fluorescence		Y
	White cell volume, conductivity and scatter	Beckman Coulter/LH 750	N (research)		U: some infections	N
	High fluorescent lymphocytes	Sysmex XE series	N (research)		U: atypical lymphocytes	N
	Neut-X	Sysmex XE series	N (research)		U: hypogranular neutrophils-MDS?	N

(continued on next page)

Table 1
(continued)

Cell Line	Parameter	Manufacturer/Machine	Reportable	Measures	Clinical Use (Yes or No or Unknown)	IQC
Red blood cells	% hypochromic red blood cells	Abott Sapphire	N (research)		U: assessment of iron-restricted erythropoiesis	N
		Siemens/Advia	N (research)			N
		Sysmex XE series	N (research)			N
	Low hemoglobin density	Beckman Coulter/LH 750	N (research)		Y: assessment of iron-restricted erythropoiesis	N
	Red cell distribution width	Beckman Coulter/LH 750	Y	Red cell anisocytosis	Y	Y
		Sysmex XE series	Y			Y
Reticulocytes	Immature reticulocyte fraction	Abott/Cell-Dyn	Y	Nucleic acid content of reticulocytes	Y: assessment of erythropoiesis	Y
		Abott/Sapphire	Y			Y
		Beckman Coulter/LH 750	Y			Y
		Horiba Medical/Pentra	Y			Y
		Siemens/Advia	Y			Y
		Sysmex XE series	Y			Y
	Reticulocyte hemoglobin content	Abott Sapphire	N (research)			N
		Siemens/Advia	Y	Hemoglobin content of reticulocytes	Y: assessment of iron-restricted erythropoiesis	Y
		Sysmex XE series	Y			Y

Platelets					
Immature platelet fraction	Sysmex XE series	N	Nucleic acid content of platelets	Y: assessment of megacaryocytopoiesis in thrombocytopenia	N
Platelet distribution width	Beckman Coulter/LH 750	Y	Quantification of platelet anisocytosis	Y	Y
	Siemens/Advia	Y			Y
	Sysmex XE series	Y			Y
Mean platelet volume	Beckman Coulter/LH 750	Y	Quantification of mean platelet size	Y: assessment of bleeding disorders and thrombocytopenia	Y
Platelets/large cell ratio	Sysmex XE series	Y			Y
	Siemens/Advia	Y			Y
	Sysmex XE series	Y	% of large platelets	Y: assessment of bleeding disorders and thrombocytopenia	Y
Mean platelet content	Siemens/Advia	N (research)		U	N
Platelet dry mass	Siemens/Advia	N (research)		U	N
Plateletcrit	Sysmex XE series	Y	Relative platelet mass	U	Y

Internal quality control is not available for all parameters and when unavailable these parameters are often for research use only. None of the parameters has an external quality control available. Part A shows detection of cellular elements normally absent in peripheral blood, and part B shows newly determined parameters of routinely determined cellular elements. For none of the parameters is external quality control available to date. Most parameters available on Sysmex XE or Beckman are also available on the new Sysmex XN or Coulter DxH800 platform.

Abbreviations: IQC, internal quality control; MDS, myelodysplastic syndrome; WBC, white blood cell.
Data from Briggs C. Quality counts: new parameters in blood cell counting. Int J Lab Hematol 2009;31:277–97.

A genuine, novel parameter can be tentatively defined as one that is difficult or even impossible to obtain with current methods. The counts of nucleated RBC, fragmented red cell, and immature granulocyte are good examples of abnormal cells or cells not normally present in peripheral blood that can be accurately enumerated with newer HA.

We provide here a selective overview of some of the new parameters, focusing on a clinical perspective. The main issues discussed in this article are suspicion and follow-up of microangiopathic hemolytic anemias, differential diagnosis of anemias caused by abnormal hemoglobinization, and suspicion of inherited thrombocytopenias. Some of these issues are also addressed in other articles in this issue (especially the ones devoted to reticulocytes and platelets).

WHITE BLOOD CELLS

Among the new WBC parameters is the neutrophil volume, which has been assessed with the VCS module of the Coulter HA.[6] Such methods were found to detect immature and reactive neutrophils, which are of interest in septic conditions. However, the new neutrophil parameters are to the best of our knowledge not widely used. Nevertheless, clinical studies bearing on their clinical utility continue,[7,8] for instance for the sometimes difficult diagnosis of neonatal sepsis. These studies use complex combinations of parameters including soluble biomarkers in plasma in addition to leukocyte indices.[9,10] Parameters derived from myeloperoxidase activity assessed with the well-established Siemens technology (formerly Technicon, then Bayer, now Siemens) do not seem to have gained wide acceptance.[11] The inherent complexity of the differential analysis of markedly abnormal WBC repartitions might be overcome with the combined use of fluorescent tags (mostly monoclonal antibodies) with flow cytometers or as an extension of the blood cell counter (Abbot Cell-Dyn and Sapphire), and/or morphologic analysis of a blood smear (Cellavision). The flag "immature granulocytes," which may be clinically relevant, is generated by the newer HA with a reasonable intermanufacturer agreement.[1]

The use of automated cell counters has been suggested for the monitoring of peripheral hematopoietic stem cells (HSC) in donors treated with mobilizing agents to facilitate the determination of the most appropriate time for HSC harvest. This has been a long quest, dating back to the 1990s[12,13] with sometimes inconclusive results; the approach has not been universally accepted, even though encouraging reports continue to be published.[14,15]

Most importantly, most modern HA provide accurate enumerations of nucleated RBCs.[16] This allows the reporting of more reliable WBC counts.

THROMBOTIC MICROANGIOPATHIES AND SCHISTOCYTES

Thrombotic microangiopathies (TMA), also known as microangiopathic hemolytic anemias, are characterized by thrombotic occlusions of small vessels with consumption of platelets and fragmentation of RBC.[17]

The human eye performs poorly in the recognition of schistocytes by microscopic examination of a blood smear. The reason is that any irregularly shaped RBC can easily be confused with schistocytes. Schistocytes have recently been better defined by consensus under the aegis of the International Council for Standardization in Haematology,[18] for a more reliable recognition by microscopic examination of a blood smear.[19]

TMA represent a critical diagnostic challenge, often with vital clinical implications. Thrombotic thrombocytopenic purpura requires prompt plasma infusion or plasma exchange.[20] Following allogeneic HSC transplantation, TMA is often difficult to differentiate from other states, such as graft-versus-host disease or sinusoidal obstruction syndrome. In this setting TMA can be caused by an immunosuppressive drug (eg, a calcineurin inhibitor), or can be associated with one of the infections that frequently occur in these immunocompromised patients. The differentiation of TMA from graft-versus-host disease is particularly important, because the therapeutic choices are completely different.[21]

Schistocytes can be identified or at least suspected by modern HA based on a refined analysis of the small RBC fraction in the context of normal global volume parameters (mean corpuscular volume and width) using proprietary algorithms.[22] As a diagnostic alert, the fragmented red cell flag has a low specificity, but its absence has a good negative predictive value.[23–25] Thus, when faced with a patient with suspected TMA, the presence of the flag should prompt careful microscopic examination of a blood smear. Other signs of TMA are elevated reticulocyte counts, chemical evidence of hemolysis (eg, immeasurable haptoglobin), and a negative direct antiglobulin test.

Automated enumeration can also help to monitor patients with the diagnosis of TMA by decreasing imprecision of the count and eliminating interobserver variability. Currently the persistence or disappearance of schistocytes from the peripheral blood is not one of the main parameters used to monitor the response to therapy, despite the fact that schistocytes are an essential clue for the diagnosis. This is because of the notoriously unreliable nature of the quantitative assessment of red cell fragments.

OTHER NEW RED BLOOD CELL PARAMETERS

Several new RBC parameters are potentially useful in the differential diagnosis of anemias with abnormal hemoglobinization, and more specifically of IRE. Generally speaking these parameters aim to detect small changes in volume and/or hemoglobin content, such as the fraction of hypochromic (low hemoglobin density[26]) or microcytic RBC. For reticulocytes these new parameters include the fraction of the youngest cells, and the same descriptive parameters used for RBC regarding volume and hemoglobin content. Given the prolonged lifespan of RBCs (normally 120 days), the additional parameters of reticulocytes, which have a short lifespan of a few days, are likely to add valuable information on recent erythropoiesis.

CLINICAL SETTINGS IN WHICH NEW RED BLOOD CELL PARAMETERS CAN BE USED

One frequently encountered clinical problem is erythrocytic microcytosis, with or without anemia. A preliminary classification of anemia based on complete blood count parameters can be useful.

Iron deficiency anemia (IDA) is common and is easily recognized in the presence of microcytosis and clear-cut peripheral chemical signs (low ferritin, high transferrin, and low transferring saturation).

For the differential diagnosis of thalassemia and IDA, it has been long noticed that microcytosis is more pronounced in thalassemia and that hypochromasia is more severe in iron deficiency.[27,28] Red cells (volume) distribution width (RDW) has been proposed as early as in the 1980s as a diagnostic criterion, with RDW being normal in cases of thalassemia without concomitant iron deficiency.[29] More recently, the ratio of % microcytic to % hypochromic determined with an Advia instrument has been successfully applied to the same issue.[30]

In addition, "unghosted cells," a parameter available on the BC UniCell DxH800, was reported to be a potential surrogate for the detection and the counting of target cells,[31] an important clue for thalassemias.

In patients with suspected hereditary spherocytosis, various indices including high reticulocyte counts without an equally elevated immature reticulocyte fraction,[32] or the mean reticulocyte volume, the immature reticulocyte fraction, and the mean sphered cell volume,[33,34] have been suggested to aid diagnosis in cases of Coombs-negative hemolytic anemia. Using a Cell Dyn Sapphire HA, it is possible to combine a flow cytometer analysis, the eosin-5'-maleimide test, to confirm the diagnosis in the presence of so called 'hyperchromic' erythrocytes, reported to be sensitive and specific.[35]

An annoying conundrum is the detection of IRE in complex conditions, such as chronic kidney disease (CKD), and other disease states with systemic inflammation and the risk of iron depletion. Causes of IRE are absolute iron deficiency, functional iron deficiency, and/or iron sequestration.[36] In these settings the diagnosis of iron deficiency can be challenging.

The fraction of hypochromic-microcytic RBC has long been considered as a potentially good index for IRE.[37] For example, post–renal transplant anemia is a frequent and multifactorial problem. IRE was associated with a percentage of hypochromic RBC greater than or equal to 2.5% in this setting.[38] Similarly IRE in patients with CKD can be reliably diagnosed using one of two methods of evaluating the fraction of hypochromic cells. The first was the %HYPO (Advia instrument, threshold of 280 g/L). The second was an index designed by the authors according to a polynomial function using hemoglobin, hematocrit, and reticulocyte hemoglobin equivalent.[39] The percentage of hypochromic RBC (%Hypo-He) is now available with Sysmex instruments.[40] More recently a good level of agreement was documented between the recognized %Hypo of Advia and a newer parameter called LHD% (for low hemoglobin density), mathematically derived from mean corpuscular hemoglobin concentration as determined by Beckman Coulter instruments.[26]

A frequent clinical question when facing complex forms of IRE is whether intravenous iron would be able to increase hemoglobin and improve clinical status.[41] This is the case in several well-characterized chronic conditions: CKD, myelodysplasia, inherited disorders of erythrocytes, and can also occur in patients hospitalized for an acute illness complicating a chronic disease. Unfortunately it remains difficult to answer this question. In anemic nondialysis patients with CKD, it has been shown that neither ferritin nor transferrin saturation performed well. The best indicator remains the assessment of bone marrow stores; RBC indices were not studied.[42] A recently published prospective study concluded that intravenous iron targeting a high ferritin level was efficacious in such patients with anemia.[43]

Following reticulocyte parameters can be used to monitor the response to iron-replacement therapy. Combinations of parameters, used as continuous measurements or after dichotomization, are proposed as more or less complex formulas for these work-ups. An example of this is the use of the standard deviation of the conductivity of the mature red cells population and the RDW-SD to discriminate IDA from thalassemia trait.[44] Another example is the red cell size factor, combining the volumes of erythrocytes and reticulocytes as the square root of their product, which has been proposed to better detect changes in hemoglobinization.[45] Finally, we failed to find data about the agreement between the hypochromic fraction of RBC and hemoglobin content of reticulocytes, the two most often proposed parameters for IRE, or the diagnostic value of their combination. In theory the reticulocyte parameter reflects what has happened in the last few days, whereas the (mature) erythrocyte parameter results from the cumulative effect of factors having acted for days and even weeks before sample collection.

In conclusion several parameters regarding RBC and reticulocytes have been established and studied for their clinical utility. By far the greatest improvement was the automated count of reticulocytes themselves. Reticulocyte parameters (mostly hemoglobin content) and the fraction of hypochromic RBC were recommended in the context of CKD,[46] although it is not clear whether the recent updates have explicitly discarded them.[47,48] Further rigorous studies must be conducted to obtain undisputable results in these settings, paving the way to endorsement by scientific medical societies and their use in clinical practice for well-defined clinical questions.

NEW PLATELET PARAMETERS
What Are They?

The proposed new platelet parameters are mainly intended to help in the diagnosis and management of thrombocytopenias. "Young" platelet can be quantified with some currently available HA. The other parameters are refinements of the assessment of the volume and indices of the cytoplasmic content of platelets.

There are well-known problems with the accurate and reliable determination of platelet volumes, as exemplified by the systematic biases between the HA of different manufacturers.[49] It is not surprising that more sophisticated parameters regarding platelet volumes, sometimes called platelet volume indices, are prone to substantial variations between HA.

Some parameters aim at a better description of the distribution of platelets according to their volume and content: this is particularly important in the case of aberrant volumes with significant platelet gigantism (see later). In cases for which the impedance method cannot identify very large platelets among the smallest erythrocytes, use of the optical method is recommended, using laser light and two angles for detection. However, there are difficulties in deriving diameter and then volume from transmitted light at low angle. One way to achieve this is to sphere the RBCs before analysis. This method has been successfully used on the Advia platform for more than a decade.

It is important to get indices regarding platelet distribution according to size when determined with a fluorescent dye,[50] even if not expressed as a volume with its unit (liter), such as an estimation of the localization of the mode (the zone with the highest number of events), or of the relative fraction of large platelets. However, the cut-offs for the fraction of large platelets are not uniform, making comparisons between instruments difficult. The width of the distribution according to volumes (platelet distribution width [PDW]) may offer additional information to MPV.[51]

Using a side angle scatter to measure diffracted light, the platelet content can be quantitatively approached with the optical method.[52] This can yield interesting information regarding platelet granules, which are influenced by biogenesis during platelet production in the bone marrow, but also by activation in the circulating blood leading to secretion, in cases with no platelet consumption. Defective biogenesis can occur for instance in myelodysplastic syndromes, as documented by a "low mean platelet component."[53]

Regarding preanalytical aspects, the anticoagulant of choice remains EDTA. There are time-dependent (after blood sampling) variations in platelet parameters. It is likely that a much tighter control of the time interval between collection and analysis (and of the temperature) than sufficient for the mere counting of platelets is required to get useful values of the new platelet parameters.

Of note all these parameters related to platelet size and volume are prone to the same possibilities of errors because of background noise, debris, and cryoglobulinemia for small platelets, and of the presence of small erythrocytes for large platelets. Finally, the accuracy of HA for the new parameters is highly questionable at very low platelet counts: MPV and platelet count (PC) themselves are much less precise and subject to greater variations between HA from different manufacturers under these circumstances.

Instrument-specific reference ranges for young platelets and PDW have been published.[54,55] It is good laboratory practice to establish local reference ranges. This is caused in part by possible differences between the same kind of instruments of one given manufacturer (including calibrations in the context of intensive use) but also by differences caused by multiple genetic influences among populations of different ethnic background, even in the same country (eg, as shown by several valuable studies carefully conducted in Italy[56]).

In our opinion it is always of paramount importance to carefully review the graphs generated by the HA and to compare them with the results of the microscopic examination of the blood smear, and not to rely only on a variety of multiple quantitative indices.

Use of New Platelet Parameters in Thrombocytopenias

Careful consideration of platelet indices, combined with careful microscopic examination of platelets, can provide clues for a hypoproliferative disease (abnormal bone marrow) or an increased platelet turnover (decreased platelet life span). Immune thrombocytopenia (called ITP when autoimmune and isolated) is notoriously difficult to diagnose because of the lack of a reliable method to detect platelet autoantibodies. International recommendations for ITP state that platelet morphology has to be taken into account.[57] Platelet size and volume are normal or slightly increased in ITP. In fact, an increase in MPV has long been considered as an indicator of increased platelet production in the face of a decreased PC, pointing to a peripheral mechanism for thrombocytopenia.[51]

When the size and volume of platelets are clearly abnormal, causes different from ITP must be sought, primarily inherited thrombocytopenias. In the setting of inherited thrombocytopenias with increased platelet volume it is important to make every effort to identify entities with significant platelet gigantism, because this finding is infrequently found in other disorders and easy to discriminate from mere large platelets. This process would refine the differential diagnosis by focusing it to a restricted number of entities, the so-called biallelic Bernard-Soulier syndrome (BSS), and MYH9-related diseases (MYH9-RD). However, there is no accepted definition of true gigantism, and only a fraction of the platelets in affected patients show gigantism. Although it is generally accepted that platelets larger than the nucleus of a small lymphocytes (approximately 8 μm) can be defined as giant, how many such platelets are required to label the platelet disorder as one with giant platelets is still debated. Some investigators have used microscopic examination, which is time consuming and highly observer-dependent, to record the largest diameter of a sufficient number of platelets (several hundred), with the help of a graduated scale or more sophisticated tools (image analysis). In control subjects the percentage of giant platelets, as defined previously, was found to be less than 1%, and in case of biallelic BSS and MYH9-RD, 6% and 16% on average.[58] In a more recent paper from an international consortium led by Italian colleagues with a long-standing and fruitful interest in this field, the different disorders defined at the gene level were consistently ranked correctly by order of increasing platelet size (mean platelet diameter and platelet diameter large cell ratio) MYH9-RD (both caused by head and tail mutations), and biallelic BSS being those with the highest values of the indices; however, there was overlap with other entities.[59] Based on such data and criteria, it would be interesting to determine the comparability of platelet parameters provided by different HA. Another approach we have recently proposed[49] is to compare the results of HA of different manufacturers for the same blood sample. We found that the failure to fit the data with a model curve of log-normal distribution despite a substantial number of events in the measurement window, with absent return to the baseline at 20 fL with a Coulter HA, or a higher count with an Advia HA and frequent events in the area of large platelets, are suggestive of platelet gigantism. However, it is infrequent in clinical practice to have instruments with differing methods for PC that can be used for such a comparison. A word of caution is required here: the platelet counts provided by the Advia platform, although more consistent with the whole picture, is not necessarily the true one and the determination by flow cytometry and specific fluorescent monoclonal antibodies can result in a significantly (from a clinical point of view) different count. Genuine gigantism would thus be a distinctive feature of both biallelic BSS and MYH9-RD, but although platelet volumes are always increased in those diseases (for reasons that become increasingly understood[60]), gigantism, as tentatively defined previously, can be less evident.

Careful examination of platelet volumes is more important to diagnose inherited thrombocytopenia when facing an isolated thrombocytopenia without available prior PC, than trying to differentiate between the two mechanisms of thrombocytopenia (central or peripheral). The clinical implications of the timely recognition of inherited thrombocytopenias are far from trivial, regarding prognosis (frequently low bleeding risk but sometimes associated risk of hematologic malignancies) and management (potentially harmful treatments of ITP can be avoided for inherited disorders).

Plateletcrit and platelet mass may be better indicators of competent hemostasis than PC, because a decreased PC is often accompanied by an increased platelet volume, whereas plateletcrit integrates both. In addition, the absolute mass of an active component within platelets whatever their number and volume could be of importance for the functioning of hemostasis. However, this remains to be proved.

Finally, some platelet parameters were investigated as potential predictors of response to thrombopoietin receptor agonists in patients with thrombocytopenia and monitoring of those treatments, such as young platelets in the case of ITP.[61]

Use of New Platelet Parameters in Thrombocytosis

No definite conclusion can be made about the value of any of the new platelet parameters to differentiate reactive thrombocytosis from clonal proliferation, such as essential thrombocythemia, although there are data consistent with a more increased PDW in case of the latter compared with the former.[62,63] Of note, the fraction of reticulated platelets was found to be greatly increased in patients with essential thrombocythemia compared with control subjects.[64] Myeloproliferative neoplasms are a setting where improvement in the prediction of thrombosis, and also bleeding, would be of interest. There are at least two reports associating the percentage of reticulated platelets with thrombosis in patients with myeloproliferative neoplasms, suggesting higher production and increased turnover.[64,65] In one study the same held true for reactive, transient thrombocytosis, and the percentage of reticulated platelets was found to be reduced during aspirin treatment.[65]

New Parameters and the Preparation and Storage of Platelet Concentrates

It is well known that blood collection and processing to prepare platelet concentrates, and their storage thereafter, lead to unavoidable functional alterations, potentially compromising their hemostatic capacity. Several studies reported changes in platelet concentrates obtained by apheresis, with decreased PDW, mean platelet component, and mean platelet mass.[66] By contrast, no changes were recorded in donors, beyond the expected marked decrease in PC.

Young Platelets: Reliable?

Problems have been reported in the measurement of "young" platelets,[67] with a poor agreement between HA.[1] Young platelets are assessed as the immature platelet fraction with the Sysmex XE and XN instruments, and as the "reticulated platelet fraction" with the Abbott Cell Dyn Sapphire instrument.[68] It remains to be shown to what extent immature platelet fraction derived from PLT-O and PLT-F (two different dyes) with the Sysmex XN HA are closely related in any clinical setting.

Platelet Parameters and Thrombosis and Cardiovascular Events in Subjects Without Hematologic Disorder

Platelets play a key role in thrombosis, especially so when it takes place in arteries, and directly or indirectly in other cardiovascular events, such as heart failure. The potential value of platelet parameters as risk factors for thrombosis and other cardiovascular events has received some attention by several investigators (for instance MPV, see review by Chu and colleagues[69]) but has not yet achieved the stage of clinical implementation (beyond the scope of this article). The same holds true for changes of those parameters during pregnancy, either normal or complicated, such as gestational hypertensive states.[70,71]

SUMMARY

New and even not so new technologies in HA have provided more and more indices. To avoid being overwhelmed or prematurely discarding promising ones, there is an urgent need for more good clinical research on topics of clinical relevance. This applies to frequent states, such as multifactorial anemias of complex patients, and rare disorders with high clinical impact, such as TMA and inherited thrombocytopenias.

REFERENCES

1. Meintker L, Ringwald J, Rauh M, et al. Comparison of automated differential blood cell counts from Abbott Sapphire, Siemens Advia 120, Beckman Coulter DxH 800, and Sysmex XE-2100 in normal and pathologic samples. Am J Clin Pathol 2013; 139:641–50.
2. Costa O, Van Moer G, Jochmans K, et al. Reference values for new red blood cell and platelet parameters on the Abbott Diagnostics Cell-Dyn Sapphire. Clin Chem Lab Med 2012;50:967–9.
3. Coudene P, Marson B, Badiou S, et al. Evaluation of the ABX Pentra 400: a newly available clinical chemistry analyser. Clin Chem Lab Med 2005;43:782–92.
4. Shu G, Lu H, Du H, et al. Evaluation of Mindray BC-3600 hematology analyzer in a university hospital. Int J Lab Hematol 2013;35:61–9.
5. Harris N, Jou JM, Devoto G, et al. Performance evaluation of the ADVIA 2120 hematology analyzer: an international multicenter clinical trial. Lab Hematol 2005; 11:62–70.
6. Chaves F, Tierno B, Xu D. Quantitative determination of neutrophil VCS parameters by the Coulter automated hematology analyzer: new and reliable indicators for acute bacterial infection. Am J Clin Pathol 2005;124:440–4.
7. Lee AJ, Kim SG. Mean cell volumes of neutrophils and monocytes are promising markers of sepsis in elderly patients. Blood Res 2013;48:193–7.

8. Park SH, Park CJ, Lee BR, et al. Sepsis affects most routine and cell population data (CPD) obtained using the Sysmex XN-2000 blood cell analyzer: neutrophil-related CPD NE-SFL and NE-WY provide useful information for detecting sepsis. Int J Lab Hematol 2014. [Epub ahead of print].

9. Celik IH, Demirel G, Erdeve O, et al. Neutrophil volume, conductivity and scatter in neonatal sepsis. Pediatr Infect Dis J 2013;32:301.

10. Celik IH, Demirel G, Sukhachev D, et al. Neutrophil volume, conductivity and scatter parameters with effective modeling of molecular activity statistical program gives better results in neonatal sepsis. Int J Lab Hematol 2013;35:82–7.

11. Bononi A, Lanza F, Ferrari L, et al. Predictive value of hematological and pheno-typical parameters on postchemotherapy leukocyte recovery. Cytometry B Clin Cytom 2009;76:328–33.

12. Yamane T, Takekawa K, Tatsumi N. Possibility of identification of hematopoietic stem cells using a conventional blood cell counter. Eur J Haematol 1995;55: 207–8.

13. Mougi H, Shinmyozu K, Osame M. Determining the optimal time for peripheral blood stem cell harvest by detecting immature cells (immature leukocytes and immature reticulocytes) using two newly developed automatic cell analyzers. Int J Hematol 1997;66:303–13.

14. Letestu R, Marzac C, Audat F, et al. Use of hematopoietic progenitor cell count on the Sysmex XE-2100 for peripheral blood stem cell harvest monitoring. Leuk Lymphoma 2007;48:89–96.

15. Mitani N, Yujiri T, Tanaka Y, et al. Hematopoietic progenitor cell count, but not immature platelet fraction value, predicts successful harvest of autologous peripheral blood stem cells. J Clin Apher 2011;26:105–10.

16. Tantanate C, Klinbua C. Performance evaluation of the automated nucleated red blood cell enumeration on Sysmex XN analyser. Int J Lab Hematol 2014. [Epub ahead of print].

17. Coppo P, Veyradier A. Thrombotic microangiopathies: towards a pathophysiology-based classification. Cardiovasc Hematol Disord Drug Targets 2009;9:36–50.

18. Zini G, d'Onofrio G, Briggs C, et al. ICSH recommendations for identification, diagnostic value, and quantitation of schistocytes. Int J Lab Hematol 2012;34: 107–16.

19. Lesesve JF, El Adssi H, Watine J, et al. Evaluation of ICSH schistocyte measurement guidelines in France. Int J Lab Hematol 2013;35:601–7.

20. Coppo P, Schwarzinger M, Buffet M, et al. Predictive features of severe acquired ADAMTS13 deficiency in idiopathic thrombotic microangiopathies: the French TMA reference center experience. PLoS One 2010;5:e10208.

21. George JN, Li X, McMinn JR, et al. Thrombotic thrombocytopenic purpura-hemolytic uremic syndrome following allogeneic HPC transplantation: a diagnostic dilemma. Transfusion 2004;44:294–304.

22. Saigo K, Jiang M, Tanaka C, et al. Usefulness of automatic detection of fragmented red cells using a hematology analyzer for diagnosis of thrombotic microangiopathy. Clin Lab Haematol 2002;24:347–51.

23. Lesesve JF, Salignac S, Alla F, et al. Comparative evaluation of schistocyte counting by an automated method and by microscopic determination. Am J Clin Pathol 2004;121:739–45.

24. Lesesve JF, Asnafi V, Braun F, et al. Fragmented red blood cells automated measurement is a useful parameter to exclude schistocytes on the blood film. Int J Lab Hematol 2012;34:566–76.

25. Lesesve JF, Salignac S, Lecompte T, et al. Automated measurement of schistocytes after bone marrow transplantation. Bone Marrow Transplant 2004;34:357–62.

26. Urrechaga E. The new mature red cell parameter, low haemoglobin density of the Beckman-Coulter LH750: clinical utility in the diagnosis of iron deficiency. Int J Lab Hematol 2010;32:e144–50.

27. Urrechaga E, Borque L, Escanero JF. The role of automated measurement of RBC subpopulations in differential diagnosis of microcytic anemia and beta-thalassemia screening. Am J Clin Pathol 2011;135:374–9.

28. Urrechaga E. Red blood cell microcytosis and hypochromia in the differential diagnosis of iron deficiency and beta-thalassaemia trait. Int J Lab Hematol 2009;31:528–34.

29. Marti HR, Fischer S, Killer D, et al. Can automated haematology analysers discriminate thalassaemia from iron deficiency? Acta Haematol 1987;78:180–3.

30. Urrechaga E. Discriminant value of % microcytic/% hypochromic ratio in the differential diagnosis of microcytic anemia. Clin Chem Lab Med 2008;46:1752–8.

31. Lee W, Kim JH, Sung IK, et al. Quantitative detection of target cells using unghosted cells (UGCs) of DxH 800 (Beckman Coulter). Clin Chem Lab Med 2014;52:693–9.

32. Mullier F, Lainey E, Fenneteau O, et al. Additional erythrocytic and reticulocytic parameters helpful for diagnosis of hereditary spherocytosis: results of a multicentre study. Ann Hematol 2011;90:759–68.

33. Lazarova E, Pradier O, Cotton F, et al. Automated reticulocyte parameters for hereditary spherocytosis screening. Ann Hematol 2014;93:1809–18.

34. Liao L, Deng ZF, Qiu YL, et al. Values of mean cell volume and mean sphered cell volume can differentiate hereditary spherocytosis and thalassemia. Hematology 2014;19:393–6.

35. Rooney S, Hoffmann JJ, Cormack OM, et al. Screening and confirmation of hereditary spherocytosis in children using a CELL-DYN Sapphire haematology analyser. Int J Lab Hematol 2014. [Epub ahead of print].

36. Goodnough LT. Iron deficiency syndromes and iron-restricted erythropoiesis (CME). Transfusion 2012;52:1584–92.

37. Goodnough LT, Skikne B, Brugnara C. Erythropoietin, iron, and erythropoiesis. Blood 2000;96:823–33.

38. Lorenz M, Kletzmayr J, Perschl A, et al. Anemia and iron deficiencies among long-term renal transplant recipients. J Am Soc Nephrol 2002;13:794–7.

39. Maconi M, Cavalca L, Danise P, et al. Erythrocyte and reticulocyte indices in iron deficiency in chronic kidney disease: comparison of two methods. Scand J Clin Lab Invest 2009;69:365–70.

40. Urrechaga E, Borque L, Escanero JF. The role of automated measurement of red cell subpopulations on the Sysmex XE 5000 analyzer in the differential diagnosis of microcytic anemia. Int J Lab Hematol 2011;33:30–6.

41. Auerbach M, Coyne D, Ballard H. Intravenous iron: from anathema to standard of care. Am J Hematol 2008;83:580–8.

42. Stancu S, Stanciu A, Zugravu A, et al. Bone marrow iron, iron indices, and the response to intravenous iron in patients with non-dialysis-dependent CKD. Am J Kidney Dis 2010;55:639–47.

43. Macdougall IC. Intravenous iron therapy in non-dialysis CKD patients. Nephrol Dial Transplant 2014;29:717–20.

44. Ng EH, Leung JH, Lau YS, et al. Evaluation of the new red cell parameters on Beckman Coulter DxH800 in distinguishing iron deficiency anaemia from thalassaemia trait. Int J Lab Hematol 2014. [Epub ahead of print].

45. Urrechaga E. Clinical utility of the new Beckman-Coulter parameter red blood cell size factor in the study of erithropoiesis. Int J Lab Hematol 2009;31:623–9.
46. Locatelli F, Aljama P, Barany P, et al. Revised European best practice guidelines for the management of anaemia in patients with chronic renal failure. Nephrol Dial Transplant 2004;19(Suppl 2):ii1–47.
47. Anonymous. KDIGO clinical practice guideline for anemia in CKD: summary of recommendation statements. Kidney Int Suppl (2012) 2012;2:283–7.
48. Locatelli F, Barany P, Covic A, et al. Kidney disease: improving global outcomes guidelines on anaemia management in chronic kidney disease: a European Renal Best Practice position statement. Nephrol Dial Transplant 2013;28:1346–59.
49. Latger-Cannard V, Hoarau M, Salignac S, et al. Mean platelet volume: comparison of three analysers towards standardization of platelet morphological phenotype. Int J Lab Hematol 2012;34:300–10.
50. Tanaka Y, Gondo K, Maruki Y, et al. Performance evaluation of platelet counting by novel fluorescent dye staining in the XN-series automated hematology analyzers. J Clin Lab Anal 2014;28:341–8.
51. Leader A, Pereg D, Lishner M. Are platelet volume indices of clinical use? A multidisciplinary review. Ann Med 2012;44:805–16.
52. Brummitt DR, Barker HF. The determination of a reference range for new platelet parameters produced by the Bayer ADVIA120 full blood count analyser. Clin Lab Haematol 2000;22:103–7.
53. Brummitt DR, Barker HF, Pujol-Moix N. A new platelet parameter, the mean platelet component, can demonstrate abnormal platelet function and structure in myelodysplasia. Clin Lab Haematol 2003;25:59–62.
54. Hoffmann JJ, van den Broek NM, Curvers J. Reference intervals of reticulated platelets and other platelet parameters and their associations. Arch Pathol Lab Med 2013;137:1635–40.
55. Farias MG, Schunck EG, Dal Bo S, et al. Definition of reference ranges for the platelet distribution width (PDW): a local need. Clin Chem Lab Med 2010;48:255–7.
56. Biino G, Santimone I, Minelli C, et al. Age- and sex-related variations in platelet count in Italy: a proposal of reference ranges based on 40987 subjects' data. PLoS One 2013;8:e54289.
57. Provan D, Stasi R, Newland AC, et al. International consensus report on the investigation and management of primary immune thrombocytopenia. Blood 2010;115:168–86.
58. Balduini CL, Cattaneo M, Fabris F, et al. Inherited thrombocytopenias: a proposed diagnostic algorithm from the Italian Gruppo di Studio delle Piastrine. Haematologica 2003;88:582–92.
59. Noris P, Biino G, Pecci A, et al. Platelet diameters in inherited thrombocytopenias: analysis of 376 patients with all known disorders. Blood 2014;124:e4–10.
60. Pertuy F, Eckly A, Weber J, et al. Myosin IIA is critical for organelle distribution and F-actin organization in megakaryocytes and platelets. Blood 2014;123:1261–9.
61. Barsam SJ, Psaila B, Forestier M, et al. Platelet production and platelet destruction: assessing mechanisms of treatment effect in immune thrombocytopenia. Blood 2011;117:5723–32.
62. Osselaer JC, Jamart J, Scheiff JM. Platelet distribution width for differential diagnosis of thrombocytosis. Clin Chem 1997;43:1072–6.
63. Song YH, Park SH, Kim JE, et al. Evaluation of platelet indices for differential diagnosis of thrombocytosis by ADVIA 120. Korean J Lab Med 2009;29:505–9 [in Korean].

64. Arellano-Rodrigo E, Alvarez-Larran A, Reverter JC, et al. Platelet turnover, coagulation factors, and soluble markers of platelet and endothelial activation in essential thrombocythemia: relationship with thrombosis occurrence and JAK2 V617F allele burden. Am J Hematol 2009;84:102–8.
65. Rinder HM, Schuster JE, Rinder CS, et al. Correlation of thrombosis with increased platelet turnover in thrombocytosis. Blood 1998;91:1288–94.
66. Ifran A, Hasimi A, Kaptan K, et al. Evaluation of platelet parameters in healthy apheresis donors using the ADVIA 120. Transfus Apher Sci 2005;33:87–90.
67. Hoffmann JJ. Reticulated platelets: analytical aspects and clinical utility. Clin Chem Lab Med 2014;52:1107–17.
68. Meintker L, Haimerl M, Ringwald J, et al. Measurement of immature platelets with Abbott CD-Sapphire and Sysmex XE-5000 in haematology and oncology patients. Clin Chem Lab Med 2013;51:2125–31.
69. Chu SG, Becker RC, Berger PB, et al. Mean platelet volume as a predictor of cardiovascular risk: a systematic review and meta-analysis. J Thromb Haemost 2010;8:148–56.
70. Maconi M, Cardaropoli S, Cenci AM. Platelet parameters in healthy and pathological pregnancy. J Clin Lab Anal 2012;26:41–4.
71. Kanat-Pektas M, Yesildager U, Tuncer N, et al. Could mean platelet volume in late first trimester of pregnancy predict intrauterine growth restriction and pre-eclampsia? J Obstet Gynaecol Res 2014;40:1840–5.

Moving?

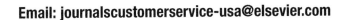

Make sure your subscription moves with you!

To notify us of your new address, find your **Clinics Account Number** (located on your mailing label above your name), and contact customer service at:

Email: journalscustomerservice-usa@elsevier.com

800-654-2452 (subscribers in the U.S. & Canada)
314-447-8871 (subscribers outside of the U.S. & Canada)

Fax number: 314-447-8029

Elsevier Health Sciences Division
Subscription Customer Service
3251 Riverport Lane
Maryland Heights, MO 63043

*To ensure uninterrupted delivery of your subscription, please notify us at least 4 weeks in advance of move.

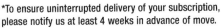

Printed and bound by CPI Group (UK) Ltd, Croydon, CR0 4YY

03/10/2024

01040494-0004